BEGINNING OF THE SCHOOL OF MEDICINE

at
East Carolina University
1964-1977

Beginning of the
School of Medicine
at
East Carolina University
1964-1977

Wayne C. Williams

Brookcliff Publishers, Inc.
Greenville, North Carolina

Published in cooperation with the The Medical Foundation of East
Carolina University, Inc. Opinions and interpretations of events and
accounts presented in this book are those of the author and do not
necessarily reflect the views of Brookcliff Publishers, Inc. or The
Medical Foundation of East Carolina University, Inc.

Photographs courtesy of the School of Medicine at East Carolina
University. Used with permission. All rights reserved.

Brookcliff Publishers, Inc.
PO Box 2428
Greenville, NC 27836-0428

ISBN 0-9626185-1-9

Library of Congress Catalog Card Number: 97-73944

Printed in the USA

10 9 8 7 6 5 4 3 2 1

Contents

Preface

In 1988, the Center for Health Sciences Communication at the East Carolina University School of Medicine video-taped two interviews of Dr. Leo Jenkins, the first with Paul Crellin as interviewer and the second with Dr. William E. Laupus. Dr. Jenkins had been retired from ECU for ten years, and was in a period of remission from the cancer that eventually proved to be fatal. The tapes, aimed at recording his memories of how the medical school came about, are vintage Jenkins, and when reviewed in 1991, provided an incentive and a nucleus for an oral history of the beginning of the school. Georgette Hedrick, former director of Information and Publications for the medical school, had compiled a detailed *Chronology of the ECU School of Medicine, 1964-1976,* which provided an initial framework.

The oral history project established a record of the experiences of the early, precarious days, when a number of adventuresome basic scientists, mostly young, gambled that they might find an opportunity in Greenville, North Carolina, to set up a new medical school. During the second half of 1991 and the first half of 1992, we made audio-tapes of a few of the original faculty and administrators. Their bias against the UNC administration was so strong that we decided that it would be only fair to ask former UNC President William C. Friday to sit for a taped interview, to give "the other side" a hearing.

Dr. Friday agreed, stipulating that before he did the interview, we should tape three of the men who had worked with him during ECU's campaign to establish a medical school. We were pleased to agree with his requirement, since it had become clear that information for an unbiased account would be difficult if not impossible to find, and the opportunity to record at length a second slant on the story was too good to miss.

In planning the oral history, we talked vaguely about the possibility that someone, someday, might use our tapes and the newspaper articles, letters, and other documents that had been saved in the medical school files to write a history of the school's beginning. When the oral history project was terminated in the summer of 1992, the tapes with their transcripts were stored in a cabinet in the building occupied by the Alumni and Development Office of the School of Medicine. Those medical school files that had not yet gone to the University Archives were stored in the attic of the same building.

Robert K. Adams II, Associate Vice Chancellor in the Division of Health Sciences, and director of development and alumni affairs, decided that writing a history of the medical school's beginnings should be undertaken while most of the major actors were still present. He talked with me about it several times during 1994, but it seemed such an insuperably big project that I hesitated to attempt it.

My only experience in historical research had been limited to the history of anatomy and medical illustration, a small backwater of even the history of medicine, which is itself a fairly narrow specialty. A handful of short papers and book reviews, and three years of teaching medical students at Duke and the University of Kentucky the rudiments of history of anatomy hardly qualified me to attempt a major piece of historical research. However, having done most of the interviewing for the oral history project, I had a foot up for doing a history of the medical school's beginning. If it turned out to be no more than a preliminary survey that might form the basis for a fuller history of the medical school, not just of its beginning, then that would still be worthwhile to do.

When I looked over the resources in the files of the office of Medical Alumni Affairs—a collection of clippings, apparently exhaustive, with the stories that appeared in all or most of the state's newspapers from 1964 through 1979 concerning the medical school, legislative records, minutes and notes of meetings, correspondence—I found that one of the most laborious and time-consuming parts of research, gathering documentation, had already been done. There were some gaps that had to be filled from the North Carolina Collection and University Archives in ECU's Joyner Library, and from the William C. Friday Records in the UNC Archives in the Wilson Library at Chapel Hill. Still, the task began to appear manageable.

My final reservation about having to go to work again, after four years of pleasant retirement, was that I had been too close to the inauguration of the medical school to have a hope of escaping partiality. I am a UNC alumnus, and worked the better part of twenty years at Duke University School of Medicine, but my interviews and reading had led me to side with ECU on the medical school issue. It seemed that Chancellor Leo Jenkins was the righteous underdog in a long and unnecessary battle with UNC President William Friday and the Board of Governors to get what was clearly needed in eastern North Carolina and, as far as I could see, wanted by the tax-paying citizens.

Before I finally made up my mind, I read again Georgette Hedrick's *Chronology of the ECU School of Medicine, 1964-1976,* along with Chapter 13 and other references to the medical school in Mary Jo Jackson Bratton's *East Carolina University: The Formative Years, 1907-1982.* Dr. Bratton's account of the establishment of the medical school provides the essentials of the story. Changing the focus to a close-up on the school of medicine would have destroyed the balance of her broader history of the university, but was precisely what I needed to attempt. Fortunately, I had already gone through much of the information in the files in preparation for the oral history project. There was still a lot to do before I could begin to make out the narrative buried in the contents of the voluminous collection of information—over ten file drawers of letters and records, fifteen years of newspaper clippings in as many albums, and other archives yet to be seen—and hope to begin writing.

In December 1994, I agreed to take on the project, and said (confidently) that I ought to be able to finish in about a year. Shortly after I began work in the early 1995, William A. Link's *William Friday: Power, Purpose, and American Higher Education* was published. This book gives the fullest account I have seen anywhere of the challenge to the UNC system from East Carolina, just after the University was restructured. Link's treatment, viewing the struggle from Chapel Hill, but avoiding undue bias, encouraged me to believe that it was not impossible to trace the medical school's beginnings while preserving a measure of impartiality.

It is inevitable that this history should revolve about a small group of dynamic individuals who were at the center of all that went on. Nonetheless, I hope I have managed to keep my eye on what it seems to me is most important in the encounter between ECU and UNC. I believe that the pivotal clash was not just between two groups of people struggling for either personal advantage or power, although doubtless these elements were present. Rather, it was between two views of the relationship that the higher education system ought to have with the public.

President William C. Friday was deeply concerned with keeping the University of North Carolina out of politics, at least out of the kind of politics in the public eye. He thought that academic questions should be settled on as nearly pure educational grounds as possible, that they were matters primarily for experts, to be dealt with administratively as far as this could be managed. He accepted reluctantly that the University, as a public institution, had to be involved in the political process, but thought it should not form its policies in response to political pressures or public opinion. In this he was a true descendent of President Frank Graham, his early mentor, though he differed from him in desiring to avoid the limelight and preferring to work in the background.

Chancellor Leo Jenkins also believed that professionals should make professional decisions in education, and that an administrator should not second-guess those he hired as experts. He differed from Friday in his willingness—he was more than willing, he positively enjoyed it—to become publicly involved in politics. He found it the natural thing to do, something to which even university presidents have a right, and he was a skillful politician. Besides, he said, the people paid his salary and those of all the individuals who made up ECU, and he thought he was obliged to give the people what they were paying for.

Going beyond this question of direct accountability, he was a populist, earnestly supporting the democratization of higher education. He was diametrically against the viewpoint he attributed to former Governor Luther Hodges, a viewpoint also held by President Friday. Jenkins said that Hodges believed in "the pyramid philosophy of education: at the top should be the very cream—that's Chapel Hill and maybe State, State as a cousin but not as a leader. And then in the middle would be Appalachian, East Carolina and the white regional colleges. And at the bottom would be the black institutions."

One thing these two major players shared, for better or worse, was their identification of the public good with the goals of their institutions. While each believed that what was good for his university was good for the state, they went after those goals differently, because their political agendas were contrary. The collision between these philosophies, although not a concern of most people involved in the conflict over the ECU medical school, raises the contest above its partisan, often petty, backbiting, and personal level. There is some excitement in the drama of personal confrontations and media battles, but the long-term suspense, it seems to me, is in the less visible drama of ideological combat.

In working through the documentation for the establishment of the medical school, I have become convinced that, while Leo Jenkins brought forward the idea, the prime mover in actually getting the school in Greenville was Dr. Edwin W. Monroe. He began to work very hard and effectively as soon as Jenkins recruited him. Then, after Jenkins became convinced that he was exposed to the possibility of losing his position if he continued to bypass the Board of Governors and approach the legislature directly, Monroe pursued unremittingly the goal they had set up. He made friends, but also influential enemies, and his success cost him dearly.

The records Dr. Monroe kept of the many skirmishes in the battle for the medical school were invaluable for the writing of this book. Also he has sat through hours of grilling, and has answered at length and in detail every question I have asked. I have found remarkable his ability to be passionately involved in a situation, and yet to be able to see and understand the disparate viewpoints others might take. This capacity must have been valuable when he needed all his wiliness to forestall attempts to block ECU's course of action.

I appreciate, also, the time Dr. Monroe has generously devoted to giving the manuscript three critical readings for accuracy and to make sure no important events were omitted.

Dr. William E. Laupus, the first dean of the School of Medicine, and ECU's second Vice Chancellor for Health Affairs, joined in my efforts to disentangle the events of 1975-1977. He had a number of useful suggestions, and his recollections enriched the account of the efforts to obtain accreditation for the four-year medical school.

Many other people have helped with this history. The persons at ECU and at UNC who were willing to submit to being interviewed were the first to contribute to it. The Vice Chancellor for Health Affairs and Dean of the School of Medicine, Dr. James A. Hallock, provided funding to complete the medical history project and some of the subsequent research.

The members of the staff of the Archives and Manuscripts Department of ECU's Joyner Library, especially Donald R. Lennon, Director, and Gene J. Williams, University Archivist (now deceased), gave me valuable assistance in searching through the Leo Jenkins archives. John White of the Manuscripts Department of the Wilson Library at UNC was similarly helpful in guiding me through the William C. Friday Papers there. Tom Fortner, Director of the Office of Medical Center News and Information, opened his files to me and furnished the photographs illustrating the text. Mr. Paul Crellin, Medical Alumni Affairs Program Coordinator, was an unfailing source of help, from interviewing Chancellor Leo Jenkins to expert advice on word processing problems.

Dr. Mary Jo Bratton encouraged me at a crucial point in my writing, gave the entire manuscript a careful reading, and provided indispensable guidance of a scholarly nature.

My wife Anne not only tolerated my habit of working in complete disregard of the clock, friends, and family, whenever I got the bit in my teeth, but made sure I remembered to eat fairly regularly. She has also given the manuscript two close readings, and detected many errors, both typographical and semantic, that it no longer has.

W. C. W.

Chapter 1
Origin of the Idea

Dr. Leo Jenkins liked to say that the idea for a medical school at East Carolina College originated with a general practitioner from Plymouth, Dr. Ernest W. Furgurson. As Dr. Jenkins described it, Dr. Furgurson came to the President's house on Fifth Street in Greenville one Sunday afternoon in the spring of 1964. He was very angry. He had just been attending a seminar at Duke University on primary health care. While in Durham, he had talked with some of his old classmates about his problems in getting another doctor to practice in Plymouth, where he had more patients than he could treat without assistance. His friends shared with him their views about the medical situation in eastern North Carolina.

President Jenkins was not at home, but Dr. Furgurson told Mrs. Lillian Jenkins about the need for a medical school at East Carolina College. She said she was not informed enough to talk about it, and suggested that he call Dr. Jenkins the next day. He did call and wanted to know why the college was not carrying through on its promises to the region that supported it. He said the college ought to do something about the terrible situation. It was their responsibility. Dr. Jenkins said that the college was not in the medical business, and never had been. Dr. Furgurson replied, "Well, you have a motto which is 'To Serve'. Why don't you live up to the motto? Who are you serving if you just sit in this cesspool?"

He said that eastern North Carolina had the worst record on health care of any section of the United States. The statistics in the east were terrible. The area led the nation in infant mortality. It led the nation in rejection from the draft for physical reasons. It was last in the nation in mental retardation programs, hospital beds, doctor-patient ratio. He wanted to know whether the college would accept its responsibility. President Jenkins told him that he would certainly take seriously the question he had raised, and would bring it to the board of trustees.[1]

When he stopped in Greenville to call on President Jenkins, Dr. Furgurson was on his way home after appearing as an invited panelist in a "Symposium on General Practice as a Career" held on Saturday, May 23, 1964, at the Duke University Medical Center in Durham. The symposium was sponsored by the Duke Endowment Foundation, under the direction of Dr. Wilbert C. Davison, former Dean of the Duke University School of Medicine.[2] Dr. Davison wrote to Dr. Furgurson in June, endorsing the idea of a medical school at ECC.[3]

Dr. Furgurson had participated in a discussion filmed for showing on television to medical students and others throughout the country. His message was that in order to assist in solving the problems of getting health care to all those who require it, doctors will have to involve themselves in politics.

He said that application lags behind discovery in medicine, and no one man can keep up with the expansion in knowledge. Specialism had resulted, causing an oversupply of physicians in certain specialties, such as surgery and internal medicine, while there is fragmentation of patient care and loss of interest in patients as human beings.

For the first time in American history, he said, everyone expected to receive adequate medical care. Having a doctor had come to be considered an inalienable right, along with the rights to life, liberty and the pursuit of happiness. The changed attitude toward medical care reflected the affluent state of our society and the improvement in living standards. "It used to be that if a man's upper leg bone stuck through his pants he might get a doctor. But he wouldn't think of seeing one for a stomach ache or because his son was an alcoholic. And in the past who ever thought of an annual check-up?"

Dr. Furgurson concluded by saying that the medical profession must accept its greatest opportunity and its greatest challenge in the next ten years. The pride and achievement upon which our country had been founded should remain our unfaltering goal.[4]

Dr. Jenkins talked to the chairman of the ECU Board of Trustees, NC Senator Robert Morgan, who later became NC Attorney General and US Senator. He told Morgan that Ernest Furgurson seemed to be a sincere man. He didn't know him too well, but found him convincing. He asked what they should do. Morgan suggested that he quietly investigate the situation, and find out what was really going on.

Dr. Jenkins had Dr. Robert W. Williams, professor of political science, verify Dr. Furgurson's statistics. Dr. Williams made a county-by-county survey, and reported back that Dr. Furgurson did not exaggerate. There was only one place in the nation that was worse than eastern North Carolina, and that was New Mexico. While the national ratio of doctors to patients was 125 per 100,000, and that of North Carolina as a whole 75 per 100,000, in the eastern counties there were less than 50 physicians for each 100,000 patients. Infant mortality in the region was indeed the highest in the nation.

"So," Jenkins said, "I told Bobby Morgan about that. He said let's bring it to our Board of Trustees and see what they want us to do. We went to our board and the board had a very simple solution. They instructed me to pursue the establishment of the medical school. That's all. Just pursue it. So, I went out and pursued it. And then the house fell in. The nasty cartoons began. The editorials began. The phone calls began. The lobbying among the doctors in Pitt County began. Some of the doctors in Greenville were very much opposed to it because they got instructions from Chapel Hill to oppose it. And we just went on. In spite of what everybody's saying, we think it's a good cause and we are going to chase it. And one by one people began to say 'You are right.'" [5]

The beginning of the School of Medicine at East Carolina College was neither as simple nor as abrupt as Dr. Jenkins's anecdote represented it. In September, 1962, Robert Lee Humber, who was State Senator from Pitt County from 1959 to 1964, had mentioned the possibility of a medical school at ECC.[6] Dr. Humber was a distinguished native of Greenville, a lawyer who attended Wake Forest and Harvard, was a Rhodes Scholar, and a prime mover in the establishment of the Movement for World Federation. He also took a leading role in founding the NC Museum of Art, and became chairman of its board of trustees in 1961. Dr. John M. Messick (President of ECC from 1947 to 1959) remembered his suggestion, but had other, more urgent projects at hand.[7]

Dr. Furgurson's provocation and Dr. Davison's subsequent reinforcement of the idea doubtless crystallized President Jenkins's interest in seeking a school of medicine for ECU. However, the idea was around before they sparked his interest. Drs. Furgurson and Davison were not originators, but were rather like the shout that dislodges the already poised snow to start an avalanche.

In 1962, Leo Warren Jenkins had been President of East Carolina College for a year, and at the school for fifteen years, having accepted the position of dean at ECTC from President Messick in 1947. Since early in his time in Greenville, he had traveled throughout the eastern area of North Carolina, speaking to civic groups and organizations, sharing his vision of East Carolina as an expanding influence and resource in the region and the state.

Jenkins was born in 1913, in Succasunna, New Jersey, near Elizabeth, where he lived until he left to attend college. He went to public school in Elizabeth, with most of his classmates the children of recent German, Italian, Polish and other east European immigrants. He was president of his graduating class at Jefferson High School for Boys, and in 1931 went to Rutgers University, in New Brunswick, NJ. Jenkins majored in political science, with enough education courses to qualify for a teaching certificate.

In 1935, he graduated from college, and began teaching at Somerville High School near Atlantic City. In the ensuing years, he taught in several other high schools, finding time to take graduate courses in education. In 1936, he took a summer fellowship at Duke University, later earned an M.A. at Columbia University, and in 1941 received an Ed.D. from New York University.

Late in 1942 came two major changes in his life: In October, he married Lillian Olga Jacobsen of Lavallette, NJ, who was also a teacher; and he enlisted in the Marine Corps in December. He was sent for basic training to Parris Island, SC. He attended Officers Candidate School, was commissioned a second lieutenant, and went with the 3rd Marine Division to Guadalcanal, Guam, and Iwo Jima. He received the Bronze Medal for heroism and two presidential unit citations.[8]

After the war, Jenkins returned to New Jersey where, in 1945, he became instructor in political science at New Jersey State Teachers College in Montclair. He had taught for only one semester when he was appointed assistant to the commissioner of higher education in New Jersey.

He met John Messick at New Jersey State Teachers College, after beginning to work for the NJ educational administration. When he accepted the position of dean at ECTC in 1947, Jenkins planned to stay in NC for only a year or two, with a view to obtaining experience which would be valuable for his career in New Jersey.[9] He never returned to live in New Jersey.

When President Messick resigned in October 1959, there was a good deal of pressure to appoint Jenkins immediately as his successor. Both the faculty and the students rallied for him. A search committee was appointed, and after due consideration of more than 20 candidates, recommended Jenkins's appointment. On January 5, 1960, the trustees approved unanimously.[10]

Jenkins chose Friday, May 13, 1960, as the day for his inauguration. UNC President William C. Friday, was the main speaker. He praised Jenkins as an educational leader, reviewing the expansion of ECC's campus and student body. He praised the college's community for its support, and recognized the college's intellectual and economic impact on eastern NC.

Governor Luther Hodges also spoke, but gratuitously mentioned the names of other candidates he would have preferred for the Presidency of the college. He suggested his reservations about the college's expansion beyond its traditional role as a teachers' college, but acclaimed its success as long as it was defined narrowly in terms of its role as a teacher-training institution.[11]

Jenkins spoke last, and promised to maintain and expand ECC's contribution to the state. He made this a pledge to the taxpayers who were paying to improve ECC's status, and accepted their authority to determine what it should do. In doing this, he was telegraphing his intentions to go to the people, bypassing the Board of Higher Education as necessary, in his efforts to improve ECC's course offerings and programs to meet discernible needs. Without being pugnacious, he challenged the educational establishment as embodied in the BHE, who had just turned down his proposal for a graduate program in business administration.

Jenkins defined his goals as including both vocational and liberal arts. He promised to expand in both directions. He promised that the faculty would offer continuing education programs throughout the region. He warned that it would be "a disservice to the people of the state" to limit the college's attempts to meet its obligations. He predicted that the institution would continue to grow indefinitely.[12]

---

[1] Interview of Chancellor Leo Jenkins by Dean William E. Laupus, October 5, 1988

[2] *Roanoke Beacon*, May 27, 1964

[3] Bratton, p. 361

[4] *Roanoke Beacon*, May 27, 1964

[5] Jenkins interview, October 5, 1988

[6] Bratton, p. 360. This chapter is based largely on Chapter 11 of Bratton's *East Carolina University*

[7] Bratton, p. 360 and note 42. Dr. Bratton interviewed John D. Messick on June 8, 1981.

[8] *Who's Who in the South and Southeast,* 12th Edition, 1971-72 (Chicago: Marquis Who's Who, Inc., 1971)

[9] Bratton, pp. 331-332

[10] Bratton, pp. 333

[11] Bratton, pp. 335

[12] Bratton, pp. 335-336

Chapter 2
Background of the Campaign

The effort to set up a second state-supported four-year medical school at East Carolina University, it has been claimed,[1] was a critical test of the viability of the multi-campus UNC system. The question should be raised whether it was as much a trial for the system itself as it was for the continued dominance of the University by the Chapel Hill campus. The effort after 1964 to establish the medical school was the continuation of a struggle undertaken years before by President John D. Messick to make East Carolina a comprehensive institution of higher learning. That endeavor was opposed by the Board of Higher Education and by its successor, the UNC Board of Governors, along with President William C. Friday, who was always wary of any effort to permit anyone outside the General Administration access to the legislature, and thus to funding he felt should be controlled by UNC.

In his crusade to raise the status of East Carolina College, President Leo Jenkins in the 1960's went directly to the people of the east and their legislators, and was prepared to do so again in the 1970's (as, after July 1972, Chancellor of East Carolina University). It did not make matters simpler or easier that the beginning of the Greenville school coincided with major reorganization of the higher education system in North Carolina.

There was no way to avoid being drawn at least into the periphery of the fundamental struggle between two contrary approaches to centralizing control of the state's college and university system, personalized between the bitterest of the antagonists, Governor Bob Scott and UNC President William Friday. North Carolina State alumnus Scott did not trust what he considered to be UNC's haughty presumption that it had the right to the dominant place in higher education in the state, in both financing and prestige. Also, he felt that Friday had misled him about restructuring the university. [2]

Robert Walter Scott was born on June 13, 1929 in Haw Fields, Alamance County near Haw River, NC, where his father, W. Kerr Scott was a dairy farmer. The Scott family had lived in this area between the Eno and Haw Rivers since the 18th century. Like his father and grandfather before him, Robert was active in the Haw Fields Presbyterian Church, founded in 1755, and became a ruling elder of the church.

Robert Scott became governor in 1969, exactly twenty years after his father, a progressive Democrat who helped bring paved roads and electrical utilities to most of the farms in the state, had become governor.

After going to grammar school in a one-room schoolhouse and to Alexander Wilson High School in Haw Fields, where he graduated in 1947, Robert Scott went to Duke University for two years, then to North Carolina State College for a bachelor's degree in animal industry. He married Jessie Rae Osborne of Swepsonville, a small mill town a few miles from Hawfields, on September 1, 1951. She attended Woman's College in Greensboro and received a BS in business education. They were married in the Governor's Mansion while Scott's father was still governor, and Robert was still in college.

Robert Scott returned to Haw Fields after his graduation from NC State in 1952 to manage the family dairy farm. He became active in the national and state Grange, and other agricultural organizations. Between 1953 and 1955, he served in the Army.

He entered politics by being elected as democratic precinct chairman, then as Alamance County vice-chairman, and eventually to the Solicitorial Democratic Executive Committee for the state party. He was national chairman of Rural Americans for Johnson and Humphrey before the 1960 convention. He served on numerous boards and commissions, including the Conservation and Development Board, the Kerr Reservoir Development Commission, and the NC Seashore Commission. In 1964, Scott became Lieutenant Governor, and was elected Governor in 1968.[3]

William Clyde Friday was born in Raphine, VA, his mother's family home, on July 13, 1920. After his birth, they returned to Dallas, NC, some three miles outside Gastonia, in Gaston County, where his father, David Lathan Friday, worked for a machine and foundry company. William Friday went to grammar and high schools in Dallas, then, in 1937 enrolled in Wake Forest College. In 1938, he transferred to NC State College, where he received a degree in textile engineering.

Friday graduated in June, 1941, and on May 13, 1942 married Ida Howell, a Meredith College graduate whom he had met on a blind date at the State-Carolina football weekend in 1940. Between his graduation and his marriage, he worked for a long summer with DuPont Corporation in Waynesboro, VA, then returned to Raleigh as the chief dormitory assistant at State. He applied for a commission in the navy, and received his call to active duty on May 11, 1942.

After three-and-a-half weeks of training, Ensign Friday was stationed at the Naval Gun Factory in Washington, DC, then transferred to the Naval Ammunition Depot near Norfolk, VA. Later that year, Ida joined him. He remained at the Depot until just before the war ended and left the service as a full lieutenant in February, 1946.

A week later, Friday and his wife went to Chapel Hill, where he had been admitted to the School of Law. At the law school, he met Dickson Phillips, William A. Dees, Jr., of Goldsboro, John R. Jordan, William B. Aycock, and others who became his friends and were allies during many of the critical events through which he later led the university. He graduated in June 1948, but after passing his bar exam and applying unsuccessfully for a position as a lawyer, he took a job as assistant to the dean of students at Carolina. Later, he became acting dean of students, then in April, 1951, he became administrative assistant to Gordon Gray, president of the Consolidated University.

In June, 1955, Gray became assistant secretary of defense under President Dwight Eisenhower, and Bill Friday was appointed acting president in March, 1956. When the selection committee for president, headed by Mr. Victor Bryant, a Durham lawyer, could reach no agreement on the candidates supported by various committee members, Friday was chosen as president on October 18, 1956.[4] It was as President of the Consolidated University that he first locked horns on a major issue with Governor Bob Scott, that issue being reorganization of the entire university system.

Jenkins's campaign, especially when it gained momentum and backing, alarmed President Friday. He was especially apprehensive of ECU's direct appeals to voters and politicians, and in spite of advocating broadened access to higher education, was opposed to decentralizing control of the public colleges and universities in North Carolina.[5]

After the end of World War II in 1945, colleges and universities in the state expanded rapidly, with little regulation. Funds for higher education were apportioned unevenly, with most of what was left after UNC received its lion's share going to the institutions with the greatest political clout, especially the regional schools, Appalachian State, Western Carolina, and the fastest growing of all, East Carolina. Detailed allocation of funds was in the hands of the General Assembly through the 1960s, with little effective intervention by the Board of Higher Education, even though the Board was charged with determining the budgets of state-funded colleges and universities. By 1972, UNC had managed to destroy that threat to its power.

From its establishment in the 1950's on the recommendation of a commission chaired by UNC champion Victor Bryant, the Board functioned effectively as a barrier against expansion of higher education outside Chapel Hill. However, its demise was practically inevitable as soon as it attempted to extend its restraints from the former teachers' colleges, whose restriction had been welcomed by the Consolidated University, to the three consolidated institutions. The UNC trustees withdrew their support of the BHE as soon as they realized it was not their vassal, but had the power to regulate the Consolidated University. It was not just a protection for the university, as it had seemed to be, against the demands for more money and expanded programs by upstart institutions outside the system, such as East Carolina College. At the point where the BHE began to make decisions affecting the University—specifically, to interfere with plans at NSCU and UNC-CH to allocate funds to build married student housing—it was clear to the trustees of the Consolidated University that the Board was a threat. At the urging of the UNC trustees and other supporters of the university, the legislature in 1959 removed the BHE's power to determine educational activities, and reduced its control over budgeting to merely giving advice.[6]

The state's higher education resources had been strained more when the veterans of World War II returned and began to attend college under the GI Bill than they were later, when ECU intensified its drive for development. During the 1940's, the university rose to the occasion, making it an opportunity for growth. During the 1960's the financial demands were not as much in issue as they had been earlier, because of increases in tax revenue and investment of federal money in education. Nevertheless, the UNC administration reacted to East Carolina's demands for growth as if they jeopardized UNC's recent successes in the consolidation battle through which it had obtained jurisdiction over most of higher education in the state. When this largest of the state's regional universities demanded the opportunity to expand further, it was also seen as a threat to siphon off part of the University's funding.

In the reorganization bill passed in October 1971, its final form largely the fruit of successful lobbying by the University and its supporters, the legislature had attempted to balance the need for planning and budgeting with the need for increased access to college and university education. The law gave the UNC Board of Governors almost complete authority in planning, program, and budget controls over the state's universities. All the powers of the BHE were transferred to the Board of Governors and the BHE was eliminated. All powers not specifically assigned to the institutional boards of trustees were reserved to the Board of Governors.

The legislature was still in ultimate control of the university and its funding, as it had been since the constitutional convention of 1875. As a result, the budgeting process could never escape political pressures. However, with the 1971 law the General Assembly gave up some of its item-by-item control of funding by allowing lump-sum appropriations for new and expanded programs, capital improvements, and increases in enrollment. At first this did little to interfere with the well-established custom of regional universities' submitting their requests through local legislators. The rancorous conflict over the ECU medical school may very well have demonstrated how big a mistake it was to divide funding authority between the General Assembly and the Board of Governors. After 1974, public battles over funding programs in the universities in the UNC system were generally avoided, though there was no lack of debate about the level of overall financial support. The Board of Governors was beginning to function as the central authority it was intended to become.

---

[1] Link, p. 221

[2] Link, pp. 172-173

[3] *Who's Who in the South and Southeast,* 12th Edition, 1971-1972 (Chicago, 1971); Beth G. Crabtree, *North Carolina Governors, 1585-1974, Brief Sketches,* (Raleigh NC: Division of Archives and History, 1974) pp. 140-42; Nancy Roberts, *The Governor* (Charlotte, 1972) p. 31.

[4] Link, Chapters 1-3; King, p. 4. The number of references to Link reveal the extent to which I have depended on his biography for information concerning William Friday's career.

[5] Link, pp. 163, 195, 221.

[6] Link, p. 160.

Chapter 3
Health Care Delivery in North Carolina

For many years before President Leo Jenkins of East Carolina College began to campaign for a school of medicine in Greenville, the lack of adequate medical care in rural North Carolina had been an issue not only for politicians, but for newspapers and the population at large, outside as well as in the most deprived areas. The members of the state's Medical Society were also concerned with the problem, but preferred that it should be solved without increasing the number of competing doctors. The physician-patient ratio in the state was among the lowest in the nation, and its infant mortality rate among the highest. Where in World War II the rate of rejection of servicemen and women for medical reasons was almost twenty-eight percent, compared to the national rate of just under twenty-four percent,[1] in 1970 in most of the state the rejection rate for young persons examined for military service had risen to over forty-five percent. In fifteen counties (fourteen of them east of Raleigh) the rejection rate was over fifty percent.[2] While various governmental efforts to deal with the state's deficiencies in health care had benefited the Piedmont and the medical school in Chapel Hill, the non-urban areas in the east and west had not gained much.

The large number of young North Carolinians barred from military service for physical causes, though not dramatically greater than in other southeastern states, was disturbing. Governor J. Melville Broughton, who served during the war years—1941-45, began to plan for improving statewide medical care. He reported to the UNC Board of Trustees on January 31, 1944 the findings of a committee of doctors that the state, eleventh in population in the country, was forty-second in the number of hospital beds per 1,000 population, and forty-fifth in doctors per 1,000. He and the committee recommended that the two-year UNC medical school should be expanded into a four-year school with a 600-bed or larger teaching hospital. The Governor said, "The ultimate purpose of this program should be that no person in North Carolina shall lack hospital care or medical treatment by reason of poverty or low income."[3]

The Board of Trustees approved the recommendation, and Governor Broughton appointed a fifty-member North Carolina Hospital and Medical Care Commission, under the chairmanship of Clarence Poe. He instructed the commission to survey the state's health situation and needs, and to recommend a program—a Good Health Program—to the next General Assembly. After eight months of study and investigation, in 1945 the commission recommended to the legislature that there should be expansion in the number of doctors, more hospitals, and more health insurance in the state. It also recommended that the state government should encourage the development of group medical care plans to enable people to purchase insurance against expensive treatment and long stays in hospital. The already established Blue Cross Plan could meet the needs of patients who could afford to pay for hospital and surgical service. The commission recommended that Blue Cross should be asked to expand services to include general practitioners and prescription drugs.[4]

Broughton's successor, Governor R. Gregg Cherry (1945-1949), did not agree with all of the recommendations of the Commission, but did support upgrading the medical school to a four-year program. William D. Carmichael, Jr., controller of the University and President Frank Graham's right hand man, began a statewide campaign to expand the medical school and teaching hospital in Chapel Hill, to set up rural health centers, and to provide loans to medical students willing to commit themselves to practice in rural communities. With the assistance of Dr. William MacNider, former dean of the medical school, and others from the university, he obtained donations from the business and industrial community. Band leader Kay Kyser, who had retired to Chapel Hill, joined in the campaign, and traveled widely across the state speaking in favor of the expansion program.[5]

The vociferous campaign to expand the School of Medicine in Chapel Hill is so full of parallels to the later struggle to establish a medical school in Greenville that it comes close to being a preview. After exploring the health care situation in other states, President Graham became convinced that if a medical school was built it should be located in Chapel Hill where the necessary basic science support was available. He helped to overcome vigorous resistance in Greensboro and Charlotte to expanding the medical school and the hospital facilities at UNC rather than in those cities.

The 1945 session of the General Assembly approved in principle the enlargement of the medical school, but left the program to be adopted in full by the 1947 session. President Graham still had to overcome the pressure to locate the school and hospital outside Chapel Hill. In March, 1946, the City of Greensboro offered the Medical Care Commission a twelve-acre tract for location of a 600-bed central hospital and four-year expanded medical school. A dozen or more cities had already made offers.[6]

On March 18, during the eleventh week of the General Assembly, the Joint Appropriations Committee took up the $44.5 million permanent improvements bill, which included appropriations for the Medical Care Commission's long range Good Health Program, including $3,790,000 for a teaching hospital at Chapel Hill and expansion of the University of North Carolina's Medical School from a two-year to a four-year institution.

The Medical Care Commission appointed a seven-member national committee, chaired by Dr. W. T. Sanger, President of the Medical College of Virginia, to do a survey of the state and recommend a site for the medical school and hospital. The committee met in Raleigh on March 17 and heard statements by the advisory committee of the State Medical Society. Then, on the next day, the committee went to Chapel Hill for lunch and a tour of the University.[7] On April 26 at a meeting in New York City, the national committee decided to make a further study of each city that had offered facilities, and compare potentialities of each with those of Chapel Hill.[8]

The Mecklenburg Medical Society, in support of the efforts of the Civic and Public Affairs Committee of the Charlotte Chamber of Commerce to have the city selected for the proposed institution, voted unanimously to ask that the proposed four-year medical school of UNC be placed in Charlotte.[9] At the ninety-second annual session of the Medical Society of North Carolina at Pinehurst, a group of Charlotte citizens presented twenty-one reasons why a medical school in connection with the University of North Carolina should be established in Charlotte. They cited the city's four general hospitals and three special hospitals with a total of 1,905 beds, and a veterans' hospital approved for construction. The total number of patients discharged from the city's hospitals in 1945 had been 32,103.[10]

The committee of out-of-state consultants toured proposed sites for UNC medical school and medical center on May 27-29, ending up in Raleigh. Following the tour of Raleigh on May 29, the committee held a meeting, but did not make their expected report to the Medical Care Commission. They announced their expectation of reporting their recommendation to the Medical Care Commission in July.[11]

Medical Care Commission officials, without any public comments, watched the progress of the Hill-Burton Senate Bill in Congress. The bill was favorably reported by the House Interstate and Foreign Commerce Committee during the week of July 15, and went to the House Rules Committee. The Committee approved the bill, and it went to the full House, where it passed by a narrow margin.

The bill provided an annual appropriation of approximately

$100,000,000 to the states for construction of hospitals. NC's share would be about $3,500,000 per year for five years. The state and local governmental units would have to provide $1,500,000 each year, for a five-year total of $25,000,000. Another requirement for annual approval would be submission of a long-range hospital plan showing existing medical care facilities and the hospital needs in the various sections of the State. Such a survey, made by five of the Medical Care Commission's field representatives, would be completed for submission to the Advisory Council of the Commission by August 1, and then to the General Assembly. If the Assembly approved the report, the Commission would submit it to the U. S. Public Health Service for approval under the Hill-Burton bill.

On the suspenseful day when the national committee's announcement was to be made, the *Charlotte Observer* publish an editorial, entitled "Virtually an Absurdity:"

Only Chapel Hill had any reasonable grounds for hoping to be recommended as a site for the proposed new University four-year medical school and 500-bed hospital. The decision was supposed to have been in the cards from the beginning, although the Commission seems to have been considerably belabored in justifying its selection of Chapel Hill. It has been the general impression of the people of the state that the idea of the four-year medical school of the University was inspired by University officials, largely upon their sentimental or prejudicial viewpoints.

In blunt phrase, the University promoters of the idea sought this development in order not to be outdone by Duke university, with which it is in deadly rivalry.

To add a third medical college to those at Duke and Bowman Gray is held by many physicians and other knowledgeable persons to be hardly more than the creation of an additional ornament for the University.

Back in the early 1920's a group of Charlotte physicians and surgeons, re-enforced by a group of local business and industrial leaders, proposed to the late J. B. Duke that he build a great hospital in connection with the possible development of a four-year medical unit here of the University of North Carolina.

Mr. Duke was instantly interested. As he did in all other of his vast adventures, he promised to give the project utmost consideration and indicated to the group that this particular kind of philanthropy strongly appealed to him.

The local group then went to Chapel Hill to consult with the authorities there as to whether or not they would cooperate in the planting here of such a four-year medical college under its auspices, together with the large hospital and other factors in the creation of a large medical center, all to be received by the state as an outright gift of Mr. Duke with essential financial endowments.

The reaction at Chapel Hill was startlingly instant and emphatic.The then President [Harry Woodburn] Chase told the Charlotte group that the University would not be interested in such a development unless it was located at Chapel Hill.

That ended the matter.

When Mr. Duke was told of this reaction on the part of the University authorities, the idea suggested continued to obsess him. Almost immediately he developed his plans for the development of the great medical college at Duke university and its large hospital along with the creation of the University there.

This is history. It seems, however, that it is history that is now in some essential respects repeating itself except that the proposed development will be financed by the taxpayers of North Carolina instead of by the long-to-be-remembered benefactor, Mr. Duke.

And, if the recommendation of the Survey committee comes to fruition, the largest city in the state with the greatest density of population within its environs and already recognized as a foremost medical center of the Southeast will be ignored with all of its admitted assets and indisputable claims as the site of this development in favor of the village of Chapel Hill, which has little to offer except intangible traditions and institutional pride.[12]

The special national committee recommended to Governor Cherry and the State Medical Care Commission on July 20, 1946, that the proposed four-year medical school and new hospital for the University of North Carolina be located on the campus at Chapel Hill. Two of the seven members submitted a dissenting report in which they stated that they were not convinced another four-year medical school would ever be needed in this State.

The Medical Care Commission voted to defer action on the reports until its regular meeting to be held early in August. The report recommended that the needed four-year medical school and hospital should be carried through only if a hospital and health center program could be developed, a practicable plan for financing medical and hospital care be established, and that the school and hospital would be an integral part of a university medical center.

The dissenting report contended that there was no evidence that another school of medicine would add a single physician to the number now practicing in the State. It said, "The principal reason that many areas in North Carolina do not attract a sufficient number of physicians and other health personnel to meet community needs is economic. The income per capita is low." (The per capita income in North Carolina in 1945 was $732 a year,[13] with only Mississippi, Alabama, and South Carolina ranking lower). The state already had two major medical schools, Duke and Bowman Gray, and would be better off without a school to produce physicians and other health personnel almost entirely for North Carolina.

The majority report recommended that if proposed expansion was carried through, the State should consider regional education in medicine and public health nursing for Negro students. This could be done, the report stated, through negotiating a contract with Meharry Medical College.

It also recommended that since citizens in the lower-income areas either would not or could not pay for public health service, the only practical solution to this problem was for the citizens of those communities to pool their resources on the insurance principle. "To anyone familiar with rural and small-town North Carolina," the report continued, "it is obvious that such a plan could not be sold on a voluntary basis to the people without some subsidy. The principal reason is economic." The report recommended that the state should use its taxing power to equalize the opportunity of every citizen to have adequate health protection. Instead of contributing from tax funds for the care of the indigent in hospitals, the State might consider subsidizing a prepayment plan for illnesses requiring hospitalization, with a subsidy in proportion to the ability of the people of each county to pay for medical care.

The problem of providing more doctors for rural areas should be attacked with a multiple approach: Improvement of social and economic conditions; overcoming the medical isolation of physicians, possibly through an integrated hospital program; selection of students from rural communities, to be partially or wholly subsidized; and guarantees of income from local communities in certain areas.

The expanded school should serve as the center from which high-quality medical care would radiate as far as possible over the geographic area. The organized medical profession of North Carolina had expressed itself in favor of the Chapel Hill location.

The majority report stated that Chapel Hill had been chosen as the recommended site because the university atmosphere provided cultural advantages for students and faculty. It would reduce difficulties in administration and in expense to the University to locate the school there. The various schools and departments at Carolina would be essential in providing necessary instruction for both medical and supporting personnel. Also, the town offered the atmosphere of a small community, and this would be favorable for training men to practice in rural communities.

The report predicted that the university would develop a philosophy of medical education, research, and medical care which would make it a facility serving the whole State.[14]

Dr. Clement C. Clay, executive secretary of the Medical Care commission announced that further study of the national panel's recommendations would be conducted by five recent past presidents of the North Carolina Medical Society, who would be asked to report their findings by August 8.[15]

The General Assembly on March 28, 1947, bringing to an end a year of uproar, especially from backers of Charlotte and Greensboro as sites for a hospital and medical school, passed legislation expanding the University of North Carolina Medical School in Chapel Hill from a two-year to a four-year school, and adding 5,000 new hospital beds statewide (500 were slated for Chapel Hill, of which 400 were actually added). The legislature appropriated some funds for the Medical Care Commission's long range Good Health Program, and $3,790,000 for the expansion at Chapel Hill and construction of a teaching hospital. They established a $6.25 million fund to underwrite grants to build health centers and community hospitals.

When the battle was over, the UNC Medical School became a center for the health services the legislature had mandated. However, increasing the number of graduating physicians and adding hospital beds benefited Chapel Hill and the Piedmont, but did little for the non-urban areas of the east and west. As the committee of national experts in health care brought in by the Medical Care Commission had reported, the failure of underserved areas in the state to attract practitioners was the result of low income. It was clear that doctors preferred to practice in areas where they could earn more for their services, where there were adequate schools for their children, and the means to a good life were available.

In eastern as in western North Carolina, the lack of access to health care was unacceptable. President Leo Jenkins of East Carolina College became convinced that the need for improvement was critical. Establishing a school of medicine at East Carolina, emphasizing primary care and catering only to North Carolinians would, he believed, help solve the problem. It would also be another step toward making the college into a university, waking the "sleeping giant" that he considered the east to be.[16]

---

[1] Lefler, p. 622.

[2] Clay, Orr, and Stuart, *North Carolina Atlas*, p. 287, Fig. 15.29.

[3] Lefler, p. 678.

[4] Lefler, p. 678; Snider, p. 230 ff.

[5] Snider, p. 231.

[6] *Raleigh News & Observer*, March 15, 1946.

[7] *Raleigh News & Observer*, March 18, 1946.

[8] *Charlotte Observer*, May 7, 1946.

[9] *Charlotte Observer*, Wednesday, April 17, 1946.

[10] *Charlotte Observer*, May 1, 1946

[11] *Charlotte Observer*, May 7, 1946; *Raleigh News & Observer*, May 8, 1946; *Raleigh News & Observer*, May 31, 1946.

[12] *Charlotte Observer*, July 20, 1946 (italics in original).

[13] Lefler, p. 637.

[14] *Raleigh News & Observer*, July 20, 1946.

[15] *Charlotte Observer*, July 20, 1946.

[16] Jenkins interview, August 31, 1988

Chapter 4
Start of the Campaign—1964-66

Once he decided that a School of Medicine was needed in eastern North Carolina, and that it should be at East Carolina College, President Jenkins set to work to build support for a two-year school of medicine. He made the project a part of his long-range plans for the College. When, on July 20, 1964, the Advisory Budget Committee of the General Assembly visited the East Carolina campus, he presented a biennial request for $12.7 million for capital improvements. The funds were to build five new classroom buildings, with top priority given a new science building, three new dormitories, an additional heating plant, a new theater, and a new laundry building. He proposed converting a building being used for music to provide much-needed administrative space, and requested funds for music and educational television equipment.[1]

At the Committee meeting, Jenkins floated his first major trial balloon on the medical school. Without asking for money to implement it, he outlined a long-range plan to provide more practicing physicians in rural North Carolina. Under this plan, a two-year medical school would be established at East Carolina, with the students going to other medical schools in the state to complete their training. Students who agreed to practice in rural NC after finishing their schooling should be offered tuition scholarships. ECC was willing to study such a proposal in concert with state education and medical officials and other experts, and to do whatever was necessary to begin the program.[2]

President Jenkins's proposal was reported in newspapers from Newport News to Charlotte. During July and August, editorials supporting the idea of a two-year medical school appeared in newspapers throughout the east, except in Rocky Mount. In the Piedmont, only the *Durham Sun* took an editorial stance favorable to the school.[3]

Later, President Jenkins confessed that the campaign to enlist support for the medical school was great sport. He said, "Frankly, I enjoyed it. I enjoyed the cartoons against us. I enjoyed the editorials because it got us friends. . . . Anyone who was slighted by a newspaper or got a raw deal and they'd find someone else who got a raw deal—there's a camaraderie that exists. Immediately, he jumps on your team. So, we've been that way to many other people. I had a whole army of folks who just didn't like the newspapers.

They came to our rescue—became our champions. As a matter of fact, our strong supporters were people who have never been to college. People who lived here and knew what they wanted, knew what they should have, and they had confidence enough that we might be the people who could deliver that for them." [4]

The Pitt County Medical and Dental Society at its August meeting approved a resolution favoring the establishment of a two-year medical school at ECC. Dr. John Wooten, the Society's president, said the resolution placed the medical and dental society "on record as favoring the establishment of a two-year basic science school of medicine at East Carolina College." [5]

At its September meeting, the five-county Pamlico-Albemarle Medical Society endorsed a proposal for the establishment of a two-year medical school at East Carolina College in Greenville. In the resolution of the medical society, it was stated that a two-year medical school could be established in Greenville for less than $4 million, whereas a four-year medical school, requiring construction of a hospital and other needed facilities, would cost an estimated $30 million.

Ashley B. Futrell, Democratic nominee for the State Senate, and Wayland Sermons, Beaufort Country Representative, endorsed the proposal. Representative Sermons, who helped spearhead the establishment of the ECC Nursing School, said that he would strongly support the proposal for a two-year School of Medicine at Greenville. [6]

In an interview televised on Sunday afternoon, September 6, 1964, by Greenville TV station WNCT-TV, Dr. Leo Jenkins said he expected his two-year medical school proposal to be considered by the legislature in its 1965 biennial session. Support for the school had begun to grow rapidly in eastern North Carolina. He said, "I think it will definitely come before the next session of the legislature." A four-year school would cost about $30 million and a two-year program around $4 million, but the ECC school could be started for no more than $250,000 by using college facilities as a foundation. Two Greenville physicians, Dr. John L. Wooten and Dr. Eric L. Fearrington, were on the program with Jenkins, both favoring the proposed school. [7]

Mr. Walter Jones, Sr., of Farmville, Democratic nominee for State Senate, told the Grifton Lions he was willing to take the leadership in the upcoming session of the General Assembly in support of a two-year medical school at East Carolina College. Jones, without Republican opposition, was assured of election representing Pitt and Greene Counties. He had been a member of the House in 1957, and introduced the bill to establish the School of Nursing at East Carolina.

Jones said he anticipated opposition to the school from certain existing institutions, even though the proposal had merit. He added, "In recent weeks I have contacted a number of legislators from the immediate area and without exception they assured me of their support." He had also sought support from Piedmont and Western legislators, and was encouraged by their sympathetic attitude. [8]

On October 1, 1964, Jenkins presented his idea to the East Carolina College Board of Trustees. They passed a resolution setting up a committee of trustees to study the proposal. The Board also elected State Senator Robert B. Morgan as their chairman. Senator Morgan was enthusiastic about having a two-year medical school in Greenville, and started working in the Senate to build support for it. [9]

Jenkins's first step was to "prepare the ground for the legislature," he said, by enlisting the interest and support of as many groups in the east as he could approach: physicians, chambers of commerce, civic organizations, and individuals. He had, in fact, already begun plowing the field months before, as has just been shown. By the time he and Walter Jones began to lobby the legislators, he had established a wide network of allies in the campaign for the medical school. Dr. Ernest Furgurson continued his support, and rallied his colleagues. The Craven-Pamlico Medical Society endorsed Jenkins's plans for a two year medical school at ECU. Senators from eastern counties—J. J. Harrington from Bertie, Sam L. Whitehurst from Craven, Carl V. Venters from Onslow—joined in the effort. Mayor Bill Flowers of Plymouth was an early and active advocate. Dr. Lenox Baker, orthopedic surgeon at Duke University Medical School, who had taught Greenville surgeon Dr. Frank Longino, took part in the campaign, which was also supported by Dr. J. W. R. Norton, the state health director. [10]

There was also opposition: Governor Dan Moore urged careful consideration of the medical school proposal. The Charlotte Chamber of Commerce published its opposition to the ECU program, and Charlotte physicians declared their intention to fight for a four-year program in that city as an alternative. Dr. William C. Archie, Director of the Board of Higher Education, said that Jenkins's program had not gone through proper channels, and was incomplete, so could not be acted on. [11]

Senators Robert Morgan and Walter Jones, who had been joined in their campaign for the school by Senator Ashley Futrell from Beaufort, Representative W. A. Forbes from Pitt County, Representative Carl Bailey from Washington, and Representative Fred Bahnson, an ECU trustee from Forsyth County, presented a bill on April 1, 1965 to establish a two-year medical school at ECC.[12] Support for the bill came from many people in the east, as well as from some in the Piedmont, including physicians.[13]

The Joint Appropriations Committee considered the bill on April 6, with supporters speaking for and opponents against it. Dr. Ernest Furgurson spoke in favor of the bill, as did Dr. Amos Johnson from Garland, a small town in Sampson County just south of Clinton, and Dr. Paul Jones of Farmville in Pitt County west of Greenville. Proponents of the medical school from ECC, Greenville, Farmville, and Bethel showed up in force for the hearing. It was attended also by Senator Robert Morgan, Senator Thomas J. White of Kinston, and Representative A. A. Zollicoffer of Henderson.

The *Raleigh News & Observer* for April 7, 1965 reported:

Opposition to the school bill came from John W. Rankin, spokesman for the Medical Center Study Commission appointed by the 1963 legislature to survey the need for medical schools in the State.

Rankin said the General Assembly should wait for results of the commission's study of "total health needs" before deciding on the school for Greenville.

He said evidence gathered so far by the study group "points to the wisdom of taking no action on a new medical school for the next two years."

Rep. Paul Roberson of Martin asked Rankin: "Is there a shortage of doctors in North Carolina?"

"Yes," said Rankin.

"Is there an way to get more doctors without building schools?" Roberson continued.

"No," replied Rankin.

Dr. George Paschal, Jr., president-elect of the N.C. Medical Society, said the group isn't opposed to the Greenville school "if the need exists."

"However," he said, "a committee of the society will recommend that the legislature defer action until adequate study can be made."

(Senator) Morgan asked him if the committee has held a meeting, and Paschal said it has not. (The *Greenville Daily Reflector* added that the members had been in contact by telephone.)

"So this will be the recommendation of a committee that has not met," Morgan stated.

Morgan also noted that the Medical center Study Commission is made up entirely of Piedmont or out-of-State people, "with not one single person from west of Charlotte or east of Raleigh."

Morgan said proponents of the ECC school "are not in opposition to a school at Charlotte or anywhere else. . . I think North Carolina's need is so great we could stand another medical school."

Dr. John Truslow, former dean of the Medical College of Virginia and a member of the study commission, said in his opinion it would be much less costly to expand present medical schools than to build a new one." There seems to be so little evidence that an increase in the number of medical schools has improved the ratio of doctors to population in rural areas of other states that we feel other roads must be taken," he said.[14]

The *Greenville Daily Reflector* reported that Dr. Edgar Beddingfield of Stantonsburg spoke on behalf of the East Carolina Medical School bill. He said he was an officer of the State Medical Society, but spoke only as an individual physician. He pointed out that the state society had taken no action on the medical school issue. "I believe the proposal has a great deal of merit," he said. "There is a shortage of doctors not only in the east but also all over North Carolina."[15] When a member of the Joint Appropriations Committee questioned him, Dr. Beddingfield said that he strongly believed that the proposed medical school should be located at ECC.[16]

Senator Ralph Scott of Alamance County (uncle of Robert W. Scott) complained that the medical school supporters should not have by-passed the Board of Higher Education, and that the bill's backers were premature in introducing it before that Board had made its recommendation. He said that if the Board was to be by-passed, then it was not needed. He commented that if the legislature tried to run higher education, students would suffer.[17] Senator Morgan replied that when the Board failed to act, the school's supporters chose to appeal directly to the General Assembly.[18]

The Senate passed the bill on June 9, 1965. The General Assembly ratified the bill on June 14, including a sum of $100,000 for the first half of the biennium, and $250,000 for the second. It was passed in spite of objections by Governor Dan K. Moore, the State Board of Higher Education, and deans of the medical schools at UNC, Duke, and Bowman Gray. The funds were designated for employing a Dean or other personnel to study the feasibility of setting up a curriculum which would meet national accreditation standards. An additional $1,500,000 was appropriated for capital improvements, contingent on obtaining up to $4,000,000 more from non-state sources.

Opponents of the bill had persuaded a majority of the House to pass an amendment, which the Senate had rejected but later accepted in a compromise to insure the bill's approval that if ECC was unable to achieve accreditation by January 1967, that the Board of Higher Education would study the proposal and decide whether the college could implement a two-year school.[19] As Dr. Edwin W. Monroe commented, this addition to the bill proved to be "a little thorn." [20]

It became an obstacle to developing a two-year school, since it made the time available to work toward that goal impracticably short. Jenkins visited two-year schools being developed at Rutgers University, at the University of New Mexico, and Michigan State University, and the four-year school being established at Pennsylvania State University. At his invitation, the Liaison Committee on Medical Education (LCME) sent two representatives, Dr. William Ruhe of the American Medical Association, and Dr. William Maloney of the Association of American Medical Colleges to ECC in July 1965. They reported that the basic science curriculum and the research facilities were inadequate as a foundation for a medical school. Also, they noted that there was no major hospital in Greenville. The LCME recommended that consultants be brought in to study the ECC situation.

In August, President Jenkins wrote to Dr. Howard Boozer, acting director of the State Board of Higher Education, informing him that he did not believe it was realistic to expect the medical school to be accredited by January, 1967. Watts Hill Jr., chairman of the BHE, told the members that Jenkins was demonstrating his wish to cooperate with the Board, contrary to earlier reports of his bypassing it. Hill said that the Board should assure President Jenkins of its full cooperation.

The Board instructed Dr. Boozer to consult with ECC on the steps so far taken to seek accreditation.

Dr. William Archie, who had resigned as director of the board, effective September 1, was gratified that Jenkins had come to the Board for its help. He suggested that ECC should bring in out-of-state consultants to assist the Board in determining what steps it should take. He said, "I wish he (Jenkins) had turned the matter over to us in the first place, but he has turned it over now. The Board belongs in the picture."

Jenkins commented that Archie was incorrect in thinking ECC had not consulted the Board in the beginning. This had been done, and the Board had turned down the request. ECC had already taken the steps Archie was suggesting, and had a list of ten consultants who had been suggested to assist with the plan. He would be picking three or four from the list. He said that he wanted the Board and ECC's supporters across the state and in the legislature to know what was being done.

Board member Dr. Hubert Poteat of Smithfield moved that they accept ECC's invitation to help in establishing the two-year school of medicine. Poteat said, "Personally I would prefer to see them shoot for the whole works and establish a four year medical school" [21]

In August, Jenkins initiated a correspondence with Dr. Isaac M. Taylor, dean of UNC School of Medicine, and on August 20 they met in Greenville for three hours. After the meeting, Dean Taylor said that he and Dr. Jenkins were in agreement in terms of their general aims and want to serve the state's needs in medical care and education in every way possible. He added, "I want to be helpful in any way I can with this very big assignment that has been given to East Carolina College." [22]

A few days after Dean Taylor met with President Jenkins, Consolidated University President William Friday announced that people from the university, including members of the medical school, would be available to give professional help to ECC on its plans to set up a two-year medical school. Friday said that since the General Assembly had decided on the policy of exploring the possibility of establishing a medical school, the university was glad to help. [23]

In November, Dr. Jenkins met with Dr. Lenox Baker of Durham, Dr. Edgar Beddingfield of Stantonsburg, Dr. Ernest Furgurson of Plymouth and Dr. Jacob Koomen, Assistant Director of the State Board of Health, who constituted an unofficial advisory committee of doctors who supported the proposed two-year school of medicine at Greenville. With Dean Robert Williams, he sought their advice concerning the evaluation team from the Liaison Committee on Medical Education whom he was inviting to look over the plans and existing facilities for the medical school.[24]

President Jenkins asked Dr. John A. D. Cooper, dean of sciences at Northwestern University, Dr. Reginald Fitz, dean of medicine at the University of New Mexico, and Dr. C. Arden Miller, dean of the School of Medicine at the University of Kansas,[25] to survey the program at ECC. They spent two days and two nights in Greenville, speaking with Jenkins, with Howard Boozer (director of the Board of Higher Education), Watts Hill, Jr. (a member of the BHE), state Senator Lindsey C. Warren, Jr., (who chaired the Committee appointed in 1971 by then Governor Robert Scott, and which recommended the restructuring of UNC), ECC Dean Robert Williams, and with the chairmen and some faculty members in ECC departments.

On January 13, 1966, the consultants made a report suggesting that rather than establish a medical school, ECC should develop curricula in allied health sciences, forming a Life Sciences and Community Health Institute. The report confirmed Dr. Jenkins's expectations about accreditation, but did nothing to turn aside his campaign. The report also did not weaken the support of legislators representing rural counties in both the eastern and western parts of the state.[26]

---

[1] Members of the Commission (who stayed overnight in Greenville after their meeting, and attended the opening performance of "My Fair Lady" at the ECC Summer Theater) were: Sen. Thomas J. White of Kinston, chairman, Sen. James V. Johnson of Statesville, Rep. David M. Britt of Fairmont, Rep. Clyde H. Harriss of Salisbury, Sen. Ralph H. Scott of Haw River, and William H. White of Jacksonville.

[2] *Greenville Daily Reflector*, July 21, 1964.

[3] *Durham Sun* (Editorial), 25 July 1964

[4] Jenkins interview by William E. Laupus, October 5, 1988

[5] *Greenville Daily Reflector*, August 26, 1964.

[6] *Washington Daily News*, September 3, 1964.

[7] *Raleigh News & Observer*, September 7, 1964.

[8] *Greenville Daily Reflector*, September 26, 1964.

[9] Bratton, p. 363; Minutes of ECU Board of Trustees, October 1, 1964.

[10] Link, p. 222; Hedrick, Chronology, p. 2.

[11] Hedrick, Chronology, pp. 2-3; Bratton, p. 365.

[12] Senate Bill 176, Chapter 986 of Session Laws of North Carolina; Extra Session 1963, Regular Session 1965.

[13] Link, 222. Hedrick's Chronology, p. 3, reports that the bill was signed by Senators Robert Morgan of Harnett, Ashley Futrell of Beaufort, J. J. Harrington of Bertie, Russell Kirby of Wilson, Carl Meares of Columbus, Stewart Warren of Sampson, Cameron Weeks of Edgecombe, Sam Whitehurst of Craven, Emmett Winslow of Perquimans, Julian Allsbrook of Halifax, Dallas Alford of Nash, and by one non-easterner, Senator Clyde Norton of McDowell County.

[14] *Raleigh News & Observer*, April 7, 1965; *Greenville Daily Reflector*, April 7, 1965.

[15] *Greenville Daily Reflector*, April 7, 1965.

[16] *Wilson Daily Times*, April 12, 1965.

[17] *Greenville Daily Reflector*, April 14, 1965.

[18] Hedrick, Chronology, p. 3

[19] Supporters of the bill "felt they could have defeated the amendment in the House too and still have passed the bill. However, to allay any fears among some who planned to vote for the bill, they agreed to accept the amendment." *Greenville Daily Reflector*, August 24, 1965.

[20] Monroe interview, January 3, 1992.

[21] The exchange about Jenkins's consulting the board is described in the *Greenville Daily Reflector, Raleigh Times*, and other newspapers, August 14, 1965.

[22] *Raleigh News & Observer, Winston Salem Journal, Greenville Daily Reflector, Greensboro Daily News*, etc. August 21, 1965. [Most reports were verbatim from the ECC News Bureau's press release of August 20,1965]

[23] *Charlotte Observer*, Wednesday, August 25,1965.

[24] *Reflector*, November 11, 1965.

[25] Senator Robert Morgan said in an interview that when he was on the Senate Appropriations Committee in 1967 he had questioned Dr. Miller about his serving on the panel of consultants on the ECU medical school, when he had been employed, or was discussing employment, with the UNC School of Medicine, where he subsequently became vice chancellor for health sciences. (Morgan interview, March 17, 1992).

[26] John A. D. Cooper, M. D., Reginald Fitz, M. D. and C. Arden Miller, M. D., *Report to President Leo Jenkins on the Feasibility of Establishing a School of Basic Medical Science at East Carolina College* (Greenville, North Carolina) January 13, 1966; also printed in Appendix I-2 of *A Plan for the Expansion*

of Medical Education at the School of Medicine East Carolina University, Prepared by the Faculty, October 1974. ECU School of Medicine Files, Folder "ECU on SOM-2."

Chapter 5
Renewal of the Campaign—1967-71

In March 1967, Senator Julian Allsbrook of Halifax and Rep. Horton Rountree of Pitt introduced bills into the Senate and House to make East Carolina College an independent university, authorized to grant doctorates and to establish a two-year medical school.[1] On April 27, after a rancorous fight in the newspapers and the legislature, the Senate rejected the legislation.

The defeat of the East Carolina bill did not end the battle. Senator John T. Henley of Cumberland County had been working unsuccessfully to have the college become part of the Consolidated University. In June, he introduced a bill (designed largely by ex-governor Terry Sanford) to make East Carolina a regional university. After vigorous politicking, especially by Governor Dan Moore, ECC Board of Trustees chairman Senator Robert Morgan, and BHE chairman George Watts Hill, Jr., the bill was amended to include Western Carolina, Appalachian, and the two mainly black colleges, NC A&T and NC Central, and the General Assembly passed it.

The requirement that the medical school program in Greenville should be controlled by the Board of Higher Education was omitted from the bill, and was never officially considered again. Authorization for a Health Sciences Institute at ECU, recommended by the BHE, was approved.[2]

When the 1967 statutes were codified, they included authorization for the board of trustees of East Carolina University "to create a school of medicine at East Carolina University, Greenville, North Carolina," meeting all requirements and regulations of the national accrediting agencies. The inclusion of this provision in the statute enabled the university to continue with the planning process, though without any funding.[3]

The granting of regional university status was not the end of ECU's campaign to be recognized as a full-fledged university authorized to award doctorates. Dr. Jenkins said that the school would use the legislation to prepare for eventually offering that degree.[4]

The recommendations made by the panel of consultants in 1966 were carried out, and a School of Allied Health and Social Professions planned. In November, 1967, President Jenkins approached Dr. Edwin W. Monroe, who was in practice in Internal Medicine in Greenville, and asked him if he would take over the direction of the allied health program. He made a point of warning him that the position would be very demanding. Dr. Monroe, a graduate of Davidson College and the University of Pennsylvania School of Medicine, had attended the two-year program at the UNC Medical School, and had returned to Chapel Hill in 1952 for his four-year residency. He was known to President Jenkins because of his work with Dean Robert W. Williams in the county-by-county survey of health facilities in the east which had helped to justify the decision to pursue the medical school idea.[5] Since Monroe grew up in the small farming town of Laurinburg, in Scotland County, he had firsthand knowledge of the eastern part of North Carolina.[6]

On January 25, 1968, the Board of Trustees requested approval by the Board of Higher Education for a School of Allied Health and Social Professions, and approved the appointment of Dr. Monroe as Dean of the School and Director of Health Affairs.[7] Dr. Monroe accepted the offer, and he was appointed in June. He worked half-time for the first six months to enable his partner in practice, Dr. Eric Fearrington, to find a replacement for him.[8]

There were many incentives at work in the drive to establish a medical school at East Carolina University. Those given public expression by its proponents were not merely slogans to rally support, as has been suggested. They were serious in intent and reacted to the lack of health care in eastern North Carolina. Dr. Leo Jenkins was not exaggerating when he said of the area:

> It had the reputation for being number one on the bottom of regions that delivered modern medical care. We led the nation in infant mortality. We led the nation in draft rejections, both medical and mental and physical. We led the nation in sparsity of hospital bed relationships. We led the nation in the lack of doctors. Our picture was a gloomy one. The only one even close to us, which still was better than us, was one in New Mexico. An Indian area in New Mexico was greatly ignored historically. They were doing something about it. But we weren't doing anything about it. And we were just saying, well the wealthy people, if they had a tonsillectomy, they'd go to Duke University or they would go to Richmond or go to Atlanta. But the poor fellow just had to wallow down here. We said that isn't right. Something ought to be done about that. [9]

That there were factual justifications is not sufficient to explain the passions that the medical school project aroused. The eastern and western regions of North Carolina, as the proposal to raise the status of the Chapel Hill medical school in 1945-1946 had made very clear, still resented the preeminence of the Piedmont (as they had from colonial times). [10] That section of the state led in education, in availability of medical care, in transportation, and in manufacturing and all other economic spheres except agriculture, tourism, and some apparel manufacturing. Perhaps worse than its actual predominance was the smug assumption of superiority that was attributed by citizens of the rest of the state to the inhabitants of the Piedmont, especially to the University in Chapel Hill, its faculty, administration, and alumni.

Dr. Ed Monroe wrote in the October, 1968, issue of the *North Carolina Medical Journal:*

> All available studies and statistics document critical health manpower shortages across the nation. North Carolina and, especially, Eastern North Carolina traditionally fare worse than most states and regions in the United States in these statistics.... In physicians in private practice, North Carolina is fifth from the bottom of all states; in total number of physicians, the state is tied with two other states at thirteenth from the bottom.... Two-thirds of the eastern counties have a physician-population ratio far below the average for the state. The same dismal facts apply to health professions in other categories—nursing, physical therapy, occupational therapy, medical record librarianships, dentistry, dental hygiene, etc. [11]

On January 4, 1969, the Legislative Committee on the Physician Shortage in Rural North Carolina completed its study. The committee had been established under the Legislative Research Commission by a joint resolution of the General Assembly on June 13, 1967. Its chairman was Representative Hugh S. Johnson, Jr., of Duplin County, and its members were Representative Horton Rountree (Pitt), Senator Albert J. Ellis (Onslow), Senator Robert Morgan (Harnett), Senator Thomas J. White (Lenoir), and Senator John T. Henley (Cumberland). (Its report was made public on February 28, but had circulated among interested groups, including the BHE, from its completion).

The findings of the committee confirmed the direst pronouncements of the supporters of a medical school at East Carolina. The physician to population ratio, near the bottom of the nation's average of ninety-seven, was sixty-nine per 100,000. The number of general practitioners was about one per 4,000 citizens. In some counties, there were no practicing physicians, and twenty-two percent of the physicians in practice in rural areas were over seventy years old.

In spite of the widespread need for family doctors, the medical schools were not doing the job of training family practice physicians, since they considered them to be relics. Instead they pointed their graduates toward specialty practice. Programs that placed medical students, interns, and residents in community hospital settings were just being started in a few areas. Medical teaching had not only failed to keep up with needs, but was also falling short in integrating advances in the medical sciences into their teaching.

The report recommended that existing medical schools increase the number of entering students, accelerate their training, and change their orientation from specialty training to primary care medicine. The UNC medical school should be given the funds necessary to carry out planned expansions. There should be closer cooperation between the university medical school and community hospitals throughout the state. A professorship in Family Medicine should be established at Chapel Hill. Referral hospitals should be planned for the eastern and western parts of the state, at which students could be given clinical experience. Though the committee was made up largely of eastern legislators, no recommendation was made concerning a program at East Carolina University.

In January, the Board of Higher Education accepted the offer of the deans of the state's three medical schools to provide information about the urgent need for more physicians in North Carolina. They also offered to spell out the financial problems they were facing. The UNC School of Medicine was represented by Dean Isaac Taylor. He described the school's plans for expansion, and discussed the need for appropriations to pay for capital improvements and increases in operating funds that would be necessary to expand class size from seventy-five students to one hundred sixty students by 1976, and to two hundred in the years immediately following.

The Deans of the two private medical schools, Dr. Manson Meads of Bowman Gray School of Medicine, and Dr. William G. Anlyan of Duke University School of Medicine, supported expansion of the existing private and public medical schools as the most economical and the fastest way to train more physicians. They warned of probable reduction in federal funding for medical schools, and described the financial difficulties being faced by all medical schools. They said that Bowman Gray and Duke were eager to expand their entering classes in order to meet the state's needs for additional physicians.

This would require financial assistance from the state for expanding faculty and teaching facilities.

Deans Anlyan and Meads asked the BHE to mount a study of the medical schools' financial problems, and to seek means of expanding their capacity to serve the state's needs. The Board agreed, and its chairman, Watts Hill, Jr., of Durham, appointed a committee to report at the Board's March meeting. The recommendations of the committee were that the UNC School of Medicine should expand its entering class enrollment as Dean Taylor had described; that the state should begin in fall 1969 to provide grants of $3,250 per medical student to Duke and Bowman Gray; that science programs should be strengthened in the state's public colleges and universities, and students encouraged to enter the health professions, especially medicine; the contract with Meharry Medical College to fund students from North Carolina should be continued; allied health science and nursing programs should be developed or expanded on some UNC campuses; the BHE should establish a medical education advisory committee, to study long-range needs and make recommendations to support the existing schools, expand programs, and create new physician training programs; and the question of ECU's two-year medical school should be referred to the Board of Higher Education. At its March meeting, the BHE accepted the committee's report, and published it as a special report.[12]

On March 18, Dr. Jenkins and Dr. Monroe presented to the legislature a $2,460,000 request to begin a two-year medical school at ECU immediately: $375,000 to plan and organize ECU's basic medical science program, recruit staff, and do preliminary planning for physical facilities; $425,000 to add staff, equipment and facilities to ECU's basic and behavioral science departments; $160,000 for planning and operating a comprehensive continuing education program at ECU for medical and paramedical personnel; and $1,500,000 to a Regional Health Authority at ECU to augment staff and facilities at eastern hospitals for teaching medical and allied health students and improve services. The new plan would use existing hospitals such as those at Greenville, Wilson, Kinston, Goldsboro, Roanoke Rapids, Tarboro, Rocky Mount, and other eastern North Carolina towns.[13]

The request was supported by a comprehensive document prepared by Monroe, presenting a detailed study of the health care system in the state, with emphasis on eastern North Carolina, and including a plan to utilize ECU's existing resources "to close the widening gap between the East and the remainder of the State." Forty maps, all but one of them (showing the location of Negro Physicians by County in 1968) prepared by the NC Regional Medical Program, provided a visual survey of the distribution of population, of hospitals, primary care physicians, specialists in all the main categories, population per physician ratios, nurses and other paramedical personnel, death rates, and families with incomes below poverty level. The distribution of the graphic symbols on the maps made dramatically visible the disparity between the Piedmont and the eastern area of the state, as well as western North Carolina.[14]

Dr. Monroe told the legislators, "[ECU] firmly believes that a basic medical science curriculum—the equivalent of the first two years of medical school—should be planned and developed on its campus now. Not to act now could find the East 10 years behind in its medical planning two years from now." He promised legislators that the medical school "would not attempt to duplicate complex medical centers such as those present in Chapel Hill or Durham." [15] However, expanding the programs at UNC, Duke, and Bowman Gray would not solve the problem for the rural counties and small towns in the state, since most of their graduates would go into specialties. The school at Greenville would produce primary care physicians, so would offer an immediate improvement in the quality of health care.

Reaction from partisans of the medical school in Chapel Hill and from backers of state support for medical facilities in Greensboro and Charlotte to ECU's drive was forceful and immediate. The issue of the school at East Carolina became even more political than it had been previously. Both educational and health care questions were largely forgotten except insofar as they provided ammunition for factional arguments.[16]

Chapel Hill, joined by most of the state's medical establishment, was a center of opposition. It had a natural group of allies in the members of the legislature who were wary of the cost of initiating a new program in medical education—the most expensive schooling of any that the state subsidized. Opponents of the Greenville school calculated that its cost would amount to a hundred million dollars or more. Of this estimate, Dr. Leo Jenkins enunciated what was to become one of his familiar rallying cries: "This is the fright figure that has been used to scare everybody relative to a medical program for the East."[17]

He and other proponents of the ECU program offered much lower estimates. They surveyed a number of new schools under development to discover their projected operating costs over the first five years of development, without building and other capital investments, and found that these schools started with amounts ranging from about a million dollars a year up to about six million dollars for the first five years. The reality was that nobody knew exactly what it would cost to develop a new school, because it hinged on such unpredictable factors as the possibility of being associated with V.A. Hospitals, and the accessibility of federal money for developing new medical schools. A good deal of unfettered guesswork was done, since the actual costs were not available anywhere.[18]

On June 27, 1969, the NC House of Representatives passed and on July 1 the General Assembly ratified a $375,000 appropriation to East Carolina University "for planning and developing a two-year curriculum for the School of Medicine authorized by G. S. 116-464" (in 1967). [19] This was a step forward, although not what East Carolina had hoped for.

The planning effort began immediately, with the invitation of consultants—experts in the basic sciences—from the Medical College of Georgia and the University of Florida in Gainesville. They were introduced by Dr. Monroe to the chairmen of the existing basic science departments at ECU, toured the city and Pitt County Memorial Hospital, met local doctors, and were questioned about curricula in the basic medical sciences. Would it be possible to develop a program utilizing the existing master's programs and facilities, with their strengths enhanced and any weaknesses eliminated?

Even though the chairmen of the pertinent ECU departments were willing to help, it was decided that it was not feasible to base the new program on existing departments. Dr. Monroe and his staff continued the planning effort, and worked through the rest of the year and the beginning of the following year to expand the Allied Health curriculum.[20]

On June 15, 1970, anticipating the approval of funding, Dr. Monroe announced the appointment of Dr. Wallace R. Wooles of the Medical College of Virginia in Richmond as Director of Medical Sciences and Professor of Pharmacology at East Carolina University. Dr. Wooles was to assist in planning and developing the two-year medical school and recruiting its faculty. He was associate professor of pharmacology and coordinator of medical education at the Medical College of Virginia in Richmond, where he had been responsible for revising the curriculum for basic sciences and clinical medicine. Wooles had been in the Department of Pharmacology at MCV and in the Health Sciences Division of Virginia Commonwealth University since 1963. In 1967 he had become associate professor of pharmacology.[21]

Dr. Wooles was born in Lawrence, Massachusetts, and earned bachelor and master's degrees from Boston College. He received his Ph.D. in pharmacology from the University of Tennessee Medical School in Memphis in 1963. At the Medical College of Virginia, in addition to being coordinator of medical education, he had taught in the schools of medicine, dentistry, and pharmacy, had given a graduate course on uses of radioactive drugs in experimental pharmacology, an undergraduate course in drugs and their action, was advisor to Ph.D. candidates, and a member of the admissions committee of the School of Medicine.

In an interview in 1991, Dr. Wooles spoke of his reasons for coming to East Carolina. After talking with Dr. Monroe, he visited the campus on at least three separate occasions, and was shown the 1969 bill that established a medical school and appropriated money for its planning. "And what I didn't realize was that we were to take this money and plan out a program, and then go and fight the battle in the legislature to get the School of Medicine," Wooles said. "That was a unique revelation, because I knew nothing about North Carolina politics. I really didn't know much about the state of North Carolina, except that it was close to Virginia." As soon as he arrived, he began to help design a curriculum, and to recruit faculty for the planned school.[22]

Dr. Wooles had recommended two basic science chairmen for consideration, an anatomist, Dr. Mike Schweisthal, who was at the University of Kentucky, and a physiologist, Dr. Robert Thurber, who had recently gone from the Medical College of Virginia to Jefferson Medical School. By the time Wooles agreed to accept the position, the two department chairman were committed, and came to Greenville shortly after he did.[23]

In September, 1970, ECU requested approval of a two-year master of medical science degree from the Board of Higher Education, and the Board referred the proposal to its Educational Programs Committee. (In March, Dr. Jenkins, in what the *Raleigh News and Observer* called "a vintage Jenkins maneuver" to gain support for getting medical school funds into the next budget, had suggested stripping the BHE of its authority for approving new degree programs.) [24]

The executive committee of the State Board of Higher Education met in September and approved a recommendation of its Advisory Committee on Medical Education that it should recognize East Carolina University's authorization to establish a two-year school of medicine. The executive committee also approved a statement that "administrators of the four-year schools were willing to accept, consistent with the admission policy of the respective school, 16 to 20 students from the two year medical school at ECU if it should be accredited."[25]

At its October meeting, the Board of Higher Education discussed the proposed medical school at ECU after Watts Hill, Jr. of Durham raised a question about its legality. It was noted that when the next General Assembly met, it would make the legality question moot, so the Board took no action.[26]

Dr. Edwin Monroe and Dr. Wallace Wooles had met during the fall with the deans of the three North Carolina medical schools and negotiated an agreement that they would accept transfer students from a two-year school. The number agreed on was sixteen to twenty students, to be distributed between the three schools.[27] This agreement generated considerable debate later on, when the deans of the three four-year schools denied that any such compact had been made.

The records of the Board of Higher Education and the minutes of committee meetings indicate that the three deans had committed themselves to accepting the transfer students from ECU. On July 17, 1970, Dr. Cameron West, responding to a request from Representative Kenneth C. Royall, Jr. of Durham, arranged for him a meeting with the deans of the three medical schools in the state, Dr. Isaac Taylor from UNC, Dr. Thomas Kinney from Duke, and Dr. Manson Meads from Bowman Gray, Dr. Edwin W. Monroe, and members of the BHE. At that meeting it was agreed that an Advisory Committee on Medical Education should be established, with Representative Royall, the deans from the three medical schools, Dr. Monroe, and Mr. W. C. Harris, Jr. representing the BHE, as members. Later, Dr. West appointed two additional physician members to the committee, Dr. Luther W. Kelly, Jr. of Charlotte, and Dr. Robert H. Shackleford of Mount Olive.

On August 18, 1970, the Advisory Committee passed a motion stating that "administrators of the four-year schools have expressed a desire to cooperate and a willingness to accept up to 16 to 20 East Carolina University transfer students whenever East Carolina University achieves accredited operating status." At the September meeting of that committee, Dr. Monroe moved that the minutes of the August meeting should be approved. Dr. William J. Cromartie, Associate Dean for Clinical Sciences at the UNC School of Medicine, representing Dean Isaac Taylor of that school, who was absent, requested that the minutes should show that the statement did not mean automatic acceptance of an ECU student. Dr. Cameron West, attending as staff representative of the BHE, suggested that there be added to the statement this phrase: "provided further that additional resources will be required by each of the three schools when the transfer classes increase beyond the 16 to 20 students."

The report was unanimously adopted as amended upon motion by Dr. Kinney, seconded by Dr. Meads.

Higher Education In North Carolina, the BHE's newsletter, in its November 30 issue contained the following statement:

> That the Advisory Committee recognizes that the North Carolina General Assembly in 1965, 1967, and 1969 authorized a two-year school of medicine to be created at East Carolina University; that East Carolina University is taking steps toward establishing a two-year medical school; that the three operating medical schools of the state have been advised of the needs of the anticipated students who will complete the two-year medical program at East Carolina University; and that administrators of the four-year schools have expressed a desire to cooperate and a willingness to accept, consistent with the admission policy of the respective schools, collectively up to 16-20 students from an accredited two-year medical school at East Carolina University.[28]

In October, 1970, a survey team from the LCME visited ECU to evaluate its potential for establishing a two-year medical education program. Their report quoted the resolution of the "meeting in August of the Advisory Committee on Medical Education of the State Board of Higher Education, of which the Deans of the three medical schools are members," except for substituting the phrase "in accordance with" for "consistent with" and "up to 16 to 20 East Carolina University transfer students whenever East Carolina University achieves accredited operating status" for the final phrase of the Board of Higher Education report.[29]

On December 20, 1970, Dr. Leo Jenkins said that North Carolina's three medical schools had agreed to accept a total of sixteen to twenty students a year from the ECU school. Other agreements with medical schools in the Southeast were being worked out.[30] Shortly afterward, there was an Associated Press report that the three deans of North Carolina's established medical schools had denied agreeing to accept a certain number of ECU graduates.[31] Jenkins immediately repudiated the AP story, which he said "purports to be a denial of any agreement on the part of the established four-year medical schools in our state to accept a certain number—a certain quota—of third-year medical students who have completed a two-year curriculum at East Carolina. This is a half-truth and is therefore misleading." He reaffirmed his earlier statement that there was an agreement by the three schools to accept a number still to be determined on the basis of available space and admission requirements.[32]

President Friday's statement in February, 1971, that there were no plans to accept transfers from a two-year program, if one should be approved later on, appears somewhat deceptive in view of the statements approved a few months before by Dean Isaac Taylor and Associate Dean Cromartie. On September 15, 1970 following a statement by Dr. Jenkins about the transfers, the *Raleigh News & Observer* reported: "Dr. Isaac Taylor, dean of the medical school at the University of North Carolina at Chapel Hill, told a reporter Monday that no such agreement exists." [33] The BHE had not yet published its transcript of the August agreement, but several state newspapers had quoted it in a news story about the BHE's action on the ECU school.

UNC was not the only institution that issued revisionist statements. At the end of December, Bowman Gray's Dr. Manson Meads said, "Bowman Gray has agreed to consider for transfer qualified students from East Carolina to fill spaces available. At our present attrition rate, that would be about three or four places each year." At the same time, Dr. Fuydam Osterhout, associate director for administration at Duke, said "Our attitude with East Carolina was one of cooperation. We'll receive applications from students in any two-year medical school and give them proper appraisal. All things being equal, we'd give the benefit to East Carolina." [34]

As Dr. Edwin W. Monroe commented in 1993, "Once those three schools realized what they had done, they backtracked so rapidly that in retrospect it's humorous. At the time it was infuriating." [35]

Drs. Monroe and Wooles attended the fall meeting of the Association of American Medical Colleges in Los Angeles. At that meeting, they were furnished with a copy of the report that the survey team, which had visited the ECU campus in October, was preparing to present to the full Liaison Committee. This was in accordance with the usual procedure in accreditation, to provide an opportunity for review and correction of factual errors.[36] The *Raleigh News & Observer* wrote that an official of the AMA, questioned by the newspaper, had said that it was unusual for a medical school to be considered by the accreditation committee before it opened.[37] The unidentified official was expressing an odd opinion, since before a medical school may open it has to be accredited by the Liaison Committee. He added that he understood the report might have been requested for public relations purposes and for the legislature.[38]

The LCME survey team commented that with North Carolina standing forty-sixth among the fifty states in the ratio of medical students to population, it was clear that the number of students in medicine should be increased. The two-year school at ECU could be expected to contribute to alleviating the physician shortage in the state, mainly through increasing enrollment of eastern NC students in medical school. They found that the faculty already in residence was adequately qualified and reasonably paid. However, there were still significant gaps in the faculty, especially for the behavioral sciences and clinical courses, but also in some basic sciences.

The committee was particularly concerned with the lack of assurance that graduates of the ECU program would be accepted in other schools to complete their training. While progress had been made in developing the medical library, the plans for making the collection adequate for a beginning medical school would not reach that goal soon enough. The team felt the Master of Medical Science degree that ECU proposed to offer would be of little, if any, advantage in being admitted to another school.

Following their detailed list of the positive factors and the areas with significant deficiencies, the report concluded:

> Finally, the survey team believes that there exists at East Carolina University the potential for developing a fully-accredited two-year school of the basic medical sciences. However, it is believed that it would be premature to begin such training in the fall of 1971, and that this date should be postponed one year until the fall of 1972. Assuming that the North Carolina General Assembly at its 1971 session provides an adequate operating budget, and assuming that there has been satisfactory progress in the areas mentioned above, it may be expected that the school will merit provisional accreditation prior to entry of its first class in September, 1972.[39]

On Thursday, January 28, 1971, according to an Associated Press report echoed in many newspapers, President Leo Jenkins said that a report by an accreditation team on ECU's proposed two-year medical school would be turned over to university officials Friday at

noon. Jenkins said ECU planned then to submit the report to Gov.
Bob Scott, who was chairman of the State Board of Higher Education. The ECU president indicated that the report's contents would
not be made available to the public until after Scott had received it. It
was to be considered by the BHE's education programs committee on
Feb. 8 and before the full board at its Feb. 19 meeting.

On January 29, 1971, Dr. Marjorie P. Wilson, Secretary of the
Liaison Committee on Medical Education formally transmitted the
report of the survey team to Dr. Jenkins. She said that the Liaison
Committee, at its meeting of January 28, had examined all the available evidence, including the survey team's report on its October 11-
13 visit in Greenville, and reports of earlier consultations. The
Committee, she said, "is of the opinion that the state of development
of the medical education program of East Carolina University does
not justify provisional accreditation to accept an entering class in
1971." A copy of the survey report was being sent to Dr. Wallace R.
Wooles, Dean of the Division of Medical Sciences. Dr. Wilson added,
"The report is considered confidential. However, it is for the use of
the University and the Medical School as dictated by their best
judgment. In general, it has been the experience of the Councils that
it is not desirable to release the report to the public press." [40]

The formal report was found not to contain the survey team's favorable conclusion about ECU's potential for developing a fully-accredited school of the basic medical sciences. There was a page missing in the report at the point where, in the team's presentation, that
favorable comment had been included.

Many people, including some legislators, who saw the report in
its two versions wanted to know what the missing page included and
why it had been removed. President Jenkins had made the report
public just as it was originally received, and made a special point of
the survey team's statement that ECU had "the potential for developing a fully-accredited two-year school of the basic medical science."
Dr. Wallace Wooles issued a statement that the developing school
had been given "reasonable assurance of accreditation" by the LCME.
The absence of any such positive statement from the report issued by
the full Liaison Committee was an embarrassment, and explaining
the apparent discrepancy to each person who inquired took a good
deal of time.

After talking at a medical education conference with Dr. Marjorie
Wilson, who was Secretary of the LCME when the report was issued,
Dr. Wooles wrote to her asking for "a simple one or two sentence let-
ter to President Jenkins stating a page was removed by committee

action and it is only an error in pagination." [41] Dr. Wilson went further, and wrote to Dr. Jenkins explaining that the recommendations of a survey visit team "were not intended to be an integral part of the report which is sent to the school," reporting the official action of the Liaison Committee, which is conveyed by the cover letter sent with the report. When the survey report was typed over and two appendices were added, the need to change the pagination had been overlooked.[42]

The sentiment in Greenville was that the Liaison Committee, ignoring as it had the overall favorable conclusions of the site visitors, was biased against the medical school. The Committee, ECU supporters agreed, had somehow been influenced, in spite of its own survey team, to take up the position of UNC and the other opponents of ECU in the medical establishment.

Dr. Wooles commented, "as soon as the LCME met—Dr. Anlyan [Dean William Anlyan of Duke University School of Medicine] happened to be a member of that group at that time—that page was missing. Everything else was intact, that page had been removed, and it ended without a summary, which was highly unusual. It put the LCME in a terrible position. In effect, they were saying that they're not going to make any judgment. This is what they found. This is a state problem. They didn't want to get involved. And I think they had a lot of medical educators from the other schools telling them the same thing." [43]

Dr. Jenkins presented the LCME report to Governor Robert W. Scott on Thursday, February 4. On that day he met with the governor in Raleigh, accompanied by Attorney General Robert Morgan, chairman of the board of trustees of ECU, and two members of the ECU administration, Drs. Edwin Monroe and Wallace Wooles. The groundwork was being laid for presenting the request for funding of the medical program to the 1971 legislature.

On February 19, 1971, the Board of Higher Education made public a report of its consideration of a proposal presented by ECU on September 23, 1970 to establish a two-year medical education program. In this report, the board held that the best approach to alleviating the shortage of physicians in the state would be to expand enrollment at the existing schools. The BHE proposed doubling enrollment at UNC, and doubling the number of in-state medical students for whom grants were being made to Duke and Bowman Gray Schools of Medicine. The state should subsidize black North Carolina students attending Meharry Medical School in Nashville, Tennessee, in the hope that they would return to practice in or near their home localities. The board objected to establishing either a two-year or a four-year medical school in Greenville, because it was too expensive and was unnecessary. What it did recommend was setting up a one-year program, like one in Indiana, which would prepare students to transfer to UNC to complete their training.[44]

J. Lem Stokes, one of Cameron West's associate directors on the BHE's administrative staff, went up to Indianapolis to study their approach to the physician shortage in Indiana. After the AMA-AAMC joint accreditation committee informed them that a free-standing two year program was not viable, the Educational Programs Committee thought the Indiana approach might be feasible in North Carolina. The committee's chairman, J. P. Huskins, Cameron West and Lem Stokes were able to convince Governor Scott on the idea of supporting a similar program.[45]

The Indiana Program for Statewide Medical Education had begun in 1967 after two years of planning, as a possible solution to the state's physician shortage, when the Indiana General Assembly approved the necessary legislation and funding. Its initial purpose was to strengthen internships, residencies, and continuing medical education programs in community hospitals. A statewide medical telecommunications system was set up, and salaries for community directors of medical education, stipends for interns and residents, visiting professorships, and many individual grants-in-aid provided for community hospital education programs. The initial phase of the program succeeded in increasing the number of interns and residents in the state and in attracting them to the smaller cities, without an increase in the number of medical graduates in the state or of foreign educated physicians. It demonstrated also that the state needed to graduate more physicians.

In the second phase of the program, the number of medical students enrolled at the Indiana University School of Medicine was increased, with new facilities constructed only on the Indianapolis campus. Many of the students were given their first year of medical education not at the medical school in Indianapolis, but on other campuses. The second and third year programs were located at the medical school. Then, during the fourth year, students were presented with the option of clerkships at teaching hospitals and clinics throughout the state. It was hoped that they would stay on at these locations for internships and residency training during their fifth and sixth years, and that they might choose to practice there after graduating.[46]

President William Friday said the Board of Higher Education's plan for East Carolina was in his judgment a sound and positive program for medical education in North Carolina. President Leo Jenkins found the proposal demeaning and a mere crumb, and wanted to have nothing to do with it. Drs. Monroe and Wooles joined Robert Morgan, chairman of the ECU board of trustees, in convincing Dr. Jenkins that they should accept the plan. They saw it as at least a toe in the door and a means of obtaining an operating budget.[47]

---

[1] *Greensboro Daily News,* March 11, 1967; Bratton, p. 295.

[2] *Raleigh News & Observer,* June 2, 3, 1967; also cited in Bratton, p. 398; *Public Laws of North Carolina,* 1967, chapter 1083.

[3] *General Statutes of North Carolina,* 116-46.4, 1967. The section refers to chapter 986 of the 1965 Session Laws, and to chapter 1038 of those of 1967.

[4] Bratton, p. 398.

[5] Bratton, pp. 403-404.

[6] *Laurinburg Exchange,* September 14, 1977.

[7] ECU News Bureau, January 25, 1968.

[8] Interview of Dr. Edwin W. Monroe, August 18, 1995.

[9] Interview of Dr. Leo Jenkins, August 31, 1988

[10] Powell, p. 7

[11] *North Carolina Medical Journal,* October, 1968

[12] North Carolina Board of Higher Education, Raleigh, North Carolina, Special Report 2-69, March 1969

[13] *Greenville Daily Reflector,* March 19, 1969.

[14] East Carolina University, *Rural Health in Eastern North Carolina— Planning and Action: A Regional Approach.* February, 1969

[15] *Raleigh News & Observer,* Wednesday, March 19, 1969.

[16] *Charlotte Observer,* March 24. 1969; *Durham Sun,* March 27, 1969.

[17] *Raleigh News & Observer,* Wednesday, 19 March 69

[18] Interview of Dr. Edwin W. Monroe, January 3, 1992.

[19] H. B. 1199, Chap. 1189, pp. 1368-9 of NC General Statutes; see also *Reflector,* Friday, 27 June 69

[20] Dr. E. W. Monroe, January 28, 1996.

[21] *Greenville Daily Reflector,* June 15, 1970.

[22] Wooles interview, November 13, 1991

[23] Dr. Monroe's comments, January 28, 1996.

[24] *Raleigh News & Observer*, March 13, 1970 (Editorial).

[25] *Greenville Daily Reflector*, September 18, 1970 AP report

[26] *Charlotte Observer*, October 17, 1970

[27] Monroe interview, January 2, 1992

[28] North Carolina Board of Higher Education, *Higher Education in North Carolina*, 5 (8) (Raleigh, NC) November 30, 1970

[29] Liaison Committee on Medical Education. *Report of the Survey of Program Under Development at East Carolina University School of Medicine, Greenville, North Carolina.* October 11-13, 1970.

[30] *Raleigh News & Observer*, December 20, 1970

[31] *Charlotte Observer*, December 29, 1970

[32] *Raleigh News & Observer*, December 30, 1970

[33] *Raleigh News & Observer*, September 15, 1970, *Greenville Daily Reflector*, September 18, 1970; Reported also in *Greensboro Record, Washington Daily News, Durham Sun*, etc.

[34] *Charlotte Observer*, 29 December 70; repeated in many other newspapers. ·

[35] Interview of Dr. Edwin W. Monroe, January 3, 1992

[36] Dr. Monroe's comments, January 28, 1996.

[37] *Raleigh News & Observer*, January 30, 1971

[38] *Raleigh News & Observer*, January 30, 1971.

[39] Liaison Committee on Medical Education, *Report of the Survey.* October 11-13, 1970. p. 17 (in the draft copy; this page number is skipped in the final report).

[40] Letter of January 29, 1971 from Marjorie R. Wilson, M. D., to President Leo W. Jenkins

[41] Letter of February 16, 1971, Wallace R. Wooles to Marjorie P. Wilson, M. D.

[42] Letter of February 18, 1971, Marjorie P. Wilson, M. D., to Dr. Leo W. Jenkins

[43] Interview of Dr. Wallace R. Wooles, November 13, 1991

[44] *Report of Educational Programs Committee as Approved by the North Carolina Board of Higher Education Concerning the Request of East Carolina University for a Master of Medical Science Degree (Two-Year Curriculum) for the School of Medicine.* Raleigh: North Carolina Board of Higher Education, September 1970.

[45] Interview of J. P. Huskins, April 2, 1992

[46] Board of Higher Education, *Report of Educational Programs Committee.*

[47] Associated Press, February 22, 1971, cited in a number of

Chapter 6
The ECU Medical School and
University Restructuring—1969-72

Dr. Jenkins, exercising the political rights which he maintained even University Presidents hold, had actively supported Bob Scott in both the primary and the general election.[1] During his gubernatorial campaign, Scott spoke favorably of ECU's efforts to provide better medical services for eastern North Carolina. When he included in his first budget message to the General Assembly a recommendation of $1.3 million for a new building for ECU, to begin a health affairs program there, Piedmont editors wondered whether the recommended appropriation could be seen as a reward for political service as well as fulfilling ECU's needs.[2]

The *Raleigh News & Observer* was later to assert editorially that President Jenkins won $375,000 from the 1969 legislature for planning and developing a medical school curriculum, by supporting Bob Scott in his gubernatorial campaign and by appealing to sectional interests of eastern legislators.[3] While this cynical observation may have contained a crumb of political insight, it ignored the fact that the Governor had long favored having a second state supported medical school, and had expressed his backing for locating it at ECU. It also ignored the central position of health care in Scott's ambitions for the state, and the attractiveness of an issue on which he could be constructive and still attack the UNC administration.

Governor Robert Walter Scott, son of a former governor, W. Kerr Scott, and nephew of Senator Ralph Scott, was by no means a devotee of Chapel Hill, but a loyal State alumnus, wary of University efforts to dominate the higher educational scene in North Carolina. He was not reluctant to put suspicions of the University, which many shared with him, to political uses.[4] He demonstrated repeatedly that he intended—though he often failed to achieve his intentions—that the University administration should be kept under the thumb of the legislature and the Board of Higher Education. It was predictable that he would collide with William Friday's stubborn determination to protect the University from political interference.

On Thursday night, March 13, 1969, Governor Scott told the North Carolina Mental Health Association, meeting in Raleigh, that the state ought to take steps to provide another medical school, possibly at ECU. He said he was not so much concerned where the school was located, but that a start should be made. He emphasized that the state must not decrease support to the medical school at Chapel Hill.[5] In spite of his disclaimers, he was accused editorially in the Piedmont of practically inviting East Carolina University to press the legislature for the establishment of a new medical school on that campus.

Representatives David Reid and Horton Rountree, both of Pitt County, introduced a bill in the General Assembly on May 23, 1969, to appropriate $375,000 for development of a basic sciences curriculum for a two-year medical school at ECU. Reid told the House that Governor Scott had clearly indicated his support of this action in his March speech before the North Carolina Mental Health Association. He was aware of the introduction of this bill, and it met with his approval.[6] Reid added a reminder that the school had been authorized since 1965. The bill being presented requested funds to implement that authorization, since the money appropriated under the original bill had reverted to the general fund on the failure of the school's efforts to obtain accreditation before January 1967.

At the time the budget request was submitted to the legislature, Dr. Edwin Monroe, dean of the ECU School of Allied Health Professions, presented a report to the lawmakers saying that the ECU administration was convinced a basic medical science curriculum which would be the equivalent of the first two years of medical school should be planned and developed on its campus now. Delaying it would postpone by many years the graduation of any medical students who enrolled in it. He took note of Governor Scott's statement that he was not opposed to the establishment of a new state-supported medical school and that he endorsed efforts by ECU to develop such a facility there. Dr. Monroe observed that Scott had gone beyond his position of four years before when he told the ECU senior class at a banquet that he would like to see a medical school on the Greenville campus.[7]

On December 29, Governor Scott published a list of what he considered to be the accomplishments of his first year in office. As he said, most of them were made possible by the tax increases he had convinced the 1969 General Assembly to enact. He gave a central place to the support for North Carolina students being given to Duke and Bowman Gray schools of medicine, to expansion of the UNC-CH School of Medicine, and the planning of a two-year medical curriculum at ECU.[8]

Then, in January, 1970, the Governor delivered a speech to the thirty-sixth annual convention of the North Carolina Dairy Products Association in Pinehurst, in which he called attention to North Carolina's crisis in medical care and called for steps to help the situation. He observed that children in forty-two other states have a longer average life expectancy than children in North Carolina, and that only ten or eleven other states rank below NC in physicians per capita. He urged further to increase enrollment in the state's three medical schools of the state, and to plan for a second state-supported medical school—he did not specify ECU—noting it would be the 1980's before graduates of any new medical school could begin practice. He also suggested a number of approaches to the health care crisis utilizing paramedical and non-medical personnel.[9]

The 1969 General Assembly, the same one which had made the Governor chairman of the Board of Higher Education, had approved seven constitutional amendments to be submitted to the voters in the election on November 3, 1970. These amendments were the final recommendations of the Commission on Reorganization of State Government, which had been busily at work since it was set up in 1953 during the governorship of W. Kerr Scott. Probably the most important of these amendments was one authorizing the General Assembly to reduce to twenty-five or less the administrative departments, agencies, and offices of the state government, which had grown to more than three hundred fifty.[10]

There was little doubt that the voters would approve, as they did, the long-studied constitutional amendments. While Governor Bob Scott had originally interpreted the mandate to his office to reorganize the state government as not including higher education, his experience on the Board of Higher Education convinced him that it could not be excluded. He had been pursuing energetically his campaign as chairman of the BHE to restructure higher education in North Carolina for some time when, on November 30, 1970, he met at the governor's mansion with President William Friday, who told him that it was time to consider placing the state's higher education institutions under one central authority, possibly under UNC's general administration. Scott interpreted this statement, and earlier conversations, as indicating Friday's agreement with him on the reorganization of the university system. (William Link, in his biography of William Friday, said of the series of talks the two men had during the fall of 1970, "The two men remembered the details of these discussions differently, yet the governor believed that Friday endorsed structural change.")[11]

Subsequent developments made it apparent that Scott and Friday had reached no clear understanding, and certainly did not agree about how restructuring should be done. The governor came to feel that Friday had originated the idea, and had later changed his mind when the UNC Board of Trustees opposed it. It was true that Friday had discussed with the Executive Committee of the Board the idea of reorganizing the university, and that they had reacted very nega-tively.[12] Governor Scott continued through the entire reorganization struggle campaign to resent what he felt to be a betrayal.

On December 13, 1970, Governor Scott held a dinner meeting with the Executive Committee of the UNC Board of Trustees, repre-sentatives from each of the regional universities, and members of the BHE. As he noted particularly at the time, there were no administra-tors present. At that meeting, Scott proposed a number of ap-proaches to reorganizing the state-funded colleges and universities, including the creation of an entirely new structure replacing both the BHE and the Consolidated University. Victor S. Bryant, Durham at-torney and member of the university board of trustees, at Scott's re-quest moved that a subcommittee be appointed to examine the ques-tion of restructuring and formulate it for presentation to the Gover-nor and General Assembly.[13]

On December 18, the executive committee of the Board of Higher Education, with Governor Scott presiding, passed a resolution in which it renewed its 1968 proposition that there should be a single agency to oversee higher education. On December 29, Scott attended a special session of the executive committee of the Board of Trustees of the Consolidated University, and told those present that the meeting's purpose was to discuss restructuring higher education in North Carolina, about whose condition he was deeply concerned. Af-ter their discussion of the problem, the executive committee thanked the Governor for his candid presentation of his views, and promised their help in finding the "best possible solution." Scott appointed a Subcommittee on the Structure of Higher Education in North Car-olina, chaired by Mr. Victor Bryant. He also announced his intention of forming a corresponding subcommittee of the BHE, to include members of the boards of trustees of the other state institutions of higher education.[14]

The Board of Higher Education subcommittee which the Gover-nor set up was under the chairmanship of Lindsay C. Warren, Jr. Mr. Warren was from Goldsboro, had served as state senator from 1963 to 1969, and was a graduate of the University in Chapel Hill. The members included one trustee from each of the nine regional universities, five trustees from UNC, and five members of the BHE. This subcommittee, labeled the Warren Committee, was weighted against the Consolidated University, or so the UNC representatives believed. The Board of Higher Education had no more members in the group than the university did, but earlier in the year while he was still in the state Senate, the chairman had publicly endorsed Governor Scott's proposal to strengthen the State Board of Higher Education.[15]

The Warren Committee, then, was divided from the start. The regional universities had experienced the results of subordination to the university, and the BHE members were quick to exploit misgivings about increasing control by the university. The UNC trustee members employed themselves in trying to protect the university's position, which they found very satisfactory as it was. As the committee proceeded, it called on the presidents of the universities not under the UNC umbrella, and on President Friday, to present their viewpoints. On March 26, Friday spoke to the Committee, with an impressive array of organizational charts, in opposition to the concept of centralization under a single governing board.

The Consolidated University administration, with President Friday at its helm, lost no time in beginning to work against the restructuring goal for which Governor Scott had set up the Warren Committee. As the Committee held ten meetings from January 15 to May 8, 1971, administrators from UNC were also meeting. Felix Joyner, Arnold King, Richard Robinson, and Ferebee Taylor were devising a strategy by which they hoped to maintain the university's preeminent position at the pinnacle of the stratified system set up by the General Assembly in 1963, on the recommendation of the Governor's Commission on Education Beyond the High School (the Carlyle Commission).[16] Above all, President Friday and his men were determined to prevent the disruptive intrusion of politicians and the public into university governance, and to prevent the strengthening of the Board of Higher Education to a point where it could effectively interfere with the detailed management of the university system.

Senator Warren arranged for President Friday and the BHE Chairman, Dr. Cameron West, to meet and attempt to work out some plan that would be agreeable to both. They proposed an intermediate position under which the prevailing structure would be left as it was except for strengthening the Board of Higher Education. Neither of the men was in favor of this arrangement, but the Committee took it for a compromise on which both agreed, and on April 3, 1971 accepted it. Both Dr. West and George Watts Hill, Jr., thought that the university had overly influenced the Committee's vote, and Hill immediately began agitating for the committee to reconsider its decision.

When the Warren Committee met on April 24, the effects of Hill's campaign became evident. Wallace Hyde, representing Western Carolina University on the Committee, moved to reconsider the earlier vote and submitted an alternative plan. Under the Hyde plan, there would be a single board over the whole system, with each of the sixteen separate boards of trustees regulating the affairs of its institution.

The UNC partisans recognized that the Hyde Plan would destroy the hegemony which their great institution had achieved in the structure set up by the General Assembly in 1963, but they were unable to prevent the Committee's accepting the new plan, and on April 24, the earlier action (which Watts Hill had called a "straw vote") [17] was reconsidered. At the Warren Committee's final meeting, on May 7-8, 1971, the university representatives made a futile attempt at reaching a compromise, but the committee approved by a thirteen to eight margin[18] a design in which there was a single board of regents coordinating budgets, programs, and objectives of the entire state system of higher education, the consolidated organization with UNC at its head was abolished, and the boards of trustees of the constituent institutions were given authority over their own campuses.

The UNC members of the committee presented a minority report in which they proposed leaving the system as it had been for the past five years. There still remained the final step of obtaining approval of the Warren Committee's decision by the General Assembly. Governor Scott campaigned for the majority report, while the Board of Trustees, the Friends of Education—a dedicated group of lobbyists for UNC, headed by trustee Jacob H. Froelich of High Point—and other supporters of the Chapel Hill university battled forcefully against deconsolidation. President Friday participated actively in the maneuvers during the early summer, but then he tactically withdrew from active campaigning. He placed his reliance on his lieutenants, particularly UNC vice president Ferebee Taylor, and on UNC trustees [Jake] Froelich and [Ike] Andrews. They reported to him "every day, on the hour, almost." [19]

The UNC trustees set up a base in a suite in Raleigh's Hilton Inn, out of which Jake Froelich and Ralph Strayhorn (a UNC trustee and alumnus from Durham) directed operations in the "holy war." They had a hard fight ahead of them, in spite of the fact that forty-five of the hundred twenty members of the House and twenty-three of the fifty members of the Senate were graduates of UNC in Chapel Hill. The legislature appeared to be swinging toward a position closer to the Warren Committee's majority than to that of the minority report. A strong central board of regents seemed to be imminent.[20]

On June 21, Dr. Cameron West, the BHE's director, came out with a statement that he could support an overall governing board. Scott called Jake Froelich in the late afternoon, and spoke with him about a "stronger regent plan." Froelich sounded out the trustees and President Friday, who said, "I can't change, but I will talk to my key trustees." Lieutenant Governor Pat Taylor said he was also bound by what the trustees agreed on.

Scott arranged a meeting that night at the Governor's Mansion, inviting Froelich, Lieutenant Governor Taylor, Dr. West, Senator Lindsay Warren, Representative Perry Martin (chairman of the House's Committee on Higher Education), Speaker Phil Godwin, Senator Russell Kirby, President Friday, and Fred Mills (the Governor's liaison with the General Assembly). The meeting went on until about 1:30 AM.

Coffee was served about midnight, and Friday, who had not budged from his position, left about 12:30. Senator Warren followed him out, and talked with him, but was unable to convince Friday to change his mind. In the end, the group agreed that it would be best to seek a consensus in the legislature—to finish the budget, the environmental bills the Governor had proposed, and the bills for reorganization of the state government—then recess for sixty days, reconvening for a special session that would discuss only the matter of restructuring higher education.

There was always the question whether East Carolina, North Carolina Central, and North Carolina A & T would agree to a stronger board.[21] Watching the contest from the sidelines, the state's newspapers chose their teams, as did civic groups and individual citizens. ECU President Leo Jenkins did not take a stand for the university position, but when in September it was rumored that he was preparing to declare his candidacy for the governorship, he expressed some of his own views. Speaking at a faculty convocation on September 7, 1971, he declared that he would keep on working for the medical facility on the Greenville campus. He also asserted he would not be a candidate for anything in 1972, but intended to continue requesting the programs he wanted for ECU, in spite of Governor Bob Scott's attempt to restructure higher education. He told the faculty, "Scott says one of his goals in the restructuring is to stop university presidents from lobbying the lawmakers for their pet programs. We expect to go to the next legislature requesting salaries commensurate with your training and ability, and at the same time, to push for a four-year medical school.

"When I speak of requests before the next session, I speak of requests that I plan to make as president of this university. I'm going to keep my hat on the shelf in 1972. But I will keep it in good condition. Most of you know I have always insisted that academic people should be involved in political life. Four years from now I hope that all of us will still be exercising our rights in the political arenas. If we abide by our obligation of keeping up with changing times, some of us may want to reconsider today's decisions not to run," Jenkins went on. "Higher education needs a re-evaluation but educators are the ones best qualified to do it. We should first of all be aware that demands for relevancy in education will often be linked to the maneuvering of administrators, faculty, students and the general public for a piece of the action," he continued. "Both myth and facts will be advanced in support of a few patterns of control. But whatever influence is felt on policy, we as professional educators will be held responsible for the results. The answers to educational problems cannot be supplied by outside agencies," he said.

He labeled as a "dangerous myth of our time" the claims of self-appointed spectators of higher education. "I am not saying that we should close our minds, proclaim our own infallibility and then continue in the same instructional patterns that we have always followed," he explained. "I am saying that the conclusion that professors are best qualified to judge the curriculum is a supportable assumption . . ."[22]

Lobbying by UNC advocates insured that Governor Scott's plan was not passed, but the final decision was postponed to the special session, as had been agreed at the June 21-22 meeting in the Governor's Mansion. The dispute continued with hardly a pause after adjournment, with Scott and Friday and others who had chosen sides for and against restructuring coming no closer to agreement. The Governor met with Friday and West a number of times early in September in an unsuccessful attempt at compromise. Scott and West were apprehensive about the role of UNC and its president in the new arrangement, and there were still personal animosities. After a meeting at the Executive Mansion on September 8, Friday decided that it was impossible to avoid having the system altered, and began to work more actively, though still not publicly, to insure that whatever restructuring took place would leave the university in a strong position. He initially directed his main efforts at the UNC trustees, and in September a committee of trustees went to the Governor and expressed their support of a governing board for the university's sixteen campuses.[23]

In spite of some differences in detail between the trustee committee's plan and Scott's, it looked as if the two sides were at a turning point. There were members of the UNC board of trustees who still held out for retaining the existing structure, however, and not until Friday met with a group of trustees at the NC State-UNC football game in Raleigh on October 2 was a compromise approached.[24]

On October 7, President Friday, secure in the support of an adequate majority of his board of trustees, told the joint higher education subcommittee of the General Assembly that he would call on the trustees at their meeting on October 18, to endorse a single governing board with the existing UNC system providing continuity while the new system was being established. He advanced the recommendation that the ten campuses not already part of the Consolidated University should be brought into the structure in two stages. A single central administration, a hundred-member board of trustees with an executive committee, and a unified code for the whole university would be retained.[25]

While the proposition Friday made constituted a major move in the direction of Governor Scott's restructuring proposal, it differed from it as to the number of trustees and about how the transition to the new system was to be handled. When the special session of the legislature began on October 26, 1971, the forces were once again arrayed opposite one another. The conflict shifted first to one side, then to the other, as political debts were called in and supporters were lost and won, and when the bill had finally been considered, reconsidered, amended, and amended again, both sides declared they had won.

The bill that was signed into law on October 30, 1971, left UNC in charge of executing the restructuring that it had originally opposed. The bill guaranteed that there would still be, though under another name, an expanded Consolidated University with the Chapel Hill campus as its flagship. Appointment of the Board of Governors—with thirty-two rather than a hundred members—was placed entirely in the hands of the General Assembly, and the Governor would no longer, once the Board was fully established, have any control of higher education beyond his right to appoint some members of the boards of trustees of the constituent schools (which retained little authority), and his influence on the advisory budget committee.[26]

The restructuring battle has been called a political defeat and an administrative victory for President Friday.[27] It seems to have been a victory both for his political skills, which were no less political for being exercised mostly behind the scenes, and for his administrative skills, displayed in his using the pattern drawn by House Bill 1456 to insure UNC-Chapel Hill's continued preeminence. In the end, perhaps in part through not taking up a clear position outside his unwavering determination to preserve UNC's leading role in the management of higher education in the state, Friday effectively defeated Governor Bob Scott's plan. It had been replaced by one which did not preserve the *status quo ante* as far as UNC was concerned, but averted the defeat which the Warren Committee's original proposal would have meant.

---

[1] *Durham Herald,* March 14, 1969.

[2] *Greenville Daily Reflector,* Thursday, May 22, 1969.

[3] *Raleigh News & Observer,* September 16, 1970 (Editorial).

[4] Link, pp. 144, 170, 195 ff.; Crabtree, Beth G., *North Carolina Governors, 1585-1974.* (Raleigh, NC: North Carolina Division of Archives and History, 1974) pp. 140-42; *Who's Who in the South and Southwest* (Chicago, 1971).

[5] *Durham Herald,* March 14, 1969.

[6] *Raleigh News & Observer,* May 23, 1969.

[7] *Raleigh News & Observer,* Wednesday, March 19, 1969.

[8] *Hickory Daily Record,* December 29, 1969 (AP).

[9] *Statesville Record & Landmark,* January 23, 1970.

[10] Lefler, p. 703; Powell, pp. 545, 546-7.

[11] Link, p. 171.

[12] Link, *ibid.*

[13] King, pp. 111-112.

[14] King, p. 113.

[15] *Durham Herald,* April 29, 1969.

[16] Link, p. 174.

[17] Link, p. 175.

[18] King, p 115.

[19] Link, p. 178, quoting interviews with the principals.

[20] King, pp. 119-122.

[21] Nancy Roberts, *The Governor* pp. 81-85.

[22] *Raleigh Times,* September 7, 1971.

[23] Link, pp. 179-80; King, p. 122.

[24] King, pp. 123-4; Link, p. 180.

25 King, p. 124.

26 King, pp. 110 ff., has a detailed account of the battle over restructuring, during which he worked closely with Friday. He credits notes made by Mr. John L. Sanders, director of the Institute of Government at UNC-CH, for much of his description of the special legislative session.

27 Link, p. 185.

Chapter 7
The Quest for a Medical School Within the New Structure

The active involvement of East Carolina University and President Leo Jenkins in the restructuring contest, as has been indicated before, was marginal, even though his objections to it were clear. The *Charlotte Observer* claimed, "East Carolina's successful fight for university status set the stage for today's restructuring efforts," [1] This may well be true, but if so the stage-setting was a by-product of Jenkins's crusade for university status for ECC. It does not appear that any other consideration ever seriously interfered with his determination to achieve this objective. Even the medical school for which he worked so diligently was no separate goal, but an element in his overall design. It was as a component of this design that he made the medical school issue into the challenge it was to the centralization of control in the new Board of Governors.

Restructuring, as proposed both by Governor Scott and the Board of Higher Education on one hand and by UNC on the other, as well as restructuring in the form the General Assembly imposed, were in conflict with Jenkins's views on competition in higher education. Whatever was done to expand or strengthen central authority and an educational hierarchy would harm rather than benefit his efforts. He derided Chapel Hill's claims to unique excellence, and the rejection of democracy in education. He never desisted from his attacks on budgetary decisions based on imputed superiority in similar programs rather than on differences in programs.[2] Placing the control of budgets and programs in the hands of a group who asserted a special position would insure that their claims to uncommon entitlements could not be effectively challenged.

To legislate and plan the restructuring the state's university system under a central board and administrative hierarchy was only the first stage of a reconsolidation in which all the regional universities were to become subordinate parts. In spite of the enactment of the 1971 bill to consolidate the institutions of higher learning in the state, and in spite of the 1970 legislative redistricting, the political coalition that had won the first skirmish in the campaign for a medical school in 1965 was still sound. President Friday was aware of this, and not inclined to make a frontal assault on ECU's forces. Noisy public battles were not at all to his taste, and clearly a political conflict between the General Administration and one of the con-

stituent institutions of UNC could only damage him and his administration. The campaign to block ECU's drive for a medical school had
to be dealt with administratively and in terms of funding and program development within the new system.

Later, when he was no longer president of an independent institution, but president of a university within the UNC structure, Dr.
Leo Jenkins was directly responsible to President Friday. To continue
directly approaching the legislature would be an act of insubordina-
tion, a violation of the rule that presidents were to abstain from approaching the legislature except as the UNC president should direct.[3]
Neither Friday's aversion to overt political involvement nor Jenkins's
disposition to be a "good Marine" and submit to lawful authority
prevented them from overlooking their adjutants' political activities.
Dr. Raymond Dawson and Mr. Felix Joyner were Friday's chief aides,
allowing him to keep his distance from the fray until almost the end.
Assisted by Dr. Wallace Wooles, Dr. Edwin Monroe took on the task
of directing political maneuvers, deflecting reprisals from Dr. Jenkins
to himself.[4]

The 1971-73 budget, released on January 13 by the Governor's
office, included no money for either the proposed two-year medical
school at East Carolina University or financial aid to the state's two
private medical schools.[5] President Leo Jenkins examined the budget
and issued a press release the following day in which he said that the
Advisory Budget Commission acted properly in leaving the matter of
funding the proposed medical school at ECU to the General Assembly. He added that any further statement by him would be premature.[6]

In February, the Board of Higher Education announced the recommendation of its Education Program Committee, chaired by Jay
Huskins, a newspaper editor from Statesville, that a one-year medical
training program be set up in the School of Allied Health Sciences at
ECU, instead of the two-year medical school, which it considered
undesirable both educationally and economically. The committee
advised making an arrangement with UNC-CH to accept all students
when they completed their year at ECU. It recommended that the
General Assembly should appropriate funds for planning and initiating the program in the 1971-73 biennium.[7]

The committee gave as its reason for the action that it would
save tax dollars and train more doctors than were already being
trained. It said further that the recommendation was "consonant
with the judgment of medical educational authorities that new two-
year medical schools are not desirable." The national trend away

from two-year programs had been encouraged by the Carnegie Commission.[8] It had been found that designing curricula for two-year schools, which would prepare students to transfer to any other school whatever for the last two years, was hopelessly complicated. The programs at different medical schools differed so greatly in the distribution of courses over the usual four years that it was almost impossible to squeeze into two years those subjects necessary to prepare for transferring to another school.

The committee recommended that the state should fund an increase in enrollment at UNC-CH from one hundred to two hundred by 1980, and support more North Carolina students at Duke and Bowman Gray. UNC's plans to expand clinical services to more hospitals in the state should be encouraged, especially in the east and west. They recommended appropriations to make it possible to begin clinical training for advanced medical students in such centers as Greenville, Wilson and Goldsboro.

It appears that the Board of Higher Education was not aware that the School of Medicine in Chapel Hill had recently revised its curriculum, making very expensive any one-year program that attempted to match it.[9] The report of the Board gave Governor Scott a fine opportunity to attack the Chapel Hill establishment, which he felt was a major obstacle to his still-crystallizing plans. On the day the report was released, he held a news conference in which he assaulted the UNC administration, accusing it of doing all it could to block approval of the ECU medical school. "Their activity in the last six months has been almost frantic and sometimes comic," he said. He pointed out that although UNC had gotten busy with plans to expand its enrollment, it did not do so until it became apparent East Carolina was serious in trying to obtain a medical school.

Scott referred to a letter from UNC President Friday to President Jenkins stating that the medical school in Chapel Hill would not accept students from the other campuses, saying it gave "further evidence of their attempts at the University to block any kind of program on another campus." He accused the officials at UNC of talking about cooperation in working out the question of the school at ECU, when all the while they were maneuvering to prevent the establishment of a medical training facility on any campus other than the university.[10]

President Friday had talked with a reporter on Tuesday, February 16, about President Jenkins's request, and about the university's response to a request from the Board of Higher Education. Friday said that he and Jenkins had discussed the possibility of seeking more funds for UNC to take East Carolina's medical school students but emphasized that there had been no official or formal request. It was not a matter of refusing a request, but of exploring an idea. He considered that he could not justify a request for additional funds to accommodate transfer students from the proposed two-year medical school.

Friday said that the university had already made a commitment to increase the size of the freshman class at the medical school in Chapel Hill. Also, he was considering the possibility of allowing some members of the first year medical class to enroll at North Carolina State University. He considered that, as president, he would have to give first priority to units within the Consolidated University structure, though there was still the possibility of developing similar agreements with institutions outside the university. Friday said the NCSU proposal originated from a long-standing arrangement in which some students from the biological sciences courses at State sometimes went to the medical school at Chapel Hill. Fourteen students already had been accepted in the current year. In a later comment, he said, "For 25 years North Carolina State has had many students go to medical school." Most of the required courses were already being offered in Raleigh, and had been for years.[11]

Friday said that the studies he had been making were in response to a request during April from the Board of Higher Education for information on the university's plans for development. "As far as expanding the entering class beyond 120, I indicated we need more time to explore cooperative arrangements in other states," he said. "We've already set up university-wide committees to examine our own resources." [12]

Governor Scott explained President Friday's action quite differently. "The reason for this is that they see this as a threat to the supreme sovereignty of the University of North Carolina," he said. "It reminds me somewhat of the so-called blue bloods of society who look down in contempt on anyone whose ancestry doesn't date back to the pilgrim fathers." He also said that the recent suggestion by the university administration to set up a one-year school at NCSU was another attempt to undercut the ECU efforts. The governor unreservedly endorsed the ECU medical school, and felt that the requirement in the proposal of the Board of Higher Education for UNC to accept transfer students from ECU was necessary, since unless they were forced to they would not do it.[13]

On Saturday, February 19, Scott and the UNC president discussed the Governor's allegations, but Friday did not respond publicly. He was clearly disturbed by Scott's attack and by the BHE recommendations insofar as they pertained to the Chapel Hill campus. At a meeting on February 22, he said to the UNC trustees that the university had been engaged in its regular mission of devising new and better means to make effective and efficient use of the resources provided by the people, for the benefit of the people. As for East Carolina, he judged the plan proposed by the Board of Higher Education to be a sound and positive program for medical education in the state.

He also informed the Board that in his February 11 letter to East Carolina's President Leo Jenkins he had specifically indicated the possibility for a cooperative arrangement with institutions outside the university system for the first year of medical training. On the morning of the trustees' meeting he had reaffirmed to President Jenkins the university's willingness to do the work necessary to get on with the necessary discussions. (On February 10, when Jenkins had come to Chapel Hill to talk with him, Friday had turned down his request to accept transfers from a two-year program, if one should be approved later on.[14] In his follow-up letter, he had reiterated that he had no plans to absorb the students from a two-year program, and had also mentioned UNC's plans to begin taking transfers from a one-year medical school program at North Carolina State University).[15]

Attorney General and ECU trustee Robert Morgan asked for a meeting on February 26, 1971, between officials from ECU and UNC so they could begin to plan how they would work together. Friday agreed, and for an hour Dr. C. Arden Miller, who until February 1 had been UNC vice-president for health sciences, Dr. Cecil Sheps, acting vice-president for health sciences, and Carlyle Sitterson, UNC President, met with Dr. Edwin W. Monroe, ECU's dean of the allied health school and director of medical education, and Dr. Wallace Wooles, dean of the school of medicine. They were able to agree on setting up a committee to direct the working arrangements between the two schools, and to prepare a joint budget request for presentation to Friday and Jenkins.[16]

In April, the ECU-UNC committee presented the findings of its study of establishing a one-year medical school in Greenville to Governor Bob Scott, to the two co-chairmen of the Joint Appropriations Committee and to representatives of the State Board of Higher Education. The study concluded that a one-year school such as the BHE suggested, was feasible. The committee proposed that students completing the year of study at ECU should be guaranteed transfer to the UNC School of Medicine at Chapel Hill to complete their training. The one-year program effectively postponed a final decision on expanding the Greenville medical program. President Jenkins and his staff accepted it, although reluctantly, as the best they could hope for at the time, and continued to push for an arrangement that would give them what they really wanted. President Friday also accepted the plan, since it gave him time to work toward blocking ECU's ambition to gain a full four-year medical school, a toehold on the climb to a full array of doctoral programs.[17]

While the joint ECU-UNC committee was doing its work, President Leo Jenkins, Dr. Monroe, and Dr. Wooles actively continued the campaign for a two-year medical school at ECU. A group of eastern physicians led by Dr. Ernest Furgurson of Plymouth held a dinner meeting on February 28 at the Brentwood Lodge in Washington, N. C., which was attended by about two hundred fifty people. Dr. Monroe and Dr. Furgurson, the moderator of the meeting, named a blue-ribbon panel of physicians (including Dr. Lenox Baker from Duke), and notable citizens from the east to advise East Carolina University officials in their efforts to acquire a medical school and to take the school's case to the General Assembly and the people. Representative Walter Jones, who spoke at the meeting, referred to it as a "rally" for the ECU medical school, and recalled that he supported ECU's medical school as far back as 1964. Dr. Leo Jenkins, Dr. Monroe and Dr. Wallace Wooles also addressed the gathering.[18]

The ECU board of trustees, meeting on March 9, 1971, in the office of Attorney General Robert Morgan, chairman of the board, postponed taking definite action on the State Board of Higher Education's recommendation of a one-year medical school. They gave as their reason the unavailability of any evaluation by medical educators of such a one-year program. They directed President Jenkins, Dr. Monroe, and Dean Wooles to ensure that East Carolina University would begin the most productive medical education program possible, in the 1971-1973 biennium. The board stated that it was not rejecting the possibility of a two-year school.

Dr. Jenkins was instructed to set up a committee to study the options available to guide the board of trustees in its decision. Dr. Monroe reported to the board that ECU and UNC officials were already working on a study of the feasibility of setting up the one-year program recommended by the Board of Higher Education.[19]

On May 11, Governor Bob Scott published a letter he had sent to

Attorney General Morgan, in which he said he believed that the best and most feasible course of action was eventually to establish a four-year medical school at East Carolina. He said there were serious obstacles to approving a two-year school. The primary obstacle was financial. "Old timers in the General Assembly say they cannot recall when funds were so tight," he said. Also, most of the people with whom Scott had talked had told him that it is not the place that a medical student takes his classroom work that influences where he will practice, but the place where he does his clinical work and internship. He concluded that this underlined the importance of making the development of clinical facilities in the east a part of the medical school program.

The Governor said that he would not undercut the Board of Higher Education, of which he was chairman, by recommending something different from what they had already recommended. He had heard from some members of the Legislature that if ECU could not get a two-year program then they did not want any at all. Scott said he discounted the rumors, but that if they were true "that is exactly what ECU would receive—nothing." [20]

Later in May, both the ECU Board of Trustees and Governor Scott accepted the one-year arrangement that the UNC-ECU negotiating committee submitted, with a joint committee managing the program and reporting to their respective Presidents and to President Friday on budget matters, and an agreement for students to transfer to the UNC medical school in Chapel Hill for their final three years. [21]

On June 30, 1971, the 1971-73 state budget was approved by both houses of the legislature, and included $1.6 million for the first year of a projected new four-year state medical school at East Carolina University. [22] Representative Horton Rountree of Greenville said that he expected the bill to create a one-year School of Medicine at ECU would receive favorable action before the legislative session was over. He said that with the money appropriated, all that was left was the implementing legislation with language that stated the intent of the appropriation. [23]

The ECU program did not get through the Senate without further controversy. On July 3, Senator Herman Moore of Mecklenburg County objected to the wording in the appropriation bill saying, "This course of action is recognized as a significant step in a statewide plan for medical education, as well as an initial step in development of an expanded medical school at East Carolina University." He moved to have the word "initial" deleted, saying that it appeared to indicate that the General Assembly was committing itself to something bigger in the future. Pitt Senator Vernon White said that the change would knock out any intent to expand that school. Moore's proposed amendment lost decisively on a roll call vote.[24]

Later that day, the Senate unanimously approved the bill to fund the one-year medical education program at ECU. That action and the ratification of the bill on July 4 were the final legislative steps in establishing the ECU program.[25] There still remained the approval of the funding for the school of medicine, which occurred on July 21, when the President of the Senate and the Speaker of the House signed the bill. The bill also referred to the "cooperative agreements between the University of North Carolina and the School of Medicine of East Carolina University whereby the School of Medicine of East Carolina University will provide training in medical education at the first-year level and the School of Medicine of the University of North Carolina will guarantee admission to all students satisfactorily completing the one-year medical program at East Carolina University." It went on, "It is the intent of this act that these cooperative agreements between the two Universities be faithfully followed." [26]

Following the session, Senator White commented, "Senator Moore tried to have it amended, but we were able to beat that down, and the bill came out of the Senate just like we wanted it. I think that in the future it (the one-year school) can grow... when the money is available... into a four-year school." He commented that establishing the school "is something all of us have been working for hard and long. We are sure that we have the appropriations now, and sure that in the future, if the need is there and we do our part quality wise, we can grow into a full-fledged four-year medical school." [27]

Before the end of September 1971, three hundred applicants had been received for admission to the first class in ECU's one-year medical school opening in September 1972. According to Dr. Wallace Wooles, the school would continue to accept applications until January 1, 1972, by which time approximately 400 total applications were anticipated for the 20 seats in the class. [28]

President William Friday's efforts to delay and maintain control of the program at ECU and to avoid dividing the state's financial resources between two medical schools were supported by the activities of the Liaison Committee on Medical Education, who sent representatives to the Greenville campus in November 1971 to assess the one-year program. The LCME site visitors came to the conclusion that the student transfer program was not completely satisfactory.

The committee decided that the ECU program could not be accredited separately, but only as part of a medical education program at the University of North Carolina. Because of the lack of clear assumption of authority and responsibility for ECU by the UNC School of Medicine, and because of some difficulties concerning the administration of the hospital in Chapel Hill, UNC was awarded accreditation for a term of only two years, rather than the customary seven years, and that award was made conditional on achieving a satisfactory arrangement with ECU. [29]

Late in January 1972, the new dean of the UNC School of Medicine, Dr. Christopher C. Fordham III, said that North Carolina was in good shape in the effort to anticipate future medical needs, but there were still improvements to be made. In one approach to the problem, UNC medical school was negotiating affiliation agreements with a number of hospitals throughout the state. He said that clinical education in community hospitals could give medical students a realistic view of practice.

Faculty members at the medical school in Chapel Hill had been assisting ECU in establishing its one-year program. Fordham said that they were frantically making plans to accommodate the 20 students who would be transferring in the fall of 1973. At the time the program was established by the legislature, there had been no planning to provide the necessary physical facilities for the transfer students.

He also said that because of the ECU program only a limited number of students could be accommodated in the second year, since UNC was assuming an obligation to provide the other three years of training. The clinical education program was a real bottleneck.[30]

There were concerns among the administrators of the UNC medical school, notably Dr. Cecil Sheps, vice President for health affairs, that supporting the ECU program could affect the status and possibly threaten the accreditation of UNC's school.[31] The reasonableness of these worries was demonstrated in the LCME's action of putting conditions on UNC's accreditation and limiting it to two years.

The decision of the Liaison Committee to withhold separate accreditation from the medical education program at East Carolina, making it a part of the UNC program, nettled President Jenkins and his staff. As the joint committee hammered out arrangements for cooperation, their discontent increased. They strongly resisted the intervention of the UNC medical school administration in what they considered their own primary responsibilities. As Dr. Wooles said, "Anyway, we got the one-year program forced upon us. We kept the right to admit our own students, to select the students that would come, to pick our faculty. We had a curriculum that was nothing like Chapel Hill's, but it covered the same material." [32]   Jenkins complained to Friday about the ECU medical school's being only a "satellite of the University of North Carolina." [33]

Consequently, dissatisfaction with the cooperative venture was no less at ECU than at UNC. However, in Greenville the vexation could be directed outward at President Friday and the Chapel Hill administration. Its effect was to strengthen cohesiveness and the determination of the medical school administration and faculty to accomplish what they had set out to do. The UNC medical school faculty members could do little more than turn their exasperation toward their own administration and chafe at Friday's measured, deliberate effort to secure control of the East Carolina maverick.

In the campaign for governor, most of the candidates spoke out about the ECU medical school. On February 9, 1972, Hugh Morton, Democratic candidate, said he would support the plan for a two-year medical school at ECU if he was elected.[34] President Jenkins met with Hargrove "Skipper" Bowles, who made no commitment, and with Lieutenant Governor Pat Taylor, whose office said he might have comments about the ECU program later.[35] Candidate Jim Gardner, a business man from Rocky Mount, said he was committed to a two-year medical program at ECU.

Democratic candidate for lieutenant governor, Jim Hunt of Wilson, endorsed East Carolina University's plans for a medical school, but said he did not know when funds would be available.[36] Roy Sowers, another Democratic candidate for lieutenant governor, said he approved the one-year medical school at ECU and felt that a good case could be made for expanding the program into a two-year program.[37]

On January 4, 1972 at UNC's Quail Roost Conference Center near Rougemont, Governor Scott assembled the Planning Committee that the law had stipulated was to constitute the initial Board of Governors, to begin the transition process to the new structure. At that first meeting, the term of service of each member was decided, and committees on personnel, facilities, and the Code were appointed.[38]

One of the critical sticking-points of the debate over restructuring had been the composition of the governing board that was to control the entire system. Dr. Cameron West and the governor had fought to retain as much control as possible in the hands of the Board of Higher Education. In the end, that Board was eliminated, its powers were shifted to the UNC Board of Governors, and their appointments were placed entirely in the hands of the General Assembly, as noted earlier. The Consolidated University group was forced to accept a thirty-two-member governing board rather than the hundred-member one they had preferred, but it was a board in which the primacy of UNC-CH was insured.

The law provided for sixteen members of the Board chosen from the UNC Board of Trustees. Two non-voting members were chosen from the Board of Higher Education, to serve until July 1973. The sixteen seats allocated to the regional universities included three for ECU, two each for Appalachian State University, North Carolina A & T State University, North Carolina Central University, and Western Carolina University, and one each for Elizabeth City State, Fayetteville State, Pembroke, and Winston-Salem State Universities. The School of the Arts had one member. Governor Scott was to serve as Chairman until July 1973, at which time the Board would elect one of its own members as chairman.[39]

The personnel subcommittee of the Planning Committee met with President Friday on March 15, 1972, at the Governor's Mansion to discuss the appointment of a black vice president to the General Administration. Friday stated that he had been for a long time associated with leading black educators across the country, and advocated consulting with the presidents of the state's black institutions, but he would not guarantee that if he became president of the reconsolidated university, he would specifically appoint a black educator.

Friday was at the time president of the Association of American Universities, made up of the presidents of the forty-eight leading universities in the United States and Canada. The question had been raised at UNC about the propriety of his representing the university, rather than having the president do so. Friday countered that it was proper for the chief administrative officer of the UNC system to represent it, as was done in the case of the multicampus university systems in California, Wisconsin, Missouri, and Texas.

A second point that was of particular concern to Governor Scott and some other members of the personnel subcommittee concerned Dr. Cameron West's role in the new structure. The sentiment at some of the former regional universities was that Dr. West's appointment close to President Friday would provide some protection against domination by Chapel Hill. The restructuring act specified that the staff of the president of UNC should include a senior vice president. Scott had specifically requested this provision, in an attempt to insure that Dr. West, who had been the governor's ally in the fray, was guaranteed a position. President Friday had already requested and the executive committee of the Board of Trustees of the Consolidated University had authorized a position of vice president for planning when the BHE and UNC staffs were merged, with Dr. West in that position. They had also authorized restoring the position of secretary of the university, and electing the associate director of the BHE, John P. Kennedy to fill it. In spite of some misgivings on the part of the representatives of the regional universities, the personnel subcommittee had approved the arrangement.[40]

At a meeting of the personnel subcommittee of the Planning Committee for the Board of Governors at the Executive Mansion on March 15, 1972, President Friday refused to make any commitment on West's position, insisting to the subcommittee that the president of a university should have the right to choose his own staff. He also would give no guarantees on the question of location of the General Administration's offices, which Scott and other personnel committee members believed should be away from Chapel Hill. Friday opposed locating the offices of the president and the Board of Governors anywhere other than within a stone's throw of the UNC-Chapel Hill campus.[41] His insistence on keeping his office there appeared to symbolize his determination to preserve the preeminent status of "The" University among the constituent universities.

After President Friday left the executive mansion, the governor and some other personnel subcommittee members expressed discontent with choosing him as president. Scott felt sure that Friday would not willingly appoint West. He also had reservations about Friday's reliability, because he believed he had gone back on agreements with him. Some thought "Friday was 'too much of a politician,' and they could never determine where he stood on controversial issues." [42]

The personnel subcommittee came up with no better candidate than William Friday. On March 17, 1972, when the Planning Committee met in Greensboro on the UNC-G campus, it announced his selection as president of the restructured university system. It also announced that the location of the general headquarters of the University of North Carolina would be in Chapel Hill for at least three years.[43]

There had been significant disagreement in the Planning Committee about the location of the headquarters of the Board. The facilities subcommittee had considered sites in the Research Triangle

Park and elsewhere in the state where there were facilities already constructed that would be suitable. They heard from the regional universities of their great concern about there being too close a connection between the old administration and the new, of being dominated by UNC-CH.

The seven-man facilities subcommittee of the Planning Committee charged with selecting the headquarters site for the Board included four former UNC trustees and three members from regional universities. Its chairman, Thomas J. White of Kinston, had been a UNC trustee. However, while the subcommittee was weighted with members naturally in favor of the location favored by President Friday, there are no grounds for doubt that it did a careful, thorough job of gathering information on the possible sites. After looking at alternatives in the Research Triangle Park, in Raleigh, and elsewhere, they decided that the most suitable building available was the almost-finished General Administration Building, located a few blocks out the Raleigh road from the UNC campus in Chapel Hill. It could be ready for occupancy in about a year, and this was the location which the facilities subcommittee recommended. The Planning Committee voted, after a heated debate in which there was a clear breach between the Consolidated University representatives and those of the regional campuses, to accept its recommendation. Wallace Hyde, supporting a rejected substitute motion he made which would have postponed the decision on the location, stated his opinion that the headquarters would remain in Chapel Hill until the building there was no longer adequate, and President Friday agreed.[44]

On April 20, the Planning Committee visited the ECU campus. Dr. Leo Jenkins stated the he would support the Board of Governors, but asked for their understanding of East Carolina's capabilities, dedication to service, and aspirations to grow. He said that ECU did not consider its situation as static. He said to the Board members, "In the future we will propose to you that we be allowed to perform the tasks that society asks us to perform and that we feel competent to perform," and added that in spite of rapid growth at East Carolina University "we have been careful to provide a sound base for our growth." He urged that the Board approve beginning a two-year medical school in Greenville. The twenty-student program was too expensive, he said.

Dr. Edwin Monroe presented the Committee with other reasons for changing to a two-year school: $1.4 million was being spent in the next biennium to provide forty students with the first year of their medical school training. With a two-year program, the same facilities could be utilized, and federal money would be available. As long as the ECU program was an offshoot of UNC-CH medical school, it would be unable to apply independently for grant money, while as a two-year school it would be a separate entity, eligible for accreditation and for federal funds.[45]

During the Planning Committee's ECU visit, one of its members, George Watts Hill, Sr., of Durham, warned that graduates of the one-year program would not be accepted for transfer to Chapel Hill if they failed to meet Chapel Hill's standards. After their visit to the ECU campus, some members of the Committee commented publicly on their views. Representative J. P. Huskins of Statesville, who had served on the Board of Higher Education before becoming a member of the Board of Governors, said that the governor and the General Assembly had made a decision, and "East Carolina is in on the ground floor." Another Committee member, Maceo Sloan of Durham, agreed with Huskins. Watts Hill, Jr., also from Durham and also a former BHE member, disagreed, noting that NC had three four-year medical schools. "The time when the state can afford a fourth medical school is so remote that I wouldn't want to speculate on where it will located," he said, and added that he believed that it would be less expensive to raise the number of doctors by increasing the number of one-year schools and expanding the existing schools, than by any other approach.

Huskins made these points in support of his position: UNC-CH is sending students to train in Greensboro and Charlotte hospitals, and plans to begin other programs in Raleigh, Greenville, Wilson, Goldsboro, Rocky Mount, and Tarboro. One-year medical programs could be set up at UNC-Charlotte and NC State, and "on as many campuses as the needs will justify." He also said, "I don't see any big medical schools springing up in any given community, in addition to East Carolina University."

Huskins and Hill agreed that the doctorate degree might be offered on some other campuses than those then permitted to offer it, UNC-CH, UNC-Greensboro, and NCSU. Hill said he hoped, however, that setting up the new Board of Governors would lead to further concentration of doctoral programs, and not expansion. Any programs added on other campuses than at present "should be limited to special competencies." Since the 1969 decision to permit doctoral programs at all of the state-financed universities had been revoked by the restructuring law, it would be up to the Board of Governors to decide which institutions would be authorized to grant them.

Representative Huskins said he could not imagine graduate programs would be "frozen forever on the three campuses of the original Consolidated University." He anticipated that there would be a time when doctoral programs would be approved at Appalachian State, Charlotte and East Carolina, and at any other institution where there were staff and background to provide such programs.

Mr. Sloan, member from Elizabeth City State University, felt that doctoral level work should be restricted to the present three campuses. He did not think the state could afford doctoral programs at all institutions. One of the purposes of restructuring was to avoid such duplication. Board member William A. Johnson of Lillington, former UNC trustee, agreed that the state did not have the resources to provide doctoral programs at all of the constituent institutions. This was the viewpoint of UNC-CH, and later, in 1976, became the policy of the Board of Governors.

The Associated Press report of the visit noted that Hill, Johnson and Sloan had agreed that during the Committee's meetings there had been no tendency for the board to split along the lines of whether the members came from the UNC board of trustees or from one of the regional institutions. Mr. Johnson had said that he believed that every member was making a conscientious effort to be objective.[46]

On May 8, 1972 the ECU Board of Trustees met in Raleigh, in the offices of its chairman, Attorney Gen. Robert Morgan. At this meeting, President Jenkins stated publicly for the first time that he was going to seek a two-year school. He planned to ask the Board of Governors for $500,000 to expand the school. He also replied to George Watts Hill's remarks during the visit in Greenville of the Board of Governors to be, saying the question of ECU's students not being qualified was ridiculous, and made merely for purposes of publicity. Evidence of the high quality of ECU instruction was that not one of the graduates of the School of Nursing had ever failed to qualify on the state nursing examination. He said he expected the physicians program to produce students of the same high caliber.[47]

In spite of the changes going on in the UNC system, the push for upgrading the medical program at ECU went on. At a luncheon meeting of the Kinston Kiwanis Club on May 26, ECU dean of medicine, Wallace R. Wooles, gave a talk entitled "What the Medical School at East Carolina University Can Mean to the People in Eastern North Carolina." He predicted that the school would graduate its first student with an M.D. no later than 1982. He said, "There is no question in my mind and the minds of most people that I talk to around the state that the decision has been made to build a second state medical school and that it's going to be at ECU." The only question that was still to be resolved was how fast it was going to be done.

He said that the one-year program was only a start. There had to be a change to a four-year school, not only because of eastern North Carolina's medical needs but also because of economic factors. The average cost of $33,800 per student in the one-year program was more than twice as much as the national average for thirty-nine medical schools, which was $16,000.[48]

In Nags Head, Dr. Ira M. Hardy II, a Greenville neurosurgeon , spoke to the Seaboard Medical Association about the school. Dr. Hardy said that a one-year school was not practical, and that efforts would be made during the 1973 General Assembly to have a two-year school funded as soon as possible.[49]

On June 23, 1972, the Planning Committee, already functioning as a Board though it would not legally become the Board of Governors until July 1, assembled in Chapel Hill. Their purpose was to make plans for carrying out the administrative merger of the six campuses of the Consolidated University and ten other state-supported institutions of higher learning, scheduled to take place on July 1. They voted to merge nine administrative agencies, including the Board of Higher Education and the Consolidated University of North Carolina. The Board of Governors would administer the NC Internship Office, the NC Educational Computer Service, the Center for the Continuing Renewal of Higher Education, the Student Educational Assistance Authority, the Educational Opportunity Information Center, and the Community Service and Continuing Education programs.

ECU's proposal for funds to expand the medical school was included in a budget request to the Board of Governors. Dr. Jenkins justified this request on the basis of the 1971 legislation that provided funding for the first-year program, as "a step in development of an expanded medical school at East Carolina University," and proposed the expansion to two years as a step toward a full four-year school leading to the M.D. degree.

Jenkins's move was a shrewd one. As Dr. Raymond Dawson observed, "If we had just put it in the budget request [from the Board to the legislature], then there would have been no examination of the larger issues, and the Board of Governors would just have found itself sort of presented with a *fait accompli.*"[50]

1 *Charlotte Observer*, October, 1971 quoted in Bratton, p. 408.

2 Bratton, pp. 408-9.

3 Link, p. 226.

4 Link, *ibid.;* Monroe interview, January 3, 1992; Wooles interview, November 13, 1991.

5 *Greenville Daily Reflector*, January 13, 1971.

6 ECU News Bureau, January 14, 1971; *Raleigh News & Observer*, January 15, 1971.

7 North Carolina Board of Higher Education, Special Report 1-71.

8 Carnegie Commission report: *Higher Education and the Nation's Health* (New York, 1970) pp. 50-52.

9 Letter of 16 March 71 from Edwin W. Monroe to Dr. M. J. Musser, Chief Medical Director, Veterans Administration Central Office, Washington, D. C., ECU School of Medicine Files.

10 *Raleigh News & Observer*, February 19, 1971.

11 *Raleigh Times*, May 3, 1971.

12 *Greensboro Daily News*, February 17,1971.

13 Link, p. 224; *Raleigh News & Observer*, February 19, 1971.

14 Link, p. 225.

15 Hedrick, Chronology, p. 14.

16 Link, p. 225; *Greenville Daily Reflector*, February 26, 1971.

17 *Greensboro Record*, April 8, 1971; Hedrick, p. 17, Link, p. 225.

18 *Greenville Daily Reflector*, March 30, 1971.

19 *Greenville Daily Reflector*, March 10, 1971.

20 *Winston-Salem Sentinal*, May 11, 1971.

21 *Greensboro Daily News*, May 13, 1971.

22 *Raleigh News & Observer*, July 1, 1971.

23 *Greenville Daily Reflector*, Tuesday, July 4, 1971.

24 *Greenville Daily Reflector*, July 20, 1971.

25 1971 Session Laws, Chapter 1052.

26 1971 Session, Chapter 1053, House Bill 1207.

27 *Greenville Daily Reflector*, July 20, 1971.

28 *Durham Sun*, October 22, 1971 (Associated Press).

29 Edwin W. Monroe interview, August 18, 1995.

30 *Greensboro Daily News*, January 30, 1972.

31 Link, p. 227.

32 Dr. Wallace Wooles interview, November 13, 1991.

33 Link, p. 227; Letter, Leo Jenkins to Robert Scott, January 6,

1972, Leo Jenkins archives.

[34] *New Bern Sun-Journal,* February 10, 1972

[35] *Winston-Salem Journal,* February 18, 1972.

[36] *Greenville Daily Reflector,* February 29, 1972.

[37] *Salisbury Post,* March 16, 1972.

[38] King, p. 155.

[39] King, pp. 153-154.

[40] King, pp. 157-161.

[41] Link, pp. 195-197.

[42] Link, p. 196

[43] Link, p. 196.

[44] King, p. 154.

[45] *Greenville Daily Reflector,* April 20, 1972.

[46] *Burlington Times-News,* May 1, 1972 (Associated Press story also appeared in several other newspapers).

[47] *Winston-Salem Sentinel,* May 9, 1972.

[48] *Kinston Free Press,* May 17, 1972.

[49] *Greenville Daily Reflector,* June 22, 1972.

[50] Dr. Raymond Dawson interview, June 10, 1992.

Chapter 8
The Jordan Committee

On Friday, June 23, 1972, when the new Board of Governors met to make plans for carrying out the merger of the Consolidated University and ten other state-supported institutions of higher learning, they approved President Friday's recommendation that a five-member committee be named to study the feasibility of funding a second-year class at East Carolina University's medical school.[1]

Governor Scott, as interim Chairman of the Board, accepted President Friday's recommendation, President Jenkins went along with it, and on June 28, Scott appointed a five-member committee to make the study. The committee came to be known as the "Jordan Committee," from Robert Jordan III, a UNC member of the Board, who was named to chair it.

The members of the Jordan Committee were Dr. Andrew A. Best of Greenville, William A. Johnson of Lillington, Reginald McCoy of Laurinburg, William B. Rankin of Lincolnton, and its chairman. The committee met several times between its organization at the Board meeting in Charlotte on July 2 and the publication of its 67-page report on December 29, 1972. It solicited the views of the deans of the medical schools and of practicing physicians in North Carolina, of the president and the director of accreditation of the Association of American Medical Colleges, of two AMA Directors involved in medical education, and of other educators. Administrators of medical schools in nine other states were also consulted.

The opinions of the medical educators and those of the medical practitioners were opposed on the point of the need for more physicians, the former holding that the expansions of medical schools already undertaken would deal adequately with the physician shortage, and the latter emphasizing the urgent and continuing need for more practitioners. The deans of the medical schools in North Carolina considered that their present number of graduates was sufficient to meet needs for doctors in the state, with only slight increases. The practicing physicians insisted that only in some of the larger cities was there no shortage, and that there was a tremendous problem of shortage in primary care physicians throughout the state. The two members of the AAMC agreed with the deans, and those of the AMA Council on Medical Education agreed with the medical practitioners.

The Jordan Committee visited ECU for one day, surveyed the space occupied by the medical school in the Biology Building, and talked to Drs. Jenkins, Monroe, and Wooles. The committee took a look at the Pitt County Memorial Hospital, and were informed about the bond issue that had been passed to build a new hospital. They did not seem to be much concerned with the possibility of an affiliation between the medical school and a community hospital.

The impression that they left with Dr. Monroe was that they had already spent a lot of time in their meetings reviewing materials presented to them by Dr. Raymond Dawson and others on President Friday's staff, that spoke to the nonfeasibility of two-year medical schools, the problems of transfer from two-year schools to four-year schools, and the lack of adequate clinical facilities in Greenville.[2] Dr. Dawson did work closely with the committee, attending most of their meetings and providing support and advice.[3]

On November 10, 1972, at the seventh meeting of the Jordan Committee, President Friday, Vice President Raymond H. Dawson, Williams Dees, Watts Hill, Sr., Watts Hill, Jr., University Secretary John P. Kennedy, Jr., and Associate Vice President J. Lem Stokes, Jr., attended. Also present were Governor Robert Scott, Dean of the UNC School of Medicine, Christopher C. Fordham III, and Dr. Edward Glazener, Director of Academic Affairs, Agriculture and Life Sciences, North Carolina State University.

Governor Scott told the Committee, "I favor East Carolina because they have worked for it." But, he said, the Board of Governors is to exercise its own judgment concerning another school of medicine in North Carolina, and where one should be located. A new school in the east would not necessarily mean more doctors in the east. He did think it was a good time to start a new school.

Dean Fordham outlined the history of the UNC School of Medicine, and mentioned that it ranked ninth in the US with regard to the national examinations given to medical students. He said the school was ready to expand. He also emphasized that if accreditation was to be assured, then the medical school in Chapel Hill must be in charge of the ECU program. The agreements reached between UNC and ECU so far were still unsatisfactory, especially in regard to faculty appointments and the promotion of students. A one-year program was not the best or the cheapest way to increase medical services.

Dr. Glazener said that a one-year program for medical studies at NCSU had been under preparation for several years. It had been patterned after a program at Purdue University in Indiana. The program would cost $199,000 during its planning year, $205,000 during its first year in operation, and $161,900 each year afterward. Most of the required courses were already being offered on the Raleigh campus. Gross anatomy and clinical instruction, which were not yet available, could be provided inside the budget estimates he had offered. There was an adequate supply of students at both the undergraduate and graduate levels.

President Friday presented the committee with a detailed proposal, first saying he was reluctant to inject himself into a complicated and difficult situation. He thought that perhaps the time was not right for a new medical school. There was a trend in the national Congress against federal funding of medical education expansion. A two-year program at ECU must carry the State's commitment to an eventual degree-granting medical school.

He made it clear that he was opposed to a second state-supported medical school, whether at ECU or elsewhere. He did not believe, he said, that setting up another independent medical education program would solve the undeniable deficiencies in medical care in rural areas. He advised that rather than a new medical school the number of students at UNC School of Medicine should be increased, and the subsidy for North Carolina students at Duke and Bowman Gray should be augmented. The one-year program at ECU should be retained until the problems about accreditation were solved. He proposed that a team of outside experts should be appointed to make a comprehensive study of the situation in health education in the state. Friday believed that it would be possible to avoid a second state-supported medical school only by keeping politics out of the issue of medical education.[4]

The recommendations of the Jordan Committee published on December 29, 1972, embodied the proposals that President Friday had placed before it in November:

> The recommendations that follow are based upon our unanimous judgment that North Carolina does need more doctors and our conclusion that when there are more graduates coming from the medical education programs of the State, more areas and regions of North Carolina will benefit from better health care.

Recommendations

> This committee has concluded that the following recommendations should be presented to the Board of Governors:

Recommendation #1

On the basis of the testimony and evidence presented to it, this committee believes that North Carolina's needs for better health care are so acute that we need, not only to support the enrollment of more North Carolinians in the Bowman Gray and Duke Schools of Medicine, as set forth in Recommendation #2, and to expand the School of Medicine of The University of North Carolina at Chapel Hill, as set forth in Recommendation #3, but also to consider seriously the establishment of a new, degree-granting school of medicine which would emphasize the training of primary care physicians. Accordingly, we recommend that the Board of Governors commission the appointment of a team of experienced and qualified national consultants to evaluate the need for an additional degree-granting school of medicine within The University of North Carolina. It is further recommended that in their study the consultants be directed to examine all possible institutional alternatives, including, specifically, the present medical education program at East Carolina University, for the provision of additional doctors in all regions of the State.

The consulting team should begin work as soon as practicable and should be requested to submit recommendations to the Board of Governors by September 1, 1973. It is recommended that $50,000 be requested by the Board of Governors to finance this study.

This comprehensive study by the consultants and consideration of their report by the Board of Governors is essential prior to the commitment of substantial State tax resources to build a second State-supported degree-granting school of medicine. For this reason the specific budget requests submitted by East Carolina University for the biennium 1973-75 to fund a two-year medical education program on that campus should not be approved.

Recommendation #2

It is the judgment of this committee that an immediate and continuing increase in the number of physicians graduating from Bowman Gray and Duke Schools of Medicine may be achieved during the remaining years of this decade. We, therefore, recommend:

(1) that the State appropriate $5,000 for each North Car-

olina student enrolled in the Bowman Gray and Duke Schools of Medicine during the 1973-75 biennium, so that these private schools may continue to increase their North Carolina enrollments;

(2) that beginning in 1975-76, the State appropriate at least $6,000 for each North Carolina student enrolled in the Bowman Gray and Duke Schools of Medicine over and above the 1974-75 base.

This recommendation is based on anticipated enrollments of North Carolina students at the two Schools as follows:

School	1973-74	1974-75	1975-76
Bowman Gray	172	178	187
Duke	105	115	129

The estimated cost of the expanded grant program to the private Medical Schools is $1,385,000 for 1973-74, $1,465,000 for 1974-75. The cost estimates contemplate that the tuition reduction portion of the grant will remain at $500 per student and that the cost of education allowances will be increased from the present $2,500 per student to $4,500 for the 1973-75 biennium.

The committee further recommends continued support of the SREB program providing spaces for 20 North Carolina medical students at Meharry Medical College. Currently this program is supported with an annual appropriation of $65,000, and this contract is negotiated periodically.

Recommendation #3

It is clear that the number of doctors graduating from the School of Medicine at the University at Chapel Hill can be increased during the remaining years of this decade. We, therefore, recommend the following action by the Board of Governors:

(1) that funds be provided in the 1973-75 biennium for the renovation of MacNider Hall and for the construction of a new laboratory-office building, as set forth in lines 18 and 32 of the 1973-75 change budget request;

(2) that the School of Medicine of the University of North Carolina at Chapel Hill be authorized to increase the size of

its entering class to 140 in 1975 and to 160 in 1976, and to proceed to the goal of an enrollment of 640 M.D. degree candidates by 1979-80; and

(3) that 20 degree candidates continue to be enrolled in the medical education program at East Carolina University, pending the completion of the action in Recommendation #1, above.

Recommendation #4

The experience of this committee in its own study of medical education in North Carolina mandates, in our judgment, that the Board of Governors establish as soon as practicable a continuing overview of institutional activity in the health sciences. Even a casual examination of the range and magnitude of programs currently offered by the several campuses under the jurisdiction of this Board makes clear that constant attention and accumulating knowledge and experiences are essential to the successful discharge of responsibility by the Board of Governors in this major field of endeavor. We, therefore, recommend that the Code Committee of the Board of Governors explore the possibility of establishing a standing Committee on the Health Sciences to advise and consult with the president on all institutional programs related to the health sciences.

Recommendation #5

Our experience, and that of the President and his staff in providing assistance to this committee during these six months, makes it quite clear that a senior-level staff officer with established competence and extensive knowledge in health sciences should be added as soon as possible to the General Administration staff. We, therefore, recommend that the president be authorized to search for and, thereafter, recommend the appointment of such a qualified person to the Board of Governors.[5]

To the people at East Carolina who read the report, its recommendations seemed clearly the result of UNC staff control over the committee's process. They were apparently unaware of the crucial intervention by President Friday himself at the committee's November 10 meeting. As Dr. Monroe saw it, the provision for the study of further development in the one-year medical school and of its being expanded to a four-year school was all that the two committee members friendly to ECU, Dr. Andrew Best of Greenville, and Reginald "Mutt" McCoy of Laurinburg "could get into that report because of all the staff control over the process. Staff meaning people like Ray Dawson, Felix Joyner, particularly those two."[6] It seems not to have occurred to Monroe or others in Greenville until later that the panel of outside consultants, while its introduction was congruous with President Friday's preference for emphasizing professional education issues over political ones, might have been a gambit proposed in the hope of derailing the drive for a four-year school.

Reginald McCoy said that he joined the majority in voting on the report only because it was clear that the Board of Governors would not proceed in any other direction than that recommended by the subcommittee. He did not think another study was needed, because there had been twelve in the previous eight years. "On the bright side though, I cannot imagine consultants coming in and studying the situation in this state without recognizing our critical needs for more doctors," he concluded.[7]

While the Jordan Committee's report urged looking into establishment of a second state-supported four-year medical school in North Carolina, it did not deal explicitly with the ECU problem, apart from the recommendation to call in experts from outside the state. However, the Board of Governors joined William Friday in welcoming the opportunity to shift the conflict about the medical school to another forum besides the mostly political one in which it had been carried on previously. As soon as the committee report was received on January 2, 1973, the new chairman of the board, Dr. William A. Dees, Jr., of Goldsboro included himself and Board member Watts Hill, Sr., of Chapel Hill in the study committee that would select the consultants. In an interview by a *Greenville Daily Reflector* staff writer, Dees said his appointment of Watts Hill, Sr., to the committee to select the medical study panel was "not in any way a move against East Carolina." He continued, "in my opinion Hill is the best informed layman in North Carolina, as far as medical education is concerned." He noted that Hill was board chairman of Watts Hospital in Durham for years, was a prime force in the establishment of the medical school at Chapel Hill. He believed that Hill's opinion of the qualifications of the consultants would be valuable to the committee.[8] He did not refer to the fact that Hill was also a champion of Chapel Hill against all challenges, and an outspoken opponent of establishing a second state-supported medical school in the state.

At a press conference, the chairman of the ECU Board of

Trustees, Attorney General Robert Morgan, said he was extremely disappointed at the Board of Governors' decision not to expand the medical school at ECU. He reacted angrily to the board's judgment, saying that they were offering the same old remedy to the physician shortage, and that doing another study was an attempt to kill the ECU proposal. When the Jordan Committee's first recommendation was viewed alone, it was apparent that the Board was dodging its responsibility by calling for an outside group to make its decision for it. This question of whether or not a second state-supported medical school was needed had been studied, debated, and discussed for more than eight years.

The only question that really faced the Board of Governors was how best to build on the steps already taken toward establishing a second state-supported School of Medicine. The legislation passed by the 1971 General Assembly clearly stated that the East Carolina program was a step in developing a four-year medical school.[9]

In a speech to the Charlotte Rotary Club on January 23, 1973, UNC President William C. Friday said that legislative interference or political meddling could weaken the structure of the sixteen-campus university system. He said that it might take three to five years for the system to adjust to the new situation and become able to navigate for itself.

"I don't know of any move to bypass the Board of Governors," Friday replied to a question about the ECU situation. He characterized his comment about "political meddling" as a reminder that "in higher education you don't make changes in 60 days, you do it in six years sometimes." He said he anticipated that Charlotte would be among the locations considered for a medical school, but would not speculate further. He said he would meet the next day with the chancellors of the sixteen UNC institutions to consider requesting expansion of the 1973-75 university budget.[10]

The UNC Board of Governors' first chairman, William Dees, was interviewed by a staff writer from the *Greenville Daily Reflector* on Sunday, February 11 in his office in Goldsboro. Dees, an attorney, was a 1941 UNC-CH graduate, who had become acquainted with Friday during his senior year through the North Carolina Federation of Student Governments.[11] After serving in the navy, Dees returned to receive his law degree in Chapel Hill in 1948, and was associate editor of the *Law Review*. He and Friday were both members of a study group in the law school, whose members, with their wives, carried on an active social life.[12]

Dees had been a member of the Board of Higher Education for

two years, beginning in 1963, and became chairman of the BHE in 1964. He had been a member of the UNC Board of Trustees since 1969. He told his interviewer that he saw the main function of the Board of Governors to be long range planning, and insuring proper execution of the plan. For example, the Board was working on an analysis of the degrees given by the various schools in the university system to locate any duplications and find out where new degree programs may be needed.

He had not found that the members of the Board ever placed the regard for any one institution above that for another. They were working on a program of higher education in North Carolina that would be the best they could develop. They worked long and hard on the tasks assigned to them. One outstanding project, he said, had been the study by the committee chaired by Robert Jordan of the feasibility of funding the expansion of the ECU medical school.

Dees said that the chancellors of the various schools in the system had cooperated closely with the General Administration and that this had not been what he expected. He had anticipated that each of the chancellors would be pushing his own school and its programs. Instead, he had found that they were working together.

When he was asked about the future of medical education in the state, he answered that it was a question that interested him particularly. As a resident of eastern North Carolina, he would like to see a medical school in the east. The more it was possible to bring to this area, the more it pleased him. He admitted a special personal interest, in that his daughter was a junior at East Carolina University. However, his position as chairman of the Board of Governors meant that he could not take sides.

He said that the Jordan Committee's report was most favorable to ECU, saying, in effect, that the medical school should be located there. He agreed that more doctors should be trained in North Carolina, which had two and a half percent of the population and trained only one and a half percent of the doctors in the United States. The question was how best to do it, and whether a plan should be chosen on the basis of successfully increasing the production of physicians.

There was the question of cost, since medical education was very expensive. The Board was trying to convince Duke and Bowman Gray to take more North Carolina students, by increasing subsidies. The student body at Chapel Hill was being increased. It was difficult to expand a program piecemeal into a full four-year one. There was nowhere for more than twenty students to continue their medical training. The ideal approach would be to take however much money was needed and build a school all at once from the bottom up.

Dees said that he would not predict what the group of five experts who were being brought in to study medical education in the state would recommend. He did know the group would be made up of five professional medical educators. He had written to deans in all the states, to the AMA, and to the AAMC for their recommendations. [13]

Chairman Dees began immediately to seek potential consultants from the list of twenty-seven names that were suggested to him. Near the middle of March, 1973, he reported to the Board that although the selection had been more difficult than he had anticipated, the out-of-state medical experts had been selected, and would be contacted shortly. He said he hoped that they would be able to begin meeting in mid-April, if all the proposed members of the panel accepted appointment. The consultants would be asked to recommend whether or not to develop a four-year medical school at ECU, and also to take a broader look at the state's medical care needs.

They would be fair and impartial medical experts, Dees said, a group of people who medical educators in North Carolina felt were qualified. The Board of Governors' chairman said the current list included four people who represented the "traditional medical school view" and four who advocated the "new medical school view." The traditional view, he said, involved internship following formal medical school study, and the new view was one which emphasized innovative educational training such as six-year study programs. [14]

In March 1973, Dr. Edwin Monroe wrote to Dees objecting to the distribution of members of the Bennett Committee among pro- and anti-traditional medical schools. He felt that the balance of opinion was markedly against ECU's goals. He also objected to the proposed inclusion of a hospital administrator, which he said was in violation of a previous agreement not to do this. In a follow-up letter, he objected to the proposed choices of particular hospital administrators, as being limited to those associated with established medical school teaching hospitals.

In his second letter, Dr. Monroe also raised questions concerning the names proposed for physicians representing community medicine. Of those proposed, only one, Dr. Kurt Deuschle of Mt. Sinai medical school, was genuinely in the field. [15]

Subsequently, the Chairman of the Board of Governors publicly claimed on a number of occasions that ECU had accepted the panel members without demur. He said, "A careful process of selection was followed in naming the membership of that panel, with the participation of ECU, Chapel Hill, and others. The majority of the members appointed to that panel were nominated by East Carolina University. ECU was given the opportunity to object to any or all of the consultants, and no objection was heard until after the consultants had reported to the Board of Governors." [16]

In April, Dees appointed a five-man committee:

Chairman, Dr. Ivan L. Bennett, Jr., Vice President for Health Affairs and Dean of the School of Medicine of New York University, a native of Wilmington, North Carolina, an academic pathologist, medical school faculty member, and career administrator; Dr. Kenneth Crispell, Vice President for Health Sciences of the University of Virginia; Dr. Kurt Deuschle, who was Professor of Community Medicine at the Mt. Sinai School; Dr. Lloyd C. Elam, President of Meharry Medical College; Dr. Robert S. Stone, Vice President for Medical Affairs at the new New Mexico medical school, resigned from the panel in May, 1973, to become Director of the National Institutes of Health, and was replaced by: Dr. F. Carter Pannill, Professor of Medicine at University of Texas Medical School at San Antonio (after June 1973 he was Vice President for Health Sciences at SUNY-Buffalo); Dr. Jules I. Levine, Director of Biomedical Studies, Center for Delivery of Health Care, University of Virginia, served as Secretary to the committee.

The Bennett Committee met in North Carolina for a long weekend each month from April to September. As its visits, interviews, and meetings continued, other issues kept the heat on ECU, UNC, the medical establishment, and interested legislators.

A five-person LCME survey team had come to Chapel Hill and Greenville on January 29-31, 1973.[17] It reported to the administrators at UNC immediately after its visit, but did not send its official report until April 9.[18] By this time, the Bennett panel had begun its work.

The LCME approved accreditation of UNC-CH for a full period of seven years, with an entering class not to exceed 130 students through 1974-75, 140 students in 1975-76, and 160 students in 1976-77, contingent upon the satisfactory development of facilities. It found the ECU program seriously lacking in acceptable quality. The material that the school had furnished to the team was deemed scanty, and it showed little evidence of progress over the preceding two years except for recruitment of an able class of students. The Committee found that the ECU medical faculty was of inferior quality, that the basic science support was weak, and that clinical training was not adequate. It questioned whether the UNC medical school was not failing to exercise authority and responsibility, while ECU was refusing to recognize its position vis-à-vis UNC, under whose accreditation they were being permitted to operate a one-year educational program. The Committee also raised the question whether the legislators and Board of Governors had not failed to delineate appropriate responsibility and authority to meet the prevailing circumstances. It concluded that without the proper exercise by the dean of the UNC medical school over the quality of the ECU program, UNC was at risk of losing its own accreditation.[19]

The ECU administration was not apprised of the report's content until it had been circulated to the Board of Governors, and its contents became public, over two weeks after it had been received in Chapel Hill. On April 25 after receiving a copy of the survey report, Dr. Edwin Monroe wrote to Chancellor Leo Jenkins (creation of the university system included the change from the title of "president" to "chancellor" for all head of the sixteen campuses). "To my knowledge it is unheard of for an accreditation survey team to write up their report and submit it to the Liaison Committee without first sharing it with the concerned institution." No opportunity had been provided to respond to, correct, or amplify those portions of the report that dealt with the one-year program at ECU. Dr. Monroe commented that although the actual program under way, the one-year medical program, was the only one that it was appropriate for the LCME to address, much of the report dealt with the issue of developing a four-year medical school. He said, "The inaccuracies, misunderstandings, and indeed the blatant editorializing in this report are unfair, irresponsible, and deserve a formal complaint directed to the Liaison Committee."

Monroe observed that no one doubted the inadequacy of the funding set up to operate the one-year program, under a budget which the Board of Higher Education had dictated, even setting the number of faculty positions that could be filled. He found "particularly unfair and unwarranted" the report's comments about the school's faculty. The committee had found no outstanding scholars among them, and described them as only modestly proficient. It was particularly galling to Monroe that the same senior faculty members had been judged highly competent in the LCME survey report only two years before. With whom, he wondered, had the committee compared the faculty in evaluating them.

The Liaison Committee's previous report had also complimented Drs. Wooles and Monroe and the East Carolina University administration. The new report judged that the administrative leadership at ECU was neither strong nor experienced by the usual academic standards, and did not provide the necessary strength for new program.

Dr. Monroe said that he and Dr. Wooles were in agreement that a one-year program was not viable, that funding was not adequate, and that they could not interest renowned teachers in joining a one-year program. In any case, the program was accredited through Chapel Hill, and could well be operated by the medical school there, as long as the intent of the General Assembly was carried out to set up a cooperative venture, and "not dictatorship." The letter concluded:

> If President Friday seriously wishes to help, he can exercise true leadership and statesmanship to insure that we get the aid and necessary resources to operate a high-quality one-year program as the base from which we can develop a four-year medical school and a community oriented university health sciences center to complement the Division of Health Sciences at UNC-Chapel Hill. [20]

On April 26, after the LCME report had been circulated to members of the Board of Governors, the newspapers related that it criticized the bickering and lack of cooperation between UNC and ECU, and blamed UNC for inadequately responding to earlier criticisms. The following day, the complete text of the report was published. On the same day, Chancellor Jenkins went to Chapel Hill to meet with President Friday. They were in accord that the report required the dean of the UNC School of Medicine to have clear responsibility for the ECU medical education program, and exert control over it, or withdraw entirely from involvement in the program. On April 30, Friday communicated their agreement to the Board of Governors.

Dr. Jenkins also met on April 27, 1973, with Dean Fordham, and Fordham assured him that UNC would provide full cooperation and assistance to ECU. Jenkins said to reporters that there was no alternative but for ECU to accept UNC's control of the medical program. While he could not avoid the hard reality of the situation, and accepted it as an interim arrangement, he was not happy with it. He and Dr. Monroe spoke with reporters, and Jenkins told them that the opposition had used "every trick in the book . . . to discredit, sabotage and destroy the effort that we have undertaken." The LCME report had already been interpreted critically and given misleading headlines in the newspapers, and had been misconstrued even before the Board of Governors had even seen it. He said that North Carolinians who suffered from insufficient health care were the real victims.

Dr. Monroe's comments were even more disparaging. He repeated to the press what he had written to Dr. Jenkins, that the LCME report had evaluated the one-year ECU program in terms appropriate only to a four-year one, rather than as an appendage of UNC. If they had compared it, as they should have, with other one-year schools, they would have found it at least as adequate, if not better than they were. Inadequate funding and the friction with Chapel Hill had made it still more difficult to operate. He said that ECU had fought for eight years to establish a medical school to meet the needs of the people of North Carolina, and would not give up the fight until the people's needs were met. Until there was a four-year, free-standing program at ECU, he observed, "we can continue to expect this kind of prejudicial treatment from the medical school establishment and from some newspapers in the state." [21]

The controversy about the medical school in Greenville became deeply entangled with the issue of the autonomy of the UNC Board of Governors. The pro-UNC and pro-ECU contestants tended to unite against one another on the question of the effect that a legislative decision would have on the still green Board of Governors.

The Associated Press polled the twenty-nine-member House Committee on Higher Education, and were told by most of the nineteen members who replied that they would be guided by the UNC Board of Governors in deciding whether ECU should have a four-year medical school. A typical viewpoint was that the board of governors should make the professional education decision, but the General Assembly should make the decisions as to the school's location and financing. Even among eastern legislators it was thought that, while East Carolina University should have a four-year medical school, the legislature should not go against the recommendations of the Board of Governors. [22]

Most legislators supported giving the Board of Governors at least a few years to get established before the legislature judged the success of the restructuring. They agreed that, apart from the merits of ECU's position, for the legislature to bypass the Board of Governors and build a medical school in Greenville would probably destroy the board in its infancy. Some of ECU's strong eastern supporters in the General Assembly accepted this position.

Senator J. J. (Monk) Harrington of Bertie County, a major

spokesman for the East Carolina position, favored waiting until the report was issued, and if it was unfavorable to ECU, taking issue with it when the legislature reconvened in 1974. He said, "We are entitled to that medical school, and we are going to get it. The Board of Governors could be the best thing for North Carolina, but they have to represent all the schools. If they get taken over by that Chapel Hill crowd, then the board would be the worst thing for the state."

He also said that he and other eastern legislators would consider a decision by the Board of Governors against the ECU medical school as sufficient evidence to prove that the Board has been taken over by Chapel Hill. Other eastern supporters recognized that it would be impossible to convince the public that a bill to expand the medical school would not be an attack on the Board.

Senator Ralph Scott, chairman of the Appropriations Committee, thought that the Board of Governors deserved at least four years before the legislature started second-guessing it. Two other members of appropriations committees, Senator Charles Dean of Richmond County and Representative Carl Stewart of Gaston, agreed with Scott.

Representative Horton Rountree said that supporters of a four-year medical school at ECU were "playing their cards close to the vest" in the General Assembly. He would not say definitely whether a bill would be introduced during the current session to bypass the UNC board of governors and expand the school at ECU. He said there was, however, a strong possibility that such legislation would be introduced. If so, it would be determinedly opposed by practically all legislators from west of Greenville.[23]

Opposition from the medical establishment of the state continued robustly during the spring and summer months. The Executive Council of the North Carolina Medical Society, meeting in its 119th annual convention in Pinehurst on May 20, 1973, considered a report recommending ECU's medical school be abolished and that no new four-year medical school be built in North Carolina. The report had been requested in May 1971 through a resolution from the Lincoln County Medical Society. Dr. John Glasson of Durham, who was then president of the N. C. Medical Society, asked the fifteen-member N. C. Joint Conference Committee on Medical Care to carry out the studies. The Joint Conference Committee, in turn, set up a four-member subcommittee under Dr. Glasson's chairmanship to prepare the report—it was, then, the report of the Glasson subcommittee, or more briefly, "The Glasson Report."

The report was officially received by the Executive Council of the House of Delegates at its first meeting, and sent to a reference committee for a recommendation to the Delegates. With the approval of the reference committee, it was to be presented later in the week to the full House of Delegates to the Society, for them to endorse, reject or accept as information only.

Dr. Edgar Beddingfield, now of Wilson, past president of the society and an ECU supporter, believed the issue might be too divisive for the society to take up. He hoped it would receive the report as information only. He did not believe a sufficient consensus existed within the Medical Society to take a corporate opinion one way or the other on the question of the medical school in Greenville.

Dr. John Gamble of Lincolnton, a Democratic state representative who supported the ECU school, said that anything other than an information-only recommendation would polarize the Medical Society. He said he hoped that people with strong feelings on the issue would accept the report just as information, and not take up an emotional stance that would divide the Society. Dr. Gamble had authored the resolution to the Society's House of Delegates in May, 1971, under which the conference committee report was commissioned. He said the resolution was not intended to ask the Medical Society to do anything beyond taking a look at the question. The report went beyond what the original resolution asked, which was to determine how many doctors the state needed and the most economical way of producing them. The subcommittee that drafted the report for the conference committee had gone far beyond the original intent. When, in late January, the report had been received by the executive council of the society, it came with the recommendation that it be referred to the House of Delegates without comment. A detailed summary of the report was published in the March, 1973, issue of the *N. C. Medical Journal.*[24]

Dr. David Welton of Charlotte, chairman of the Joint Conference Committee on Medical Care, declined to express an opinion on whether the committee members or anti-ECU forces in the Society could be expected to urge an endorsement of the report. Another member of the conference committee, Dr. Charles Styron of Raleigh, a former president of the society, said he would oppose rejection of the report. He said he would favor having the House of Delegates either endorse the report or accept it as information only.[25]

On Tuesday, May 22, a majority of the House of Delegates adopted the subcommittee report. The one-year medical school, it was agreed, should be phased out and replaced by an area health education center. In a separate action, the delegates also passed a proposal for the General Assembly to provide funds to expand the entering class at UNC-CH to 140-150 students by 1976. The delegates also approved a suggestion that financial support to Duke and Bowman Gray be increased for NC students in these schools.

Dr. Edgar Beddingfield predicted the House of Delegates' action would not effect ECU medical school expansion plans. There would be no consequence for the medical school's ultimate fate, but the Medical Society would be temporarily harmed.

A spokesman for the reference committee, which had met secretly Monday night and split two-to-one in favor of endorsing the report, said they rejected the information-only position because they felt it was important for the Medical Society to take a stand on this issue, even though it was an emotional one.

Floor debate on Tuesday was about equally divided between ECU supporters and opponents. Dr. Lenox Baker of Durham said, "If we approve this report, we will be telling the people of North Carolina that we doctors don't want any more doctors to practice in this state. This society is split. And I don't believe that it can speak for a majority of the people here. There are too many on each side of the question and too many undecided."

Dr. Robert B. Hodgson of Perquimans Country said that the ECU question was the most political issue that he had ever heard discussed in a medical group. He believed that whatever stand the Society took, it would be a source of criticism. There was no way it could win. "The politicians will only make fools of us."

Dr. John Gamble spoke out strongly against the report. If it was adopted, he said, the Society would be "saying no to the qualified young men and women in North Carolina who can't get into medical school," and to the state's citizens who were concerned with improving medical care.

The doctors who spoke in favor of endorsing the report were generally from the state's urban areas, with a few Eastern doctors also in favor of it. Dr. Charles Styron said, "The House of Delegates ought to take a position. We owe it to ourselves, to the citizens and to the politicians to tell them how we feel on this. We shouldn't dodge the issue." Dr. John Glasson spoke out strongly in favor of his committee's report. He said, however, that an endorsement would not indicate a consensus of the Delegates. He did not believe that it would be possible to arrive at a better estimate of the need for doctors in North Carolina.[26]

After the meeting, a number of physicians expressed their opinions about the House of Delegates' action: Dr. J. Elliot Dixon of Pitt County, supporter of the ECU school, said of the society's vote that it wouldn't affect the state legislature's decision. Dr. Marvin N. Lymberis of Charlotte, who opposed the ECU school, said he hoped the vote would have an effect on the legislature's decision. He did not think, however that the legislature was likely to expand the school, because of the cost and the difficulty of recruiting faculty.

Dr. Lenox Baker commented after the vote in the House of Delegates that the decision had set medicine back twenty-five years in North Carolina.

William A. Dees, Jr., UNC Board of Governors' chairman, interviewed by telephone from the Medical Society meeting, said that the General Assembly was not likely to be influenced very much by the NC Medical Society's vote to abolish the ECU School of Medicine. The September report by the consultant panel would be more influential, because the panel members were medical educators, not practitioners. The medical society's decision would be interpreted, Dees said, to mean they did not want more doctors trained.

The Board of Governors, he said, would recommend to the 1974 General Assembly, whose relationship with the state's medical society had not been good, whether the ECU school should be expanded, after the panel of out-of-state consultants had completed their study of medical care and education in NC.[27]

On returning to the House of Representatives on Wednesday, Dr. John Gamble told his colleagues that the state medical society Joint Conference Committee on Medical Care, which recommended abolition of the ECU medical school, had been stacked against ECU, and completely biased. He said that eight of the fifteen members of the committee were directly tied to the three existing schools which would benefit if the ECU school was eliminated. Among these were Dr. William Anlyan, Vice President for Health Affairs at Duke and Dr. Manson Meads, Dean of Bowman Gray medical school, who had served with Dr. Glasson on the subcommittee which did the actual study. Also, there were Dr. Christopher Fordham, Dean of the UNC-Chapel Hill School of Medicine; Dr. Cecil Sheps, UNC Vice Chancellor for Health affairs; and Alexander McMahon, a former Duke trustee heading Blue Cross-Blue Shield of North Carolina. Three other committee members held faculty position at Duke, UNC, or Bowman Gray. Only one committee member, Dr. Edwin W. Monroe, Vice Chancellor for Health Affairs at ECU, voted against the report.

Gamble said that doctors attempt to protect their high incomes by restricting entrance into the medical profession, and that they do this by restricting the availability of medical training.

In Greenville, Dr. Edwin Monroe said that the action of the medical society would in no way influence the operation of the one-year program at ECU or its possible expansion to a four-year medical school. He was disappointed that the leaders of the State Medical Society failed to recognize what was a clear and irrefutable fact to everyone else in the state, that there was a severe shortage of doctors in North Carolina and the rest of the nation. He suggested that the people of the state, when they read about the actions at the State Medical Society meeting, should remember that forty percent of the delegates to the Society came from seven cities in North Carolina—Charlotte, Asheville, Greensboro, Winston-Salem, Raleigh, Durham, and Chapel Hill.[28]

At a meeting of the joint health committee of the General Assembly July 23, 1973, the deans of the UNC and the ECU medical schools presented conflicting opinions about the effect medical schools have on the number of doctors in neighboring areas.

Dr. Christopher Fordham III presented a map of the United States showing medical schools and the physician distribution around them. "This map clearly shows that medical schools have no impact on the number of physicians in nearby counties," he said. While the number of doctors increased in the county in which a medical school was located, adjoining counties were not affected.

The UNC dean said that the Chapel Hill school had set up five Area Health Education Centers across the state, mostly at local hospitals. Medical students could take residencies and training under these centers. He considered this a preferable alternative to new medical schools.

ECU Dean Wallace Wooles replied, "The medical needs of rural areas could most readily be met by the establishment of medical schools in the larger communities in these areas." There was a seven-year lag between a student's starting medical school and the time he or she entered practice. He argued that "medical schools drawing on local population and providing residency training is the best way of providing doctors in a given area." He also said that the longer the legislature delayed starting new medical schools, the more the problem of doctor shortages would be compounded.

To the same committee, Dr. Thomas D. Kinney, director of medical education at Duke University Medical School, proposed setting up a special medical scholarship fund to encourage North Carolinians to attend medical school in the state rather than going out of the state to medical schools.

"The projected increase in physician supply nationally and in North Carolina approximates three per cent per year during the latter half of the decade, while the population is growing at a rate of one per cent," Dr. Fordham added. Merely increasing the number of physicians, however, would not improve access to medical care for all citizens because physicians tend to settle in urban areas.[29]

Following Fordham's presentation, Representative H. Horton Rountree of Pitt County sharply questioned him on the number of North Carolina students in the state's four-year medical schools, how many graduates practiced medicine in North Carolina, and the availability of programs in family medical practice at the UNC medical school.

Fordham answered that there was no question of a shortage of family practitioners, since more students were expressing interest in this field and more courses were becoming available to them. He also noted that a number of different factors went into a student's decision on where he would practice medicine. Among these were his family's influence, his ties to his home state, and where he took his training and residency.[30]

In May, the General Assembly's reservations concerning the Board of Governors' handling of the ECU medical school question came into focus with the adoption of two resolutions about health care. One, House Joint Resolution 1106, directed the legislature's joint committees on health to study the shortages in the state of medical manpower and facilities.[31] A second resolution, House Joint Resolution 1133, established still another group, the Medical Manpower Study Commission. The Commission was set up to study the continuing physician shortage in North Carolina, to hold hearings, and to review relevant materials, including the report of the Bennett Committee. After their investigations and deliberations, the Commission was to make recommendations to the 1974 session of the legislature, aimed at solving the state's problem of inadequate medical care.

As the Commission's co-chairman, Representative J. P. Huskins of Iredell County later told the Joint Appropriation Committee of the General Assembly:

> We set out in earnest to discover the extent of the doctor shortage, its impact upon the health and economic well being of the people, and the adequacy of efforts being made to solve it. We held public hearings all across North Carolina and thus gave the people at large their first opportunity to

have a voice in plans being made to serve their health care needs. The people had little or no voice in the work of the Jordan committee, the deliberations of the panel of outside experts or the formulation of the Board of Governors' statewide proposal. But they did have an opportunity to tell our commission of their needs, their fears and their frustrations.[32]

Huskins was highly respected in the General Assembly for his intelligence and his objective, meticulous approach to problem solving. He did not admire the way the administration at UNC-Chapel Hill did business.[33] His knowledge of both sides of the controversy about the medical school was unmatched in the legislature. He had been a member of the state Board of Higher Education, and until June a member of the UNC Board of Governors.

Representative Joseph Patterson "Jay" Huskins was editor—he had an A. B. in journalism from the University of North Carolina in Chapel Hill—of the Statesville *Record and Landmark* when he was appointed by Governor Dan Moore to the Board of Higher Education in 1965. At that time, the legislature had just authorized the establishment of a two-year school of medicine at East Carolina College. UNC supporters in the legislature had added to the law a requirement that unless the school was accredited by the Liaison Committee on Health Education of the AMA and AAMC the Board of Higher Education would reconsider its establishment. When accreditation was not granted, Huskins was chairman of a the board's New Programs Committee, and it was after carefully studying the situation that his committee recommended against a two-year medical school at East Carolina.

Huskins's subsequent experience in the House of Representatives, which he joined in 1971, and as a member of the UNC Board of Governors, where he was on the budget committee, convinced him that the action taken on the BHE's recommendation had been wrong. He said that he had come to believe that, "had statesmanship rather than envy and rivalry, prevailed back in 1970, the legislature would have been advised that East Carolina University could mount a successful, accreditable two-year basic medical science program with $11 million in capital and $2.5 million in operating funds." It was his opinion, he said at the first meeting of the Medical Manpower Study Commission, that the Board of Governors did not want a confrontation with the legislature over the ECU medical school.

By the time the Bennett Committee's report was received by the

UNC Board of Governors, the Joint Health Subcommittee and the Medical Manpower Study Commission had agreed to join forces, because their agendas were so close together. The Subcommittee had heard from sixteen people, including deans of medical schools. The Commission was half through its investigation. It had held its nine public hearings, was investigating the cost of establishing new medical schools—costs were obtained from eleven of twenty new schools—across the country, and studying the recommendations of the out-of-state consultants. By the time the legislature met in 1974, both the Subcommittee and the Commission were ready with their findings, which they presented in separate reports to the General Assembly.

---

[1] *Greenville Daily Greenville Daily Reflector,* June 24, 1972.

[2] Monroe interview, January 3, 1992.

[3] Link, p. 227.

[4] Link, p. 228; William C. Friday Papers, Subgroup 1, Series 1, "Medical Education Aug.-Nov. 1972," (Friday's presentation to Jordon Committee, November 10, 1972).

[5] *Report of the Committee to Study the Request of East Carolina University for a Second Year of Medical Education,* Board of Governors, The University of North Carolina, Dec. 29, 1972; see WCF Papers, Subgroup 1, Series 1, "Medical Education," Dec. 1972.

[6] Monroe interview, January 3, 1992.

[7] *Greenville Daily Reflector,* January 14, 1973.

[8] *Greenville Daily Reflector,* February 11, 1973.

[9] *Greenville Daily Reflector,* January 16, 1973

[10] *Charlotte Observer,* January 25, 1973.

[11] Link, 57.

[12] Link, 58.

[13] *Greenville Daily Reflector,* February 11, 1973.

[14] *Greenville Daily Reflector,* 16 March 16, 1973.

[15] Letters from Edwin W. Monroe to William A. Dees, March 6, 1973 and March 14, 1973, Jenkins Archives.

[16] Statement given by Dees to the Joint Appropriations Committee, February 19, 1974, in ECU School of Medicine files, folder "Joint Appropriations Committee, Public Hearings Feb., 1974." He made similar statements to various civic clubs during December 1973 and January 1974 (texts in ECU School of Medicine files,

folder "Bennett Committee").

[17] The members of the survey team were Drs. James L. Dennis (Chairman), Emanual M. Papper, Allan D. Bass, T. Stewart Hamilton, and Marjorie P. Wilson (Secretary). See Liaison Committee on Medical Education, *Report of the Survey, The University North Carolina, Chapel Hill, School of Medicine, Chapel Hill, North Carolina,* January 29-31, 1973.

[18] Link, p. 228.

[19] Liaison Committee on Medical Education, *Report of the Survey,* January 29-31, 1973, with letter of transmittal to William C. Friday, LL.B. President, University System of North Carolina, April 9, 1973. Copy in ECU School of Medicine Files, Folder, "Accreditation."

[20] Memorandum from Monroe to Jenkins, April 25, 1973, Jenkins Archives and ECU School of Medicine files.

[21] *Raleigh News & Observer,* April 28, 1973.

[22] *Charlotte News,* March 5, 1973; *Greenville Daily Reflector,* March 5, 1973.

[23] *Raleigh News & Observer,* Monday, March 5, 1973.

[24] *N. C. Medical Journal,* Vol. 34, No. 3 (March 1973) pp. 210-215.

[25] *Raleigh News & Observer,* May 21, 1973.

[26] *Greensboro Daily News,* May 23, 1973.

[27] *Charlotte News,* May 23, 1973.

[28] *Greenville Daily Reflector,* May 23, 1973.

[29] *Chapel Hill Weekly,* July 23, 1973.

[30] *Raleigh News & Observer,* July 26, 1973.

[31] The Joint Health Committees were chaired by Senator Kenneth C. Royall, Jr., Chairman of the Senate Committee on Public Health, and Representative Mrs. John B. Chase, Chairman of the House Committee on Health, who also served as ex officio members of each subcommittee. The joint committees consisted of four subcommittees, (1) Health Care Facilities and Services, (2) Health Costs, (3) Health Manpower Training and Education, and (4) Health Manpower Utilization and Licensing, with each subcommittee chaired by a Senator and a Representative.

[32] Address by Rep. J. P. Huskins before the Joint Appropriation Committee of the General Assembly, in Raleigh, February 19, 1974 (Copy in ECU Medical School files, "J. H. Huskins" folder); see also Greensboro *Daily News,* July 28, 1973.

[33] Huskins interview, April 2, 1992; Monroe interview, Jan. 2, 1992.

Chapter 9
The Bennett Committee—
Summer and Fall 1973

The Bennett Committee continued to visit North Carolina each month through the summer and fall of 1973. They interviewed medical educators and administrators and practitioners. During their six-month investigation, they spent an aggregate of about three weeks in the state, visiting and talking with the faculties of UNC and ECU. They visited Duke and Bowman Gray. They spent one afternoon and evening in Greenville, and toured the Biology Building where the medical school was located. They made a short visit to Pitt County Memorial Hospital, but took no note of its impending expansion.[1] They made two other brief visits to Greenville. They talked with Dr. Ed Monroe, Dr. Wallace Wooles, and with Chancellor Jenkins, as well as other members of the ECU medical program faculty and administration.

Chancellor Jenkins and other ECU officials who had not been able to meet with the panel of consultants when they came to Greenville later met with them privately on the N. C. State campus. Jenkins seized the opportunity to give forcible expression to his point of view and aims. He opined that during their months of study, the panel had doubtless been impressed by the strength of the public's demand for more doctors. He hoped that they had become aware, as he had been for a decade, of the need for more doctors and the absence, so far, of any solution.

He was confident that they had been given a sampling of the newspaper articles and editorials on the issue of expanding the East Carolina University Medical School, some of them implying that the school was an example of ECU's and his own empire building. However, ECU had no need for a medical school in order to continue its major role in higher education in North Carolina. It could have saved itself and its faculty and administrators frustration, hard work, criticism, and insults in the news media if they had ignored the medical manpower problem. But they could not ignore it, when those in a position to attack the problem most effectively did little about the physician shortage. The history of ECU during the previous ten years was the history of an effort to deal with that problem.

Finally, the people were aroused and had communicated this through their representatives in the General Assembly. It had been made clear by polls taken by legislators and by a statewide poll by a marketing service that a large majority of people supported the clear objective of ECU, a new degree-granting medical school whose emphasis was on training primary care physicians.

According to Jenkins, the old cost figure of $100 million used by some opponents of adding a medical school to scare potential supporters away had been laid to rest, replaced by reasonable and realistic cost estimates obtained from the Association of American Medical Colleges. The need for more medical care in North Carolina had been documented, there were qualified students, and the money was available to build a new school.

Chancellor Jenkins told the panel he had attempted to outline why and how East Carolina University's School of Medicine came to be, and how the majority of the people across the state viewed its future. They should be aware of the unmet need, the growing frustration, and the public demand that the state's medical manpower and health care needs are met. The people of the state were looking to the consultants and to the state's leaders to insure that the commitment and the beginning at East Carolina were realized.[2]

This presentation to the Bennett Committee was a typical Jenkins articulation of his populist viewpoint, so diametrically at odds with the approach to governance taken by UNC, and largely shared by the panel of medical consultants. There is no evidence that his oratory swayed the panel to the slightest degree. It is doubtful whether he expected it to: his remarks were printed in their entirety in the *Greenville Daily Reflector* on the day he delivered them.[3]

Dr. Monroe and others at the ECU medical school were convinced that the Bennett Committee, chosen with little attention to input from Greenville, was a setup designed by the UNC administration to give credibility to their push for control of ECU's program. They took the choice of Dr. Ivan Bennett as evidence for their belief, since they were sure even before the committee's work began that he would be against establishing a second state-funded medical school. Dr. Kenneth Crispell, dean of the medical school in Charlottesville, Virginia, had fought against state support for the Eastern Virginia Medical School in Norfolk, while Dr. Jules I. Levine, Executive Secretary of the Committee, worked for Crispell.

Monroe wrote on January 29, 1973, to the Board of Governors: "Dr. Deuschle is very knowledgeable in community hospitals. . . Dr. Stone recently completed his school and it is approved." Dr. Monroe said he felt obligated to give the nominations to the Board of Governors. "I am very hopeful that the state and ECU can get a fair and objective treatment and deeply hope the consultants will not allow themselves to be influenced by public feelings (toward ECU) of existing medical school officials." [4]

Dr. Monroe said he had some "concerns" about some of the panel's members, but would not make any individual or specific complaints. In his March, 1973, letters to UNC Board of Governors' chairman, William Dees, he contradicted himself about this. In these letters he complained both specifically and about individuals.[5]

April, 1973, was a busy month for ECU partisans. On the fifth, Senator Jesse Helms wrote a letter to NC Republicans, supporting the four-year, degree-granting school, and criticizing the report of the Jordan Committee. He said, "In all candor, I have hesitated to write this letter for fear that I might be misunderstood. I want to discuss what I have viewed, for years, as a critical human need—the need for a four-year medical school at East Carolina University.

"I am not suggesting the dissolution of the new system of higher education, the Board of Governors, however it is the feeling of many, many people across the state that the Board is not acting fairly and responsibly in this issue. I and my staff have studied the recent Report of the Board of Governors carefully and have gleaned from it some important facts that the major newspapers have ignored up to now."

Helms then pointed out that NC was producing far fewer doctors than other states. "The United States has one M.D. per 613 people; North Carolina has one per 1,063 people." In the state, only twenty counties were at or above the statewide average of physicians to population. Forty-three percent of the doctors were located in six counties which contained only twenty-five per cent of the state's population.

If the state had wanted to raise the number of physicians to the national average of physician/population ratio in 1970, it would have needed 1,950 more doctors. In 1973 even more were needed.

He continued, ". . . after clearly pinpointing this dismal situation, the Report makes several recommendations that have now been presented to the 1973 General Assembly for approval and for supplemental funding. One recommendation calls for virtual doubling of state funds to Duke and Bowman Gray medical schools, in order to get them to accept more North Carolina students. In return for several million new dollars over the next seven years, Duke will graduate three more North Carolinians annually beginning in 1980 than Duke is now committed to produce at the current level ($3,000 per student) of state funding; Bowman Gray will graduate seven more." Increasing enrollment in the UNC medical school would bring only twenty-seven more graduates, and cost more than $30 million.

"Our friends, the Democrats, are caught in a dilemma. They recognize some of this, but do not wish to appear critical of the Board since they and their Governor created it insofar as the public is concerned. On the other hand, they also claim the credit for starting the East Carolina Medical School. The East Carolina University School, too, is viewed by the public as an eventual four-year medical school.

"Looking purely at the political situation—and, I repeat, this is not my motivation for supporting the ECU position, I honestly do not see how our party could gain more support and strength now and in the years ahead than by seizing the initiative. Let us at least put all of the facts across to the people and let them make an informed judgment."

Helms concluded, ". . . though this letter is not politically motivated, I do suggest that the people of Eastern North Carolina are hopeful that the Republican Party will take the lead in giving that section of the state consideration which, ironically, it has so often been denied heretofore. The hopes of building, in good faith and on sound principle, a two-party system in North Carolina rest in Eastern North Carolina. A look at last year's election returns clearly shows that the tide was turned there—in Eastern North Carolina."[6]

UNC Board Chairman William Dees commented that supporting the four-year school "is the politically popular thing to do. Witness Senator Helms. Obviously he's not too informed. But that's encouraged the Democrats to take a look at it."[7]

On April 16, Lieutenant Governor Jim Hunt, Democratic party leader, said that if the Board of Governors' panel of consultants did not recommend location of a four-year medical school at ECU, "There will probably be an effort to establish a med school at ECU anyway, and the chances for such a bill would be reasonably good." He said he personally supported expanding the school at ECU. Hunt said that the legislature had a clear right to make the decision, and not just accept the Board of Governors' recommendation. It would not be interference in the powers of the Board to make decisions regarding education, since the question of health care was a much broader question than just education. Location had more effect on health care than it did on education, and eastern North Carolina had the greatest need for physicians of any area of the state.

He said that the force behind ECU's medical school proposal was not just political. ECU had raised political support, but the desperate need has been the main motive, not the glorification of ECU. "The great strength is from the people who see a great and pressing need.

Look who signed the Senate bill (a resolution calling for another med school). They are from all over North Carolina." He recognized that whenever something was wanted by a great many people it became a political issue.

Hunt agreed with the statement by House Speaker James Ramsey that the legislature would not deal with the ECU question in the current legislative session, but felt that passage of Representative Dr. John Gamble's proposal to establish a $25 million reserve fund to train medical personnel was entirely possible. Because of the $250 million surplus there were no plans to make tax cuts, and this made it likely that Gamble's bill would be passed.

Hunt said that if the Board of Governors did not endorse the ECU proposals, there would be an effort in the next General Assembly to build the school. He disagreed with the charges that some had made that the new board's authority would be threatened if the ECU partisans sought funding directy from the General Assembly. That view made things too simple, because so much more than just education was involved. He considered that health care was one of the really big issues in North Carolina, and hoped that the Democratic Party would take a position on health care.[8]

In Greenville, the Jaycees prepared a brochure and fact sheet summarizing data on the comparative costs of various approaches to solving the shortage of health care workers in North Carolina. They planned to send it to each Jaycee organization in the state, and urged Jaycee members to make the facts known to their legislators.[9]

The North Carolina Democratic Party polled its executive committee members—about 300 of them—on whether the General Assembly should decide on the proposed four-year ECU medical school this session, or leave the decision to the UNC Board of Governors. State Democratic Party Chairman, Jim Sugg, said he began the poll because he was anxious to find out how the executive committee members felt about the medical school question. He did not think that the polling would interfere with the Board's authority, and doubted that it would undercut the Board if the legislature went ahead with the four-year ECU medical school. He had not discussed the poll with party leaders, but had discussed it with staff members at the party headquarters.

The state's highest-ranking Democrat, Lieutenant Governor Jim Hunt, told newspaper reporters he knew nothing about the poll. He said, "I certainly would not urge that such a poll be taken" but added, "wouldn't want to criticize anyone for it." He said also, "I don't know if a legislative decision this year would undercut the board. I don't think it was intended to undercut the board."

William Dees was sure that the legislature would undercut the board if it made a decision on the controversial ECU expansion. He declared that the Board was established to take issues such as the medical school at ECU out of the partisan battleground of the legislature. This issue was the first test of whether the Board could run the university system without legislative interference, Dees said. He also said that if the Democratic Party adopted a policy on the medical school, it wouldn't bother him, but legislative action before the consultants' report in September would. [10]

ECU medical school dean, Dr. Wallace Wooles, said the poll indicated that there must be a lot of support for adding a four-year medical school at East Carolina University. He said he had encountered a great deal of support for the expansion, all over the state. It was common knowledge that there was a terrible shortage of doctors and that something had to be done. He thought the poll indicated the public had started communicating the urgency of the matter to the state's Democrats. He expected that the poll would bring Democratic support for a four-year medical school on the Greenville campus, and hoped that the General Assembly would take action as soon as possible. "Every year we delay, we make the problem that much worse," he said. [11]

ECU backers retained a professional advertising firm, Productive Communications of Greenville, to place ads in major newspapers. A full-page advertisement appeared Wednesday in the *Winston-Salem Journal*, *Twin City Sentinel*, and *Raleigh News and Observer*, with the text of Senator Jesse Helms's April 5 letter.

The *Journal* called to ask Mr. Tommy Payne, one of the owners of Productive Communications, if ECU played a role in the ad. He said: "No more than—let's leave it at the point that this was a peoples' idea. This whole thing has sprung up outside the official family." The reporter repeated the question, but Mr. Payne continued to refuse a direct answer. "This is one of the teeny expressions of grass roots sentiment on this," he said.

Mayor William Flowers of Plymouth, a sponsor of the ad and a longtime friend and supporter of Chancellor Leo Jenkins, said that the funds for the ad were raised by people in nineteen eastern NC counties. He said no ECU officials were involved in placing the ads. In September 1972, Flowers had set up an organization, the Eastern Health Improvement Group to support the four-year school at ECU. He and others of its founders had traveled widely in the east encouraging community leaders and civic groups to join in the campaign.

Earlier in the month, he and other Democrats in eastern North Carolina had distributed 150 to 175 petitions through civic clubs and municipal government officials across the area, seeking signatures backing expansion of the ECU medical school.[12]

Senator Jesse Helms told reporters that two or three people had called him after his letter was made public and asked whether he would object to having it published in an ad, and he told them to go ahead. He said, "I don't know who's responsible for it, or who's paying for it. I know the people down there are all exercised about the medical school issue, and I think a group of them just got together and got up a kitty to publish the ad." He also said the Winston-Salem newspapers may have been chosen because of a recent *Journal and Sentinel* editorial criticizing his stand on the ECU issue. He said the editorial misrepresented what his letter said.

Helms said that the medical school issue was none of his business, except from a personal standpoint. He had been forced by the public position he took in favor of the medical school to break ranks with some of his doctor friends whose opinions differed from his. However, he felt he had to say and do what he thought was right. He said he had not intended for the letter to be made public when he sent it to members of the state republican Executive Committee and local party chairmen throughout the state. On the other hand he hadn't tried to hide it either, and he did not object to its being used in a publicity campaign. He said his staff had done some checking and found that a copy of the letter was given to the *Greenville Reflector,* which first published its contents, by Bill Dancy, a member of the Greenville city council. His own office had not sent the letter to any newspapers.[13]

On April 12, 1973, Representative Gerald Arnold of Harnett County introduced a bill to set up an eight-man commission—four members from the House and four from the Senate —to study the state's medical manpower needs. (This was the Medical Manpower Commission mentioned before, which was set up on May 24 by a Joint Resolution of the House and Senate, with Senator William D. Mills and Representative J. P. Huskins as co-chairmen). Arnold favored expansion of the ECU medical school, and said he would not be opposed to legislation asking for an outright appropriation for expansion of the school. He said he felt a study was needed "to bring all the facts out" because the proposal had aroused so much controversy.

Arnold proposed that the commission would review all the reports and documents pertaining to the state's need for medical manpower, including the findings of the consultant panel working for the Board of Governors of UNC. The commission would report to the January 1974 session of the General Assembly, and make specific proposals for legislation to solve the medical manpower problem. He said that the need for doctors was already present, and the medical school at ECU a reality. Neither of these facts changed when the legislature created the UNC Board of Governors. He said that he hoped the manpower commission would put an end to the consultants' report, unless it told the Board and the legislature how to set up another medical school.

Dr. Edwin W. Monroe said that Representative Arnold was simply proposing that the legislature would review not only the report from the panel of consultants, but also all other reports and laws produced over the previous few years that were related to medical manpower needs. Then, he hoped, the commission would recommend some comprehensive approach to the problem and not a piecemeal, partial attack. Experience had already shown that a fragmented approach did not produce any meaningful results.[14]

In May and June, the panel of medical consultants spent some time in Raleigh, talking with politicians and physicians. Bennett's letter to those invited to speak said that the panel's members would like to hear their views concerning the health care needs of North Carolina in general and the possible need for a new degree-granting school in particular. The consultants were earnest in their search for a broad spectrum of information, but as scientifically-oriented investigators, naturally emphasized objective factual data both in their inquiry and in their eventual judgment. While they met with and listened to many people with varying viewpoints, they appeared to discard evidence that was arguably merely anecdotal, even though it presented individual views of and experience with the health care system, in favor of statistical reports and previous studies. Also, they evinced an unmistakable partiality for expert testimony, such as that of LCME survey teams and the local medical and medical education establishment.

At a meeting on July 13, Representative Robert Jernigan of Ahoskie told the panel that eastern North Carolina very much needed the medical school, and that it was extremely important to that part of the state. He hoped that they would advise the Board of Governors to go ahead with building a four-year medical school at East Carolina University. After he talked with the committee, Jernigan said that its members were very concerned about internship posts in the east, because doctors were likely to return to the area in which they served as interns. They considered it was probably more important in influencing where they would practice than the location of the medical school which they attended.

Representative Jernigan did not think this affected the need for a medical school, but it did mean that in conjunction with the school, it was important to identify hospitals within twenty-five to thirty miles of Greenville that would offer internships for graduates of ECU and of any other medical school. He told the panel that the people of the east had been working on this problem for a long time, and believed they had the support of the people of the state. He said there was a great need for doctors, and he was willing to begin building still another medical school in the western part of the state when the one at ECU was well established.

Representative Horton Rountree said that the study group listed five hospitals in the area around Greenville, and one being constructed (Pitt County Memorial). However, they did not seem to believe these had the necessary qualifications to provide residency and internship training. The lack of hospital facilities appeared to be a big drawback as far as a degree granting school was concerned. He said he had emphasized to the panel that the Legislature was going to take action on its own if the Board of Governors did not recognize the need that existed.

Senator Hamilton Horton, Jr., of Forsyth County told the consultants the question was not whether to establish a medical school at ECU or not. "We already have one there." The question was no longer whether to establish, but whether to break up an existing institution, with the attendant breach of faith, or to expand the medical school into a full-fledged degree-granting program.[15] He said, "The entire history of the ECU medical school has been attended by criticism, second thoughts as to its advisability, academic in-fighting, and political power plays." But, he said, the General Assembly had repeatedly shown its intention to locate a school of medicine at ECU.

President Friday was embarrassed by Horton's remarks, and on July 17 wrote to Archie K. Davis, a member of the Board of Governors, "I am going to talk with him right away because he obviously is creating profound difficulty for us.[16] On the same day, he wrote to Senator Horton, defending the Bennett Committee as a panel of "exceedingly competent national figures in medical education." [17] It was apparent that the UNC administration was more concerned with the opinions of medical education experts than the legislators were.

Senator Ralph Scott was also invited to meet with the panel, but declined to attend, sending a letter saying the state should proceed with its plans to start a two-year medical school at East Carolina University, with the expectation that it would become a four-year school. Others invited to the meeting included Representative Carl Stewart, Senator Russell Kirby, Representative Liston Ramsey, and the co-chairmen of the committee on higher education, Senator Tom Strickland and Representative J. P. Huskins. At Hunt's request, the panel included Representative Kenneth Royall, chairman of the Senate's committee on health affairs.

Lieutenant Governor Hunt requested a postponement or a second meeting. He had made it clear he supported expanding the school, and had predicted that the 1974 legislature would establish it, regardless of what the Board of Governors and its panel recommend.

Governor Holshouser's office announced that the panel had not asked to meet with the governor, who had already said he would support the governing board's decision.[18]

On August 9, the panel met with students at the medical school in Chapel Hill. Among the students who attended the meeting was John W. Uribe, who had transferred from the ECU one-year program. Uribe was a graduate of The Citadel, and was one of only two first-year students present. On August 20, he wrote a letter to Dr. Ivan Bennett , who had chaired the meeting, registering his dissatisfaction with what he considered a "most biased affair." He said that he had debated writing, "because I felt it might exacerbate your already negative view of East Carolina School of Medicine." He had come to the conclusion that he ought not to suppress his feelings, even in the face of a possible adverse response.

Uribe protested that Bennett had allowed the students who had attended their first year of school at Chapel Hill to state their views freely, without objection. The questions then directed to them did not judge the worth of their remarks, but instead accepted them without reservation, and tried to expound on reasons for not establishing a four-year medical school at ECU. The entire committee responded favorably to the students' remarks, whose objectivity was not questioned, even though they presented the viewpoint of an institution publicly opposed to a new medical school at East Carolina.

He went on to contrast Bennett's reactions to the Chapel Hill-oriented students with his reactions to a speaker favoring ECU. He said, "I was interrupted on several occasions by comments and questions disputing and discrediting statements that focused on positive reasons for the establishment of a new school." The panel, he wrote, had succeeded in discouraging him from saying what he meant to say, as though they were trying to convince themselves that a new school was unnecessary because the establishment, of which they were members, opposed it.

While Uribe was replying to the panel's initial request for views on relieving the physician shortage, with particular reference to the Greenville school, their questions after he spoke did not consider this. Instead, they asked him about his evaluation of the first year program at East Carolina and the qualifications of the transferees to enter the second year at Chapel Hill. They did not direct such biased (and "in some respects demeaning") questions to the other first year student.

Uribe ended his letter by saying "You further emphasized your partiality when you closed my statement with the remark, 'In your situation, you are not capable of making an objective evaluation.' Gentlemen, I am quite willing to concede this point. The question is, are you?" [19]

From the start, the Bennett panel experts agreed with President Friday's point of view, which was based on the best advice that he could obtain from the medical establishment inside North Carolina, including from his own medical school administration. He was justified to be confident that the Committee would support the medical establishment and UNC's stance, even if they were not specifically informed what it was. According to the panel's final report, they consulted him only twice, and he limited his active participation in their proceedings to administrative support, under the direction of John Kennedy, a former member of the Board of Higher Education staff who had become UNC secretary. Friday scrupulously avoided taking up any public position, although he continued to be convinced that it would be a mistake to establish a second state-funded medical school.[20]

Such a school would unavoidably drain off resources that the Chapel Hill medical school needed in order to carry out its mandate to expand admissions and improve its clinical facilities. Financial considerations aside, there was also the threat to the General Administration's control over the regional universities. In a political confrontation between UNC and ECU, with Leo Jenkins's demonstrated skills in arousing public support and dealing with the legislature, there was a fair probability that Friday would fail. The indirect approach to the issue, through the Bennett Committee and other nonpolitical avenues, was more suited to his style of operation, and his preference for bureaucratic over popular decision making.

The panel had accepted two main charges in their initial discussions with William Dees, the chairman of the Board of Governors, and with President William Friday. First, it was to evaluate the need for an additional degree-granting school of medicine within UNC. Second, it was to "examine all possible institutional alternatives, including, specifically, the present medical education program at East Carolina University, for the provision of additional doctors to all regions." As the months passed and the Committee repeatedly visited North Carolina but spent only a small part of its time in Greenville, the people at ECU became increasingly impatient. Their suspicions about bias against the medical school appeared to be confirmed. In September, Dean Wallace Wooles's frustration surfaced in a letter to the Committee's executive secretary, Dr. Levine, in which he complained that the consultants had been to Greenville only twice. The panel had also failed to obtain information about ECU's plans for a four-year school. Their actions hinted at bias, Wooles thought.[21]

Chairman Bennett replied to Wooles that his letter could have had only one purpose, which was to distort the panel's dealings with ECU. He said that the Committee had visited Greenville not two but three times, once for a whole day. He insisted that they had not only not failed to review any plans about which ECU had furnished them information, but had worked diligently to get as much data as they could.[22] The final report said that the Committee's efforts at ECU "to obtain more specific information or even ideas have been turned aside with the assertion that one cannot realistically plan a project without having received the authority to implement it."[23]

In April, when the panel had barely begun to meet, Representative Larry Eagles of Edgecombe County introduced a bill calling for a referendum on the proposed four-year medical school at ECU, with seventeen co-sponsors. When Eagles said he had not discussed his bill with Chancellor Leo Jenkins, he was inundated by the chuckles of his fellow legislators. In fact, Jenkins was not in favor of the bill, nor were other legislators from the east. Eagles said there was no reason to wait for a study by consultants, as proposed by the Board of Governors. "The people of North Carolina have enough sense to know we need doctors and where the school ought to be better than somebody from Chicago or someplace," he said. "This gives the people the right to vote $50 million to establish a four-year medical school at ECU and what's wrong with letting the people vote on it? I'd like to give them a chance to vote on this just like we do for roads, schools, or a zoo."[24]

In May, Dr. Leo Jenkins had said that putting East Carolina's one-year medical school under the direction of the UNC medical school had no bearing on plans to expand the school. On ECU Alumni day, he expressed his hope that the legislature would support ECU's development to meet the needs of the people of North Carolina. During the same month, Dr. Ed Monroe said he did not believe that the committee of outside consultants would decide in favor of the expansion of the ECU medical school.[25]

Supporters of the ECU school said that they had successfully approached the General Assembly, and that it was prepared to grant funding to the school in the 1974 session. Senator Ralph Scott of Alamance County, who had been a prime mover in the restructuring of UNC, said that he felt the time had come to expand the medical program at ECU. The Reverend Marse Grant, editor of the *North Carolina Biblical Recorder*, published an editorial in the periodical in which he praised the General Assembly for setting up the $7.5 million reserve, and favored anything that could be done to improve medical care in the state.[26]

Phillip Kirk, Jr., administrative aide to Governor James Holshouser, told the Salisbury Kiwanis Club that he was opposed to expanding ECU's facilities. He said he was expressing his personal opinion, and not necessarily reflecting the Governor's viewpoint.[27]

On June 5, 1973, Dr. William Cromartie was designated administrator for the conjoint UNC-ECU medical education program. He had been at UNC School of Medicine since 1951, and was associate dean for clinical sciences. Dr. Cromartie stayed in Greenville two or three days during the week, and went home on weekends. He seemed to the younger faculty members to be quite grandfatherly, with his white hair, horn-rimmed glasses and benevolent expression. He would meet with the faculty now and then, but most of them could not work out quite what he was doing. It appeared to them that he had been called an administrator but was actually present to oversee the program's demise.[28] "My job then," Dr. Cromartie himself said, "was to see that the students here had a good education experience— that the program was similar enough to that of UNC first-year medical students to permit easy transfer. Since the curriculum had been planned that way from the start, this was not too difficult." [29]

One faculty member said, "Dean Christopher Fordham III of the UNC medical school would come down now and then and call a meeting in the library. The faculty would all go in, and Dr. Fordham would sit at a table, hardly ever looking directly at anyone. He would sit there, and take his pipe tobacco and put it on the table, and clean his pipe and rub his chin. He had nothing positive to say. Occasionally, Dr. Cromartie would call in medical educators from other states.

These were not physicians nor basic science teachers, but medical educators from Florida State and one or two other places, educators that did not actually do any medical education, but only wrote papers about it." [30]

In July, Dr. Fordham and Dr. Wooles appeared before the state House and Senate health committees to discuss the new medical school. Dr. Fordham maintained that locating a medical school in a certain area did not necessarily mean more doctors for that area. Dr. Wooles argued that the best way of providing doctors to an area is to locate a medical school there that draws on the local population for its students and provides residency training.[31]

Also in July, an arrangement was worked out for ECU medical students to receive clinical instruction at Cherry Hospital in Goldsboro. Negotiations were going on with Pitt County Memorial Hospital in Greenville and Lenoir Memorial Hospital in Kinston.

There were widely varying estimates of the cost of a new school. Dr. Leo Jenkins cited the figure of $10 million to start the school. Dr. Edwin Monroe cited a figure of $16 million. Dean Wallace Wooles had developed a detailed plan with an estimated cost of $60.9 million. Opponents of the ECU school estimated that it would cost at least $100 million.

In August, President Friday asked the Bennett Committee to submit their report by the last week in September, and on September 14, 1973, the panel sent its report to the Board of Governors. The 285-page summary, *A Statewide Plan for Medical Education in North Carolina*, was published on September 21, 1973.[32] The panel found North Carolina's rejection rate of draftees for medical reasons "outstandingly good," contradicting a major factor in the justification that had been given, since the immediate post World War II period, for beginning with a plan to improve health in the state. The census figures cited in the report showed that North Carolina was the best of twenty southern states in this respect in the 1968-71 period, but showed the least improvement during that time. The panel concluded that the state was not in the midst of a health crisis.

As for the medical school issue, the panel concluded that another medical school would not ease the shortage of primary care physicians. Contrariwise, additional physicians would aggravate the problem, by widening the gap between the affordability of medical care in relation to location and income. Increasing the number of physicians would bring an increase in the cost of medical care through raising professional fees and multiplying expensive procedures for diagnosis and treatment. The best way to increase the productivity of practicing physicians would be to utilize more allied health professionals.

ECU was not the best place to locate another school. The conclusions of the LCME report were substantially correct, and the only way Greenville's program could continue would be to have it managed completely by UNC-CH. For it to become viable, it had to be dealt with realistically as what it actually was, a UNC-CH undergraduate program. The Chapel Hill medical school should firmly and decisively control curriculum, faculty and student selection, administration, and planning. ECU's school was premature and ill-conceived. It had been made impractical by ECU resentment and UNC lack of enthusiasm for a program it had not designed.

The state should give high priority to expanding the number of teaching hospitals. A network of AHEC's would better provide primary medical care than a new medical school. The Board of Governors should strongly support Glenn Wilson's community medicine program and "provide for a mechanism to enable the two private medical schools to share with UNC-CH the burden of development of regional centers using their expertise and educational resources in an organized, integrated, statewide effort." [33] The AHECs were the most important possibility available to increase the number of doctors, improve their skills, and make their services more available all over the state.

Chancellor Leo Jenkins, who was in Pitt Memorial Hospital undergoing treatment for high blood pressure, made a statement after the panel's report was accepted by the Board, commenting that the Bennett Committee recognized no crisis in the availability of doctors in the state. He said that the medical school issue was before the people of North Carolina, and that the public would hold the Board of Governors accountable for their decision. In the end the people would decide the issue, not he nor the panel nor the Board of Governors. He would postpone any decision about continuing his campaign for a full-fledged medical school until he had met with the ECU Board of Trustees. [34]

The chairman of the ECU Board of Trustees, Robert L. Jones, a businessman from Raleigh, wrote to the Board of Governors in even more forceful terms. He said that nothing could be gained by procrastination or postponing the inevitable development of a medical school at ECU. He said he believed firmly that it was time to proceed with the four-year medical program mandated by the legislature. He disagreed with the findings of the consultants, said that they had not sufficiently investigated the medical school operating at ECU, and had overestimated how much it would cost to expand it. He objected to discrepancies and inconsistencies in the consultants' report, and raised a number of questions about its conclusions. He said, "To suggest creating 300 new residency positions immediately, when we had an eleven percent vacancy in existing residency slots this year, seems to get the cart before the horse. It is suggested to get out and recruit medical students from other states as a fast way to improve our doctor ratio. Is it conceivable to think that other states are so naive? What if they recruit our graduates?"

Jones challenged the report's contention that the best statistics available supported the conclusion that there was no health crisis in North Carolina , and that more doctors would not improve health care. He asked, "If there is no crisis, why are we rated forty-third in the nation in a ratio of doctors to population? Surely if there is no crisis here, then there would not be one in the forty-two states ranked higher than North Carolina. The report makes note that the rural areas are losing doctors by death and retirement and that replacements are not forthcoming. These areas find themselves with ratios as low as five per 100,000 population and I cannot help but think that this is a critical situation."

Jones also argued that the panel had not adequately investigated the ECU program, and had distorted the statistics on the cost of establishing a degree-granting school. He wrote, "It is ridiculous to take total capital expenditures plus total operating cost from now until 1982 and divide by the number of graduates at that date to come up with a cost per student."

Jones strongly recommended that if the four-year status was not approved, then the one-year program should be abolished "for it could only add confusion to the centralization theory." He sent copies of his letter to the members of the General Assembly.[35]

Dr. Edwin W. Monroe, ECU Vice Chancellor for Health Affairs, said the recommendations of the panel were weak and did not call for any significant increase in the number of medical students in North Carolina. He asked, "How can you get more doctors if you do not produce more doctors?"[36]

Governor Holshouser held a meeting at the Governor's mansion on the day before the consultants' report was made public to brief state legislators on its contents. It would be up to the 1974 General Assembly whether to accept the recommendations of the medical experts, or ignore them and allocate funds to expand the ECU program from one year to four years.[37]

The Board of Governors convened on September 27 to discuss

and vote on the consultants' diagnosis and recommendations. There was a violent rupture between the two factions, and an acrimonious three-hour debate between the members of the Board who supported the proposals and those supporting the ECU position. Robert Jordan made a motion, seconded by Jake Froelich, to adopt the recommendations of the Bennett Committee and call on President Friday to carry them out. Led by Reginald E. "Mutt" McCoy of Laurinburg, former ECU trustee, the partisans of the Greenville medical school championed a substitute motion to send the Committee report back to a committee with more equitable ECU representation than the Jordan Committee had. The motion was rejected by voice vote, and the original motion was passed by a margin of twenty-two to eight.[38]

W. W. Taylor, Jr., of Raleigh, a member of the ECU Board of trustees for fifteen years before becoming a member of the UNC governing board, said that the final decision would be made by the General Assembly, and that no matter what action the Board might take there would be a four-year medical school at ECU in a few years. He attacked the consultants' report as "an obvious and studied effort to kill off any plans for a four-year medical school at ECU." He said the report was susceptible to criticism on a factual basis. New medical schools had been built recently for a great deal less than the $40 to $60 million the consultants estimated, he said. The estimate that ECU had made of $25-30 million to build the school and $40 million more for a teaching hospital was as well-founded as the consultants' calculations.

After voting to accept the panel's report, the Board instructed President William Friday to prepare a plan for medical education consistent with its recommendations. His plan was to include cost estimates, and was subject to revision by the board.

The report's supporters repeatedly contended, in agreement with its findings, that the most urgent need in North Carolina was for clinical teaching facilities, and that these should be put in place before expanding existing medical schools or building new ones.

The ECU backers continued to protest, and were joined by black board members who were of the opinion that the number of black physicians in the state could be increased by opening a second state-supported medical school. They opposed accepting the report, which they said was unsatisfactory and did not deal sufficiently with getting more minority members into the medical profession. Rather than continuing to pay Meharry Medical College in Tennessee to train black medical students, North Carolina should be training its own, Dr. E. B. Turner of Lumberton argued. He said eleven percent of the

451 students in the UNC-CH school were black, and this was within one percent of the national goal for 1975. However, he found the report generally unsatisfactory.

The recommendation to change the state's requirements for licensing foreign medical graduates was also attacked. Dr. Wallace Hyde of Asheville accused the panel of saying that the state should lower its standards. He did not believe that most foreign doctors who came to this country had been properly trained.

Reginald McCoy complimented the panel on its work, and said the report was excellent in many respects, but needed other data to supplement it. It was not a strong and enduring solution for North Carolina's problems.

David J. Whichard II, a strong ECU supporter, called the report fine, but said it dealt with the doctor shortage only through 1980. He argued that it was time to start another medical school that would be turning out physicians for the 1980's. Whichard pointed out that there are more than 7,400 vacancies in residency positions already established and funded, because there are not enough medical school graduates to fill them. He questioned adding 300 more residencies in state hospitals, even though physicians tend to stay where they take their residencies. One-third of the residencies and internships are filled by foreign medical graduates already, and it would not be likely to help the situation unless more students are put in "the beginning of the pipeline" of a new four-year medical school. Both Whichard and McCoy stressed they were UNC-CH alumni, but strongly supported ECU.

William A. Johnson of Lillington, who had served on the Jordan Committee, cited against the report's conclusions its own statement that eighty-nine percent of the NC residencies were filled, well above the national average. He wondered where more residents would be obtained, if not from training them inside the state? [39]

On October 22, Dr. Edwin Monroe sent Chancellor Leo Jenkins and each member of the ECU Board of Trustees two documents prepared by the medical school's faculty. One was titled with a quotation from the Bennett Committee's conclusions: "North Carolina is not in the midst of a health crisis." The second was a copy of the medical faculty's plan for developing a degree-granting medical school. In the first paper, a tightly argued analysis of the report of the Bennett Committee, each of its main conclusions was examined. The judgment about North Carolina's non-crisis in health care, "must have been formed without reference to easily available data," the faculty said, and went on to cite some of the information contrary to the panel's findings:

> The state ranked 43 out of 50 in the ratio of population to physicians.
> The US ratio was 613:1, the NC ratio 1063:1.
> Only seven other states were worse off than North Carolina.
> Sixty out of 100 counties were worse off in 1971 than in 1963.

The statistics, the brief continued, did not reveal the human dimension of the health care crisis. Without increasing the actual number of physicians in training, adding residency training programs would do nothing to alleviate the problem. There were already more slots for post-graduate medical training in the state than could be filled from outside or within North Carolina. Importing physicians from foreign countries would not be acceptable, in part, because of differences in their training backgrounds. In addition, the United States already in 1972 absorbed 11,416 foreign medical graduates, compared to 9,551 graduates of American medical schools. The foreign graduates represented twenty-five percent of the world's supply of new physicians outside China and the Soviet bloc countries. The inequitable situation was compounded by the lack of opportunity for qualified students in the U.S. to obtain admission to medical schools.

The brief continued by asserting that the panel of consultants failed to examine the ECU School of Medicine thoroughly, and directly contradicted the General Assembly's mandates that a degree-granting medical school should be established in Greenville. The consultants failed completely to recognize the contrasts between family practice and other medical specialties in the area of providing primary care to patients.

According to the faculty, the panel made unwarranted generalizations, or merely repeated the LCME surveys on student selection (contradicting, without additional data, the 1973 survey report's conclusions as to the quality of students), curriculum, faculty, administration and planning. The faculty stated the consultants' basis for estimating the cost of establishing a new medical school in North Carolina was flawed.[40]

The second document Monroe submitted to the trustees, *A Plan for the Expansion of Medical Education at the School of Medicine of East Carolina University, Prepared by the Faculty,* dated October 1974, was a study of the entire project of justifying, designing, and establishing a four-year medical school in Greenville. This 144-page study examined the history of the campaign, presented a proposed timetable for expansion, outlined the curriculum, administrative structure, faculty, facilities, admissions policy (emphasizing disadvantaged and minority students and students interested in family practice), and devoted its last thirty-two pages to a demographic profile of eastern North Carolina, its educational resources, and the area's shortage of primary care physicians.

As a direct reply to the cost estimates of the Bennett Committee, the Plan recommended a specific allocation of appropriated funds:

$338,100 for purchase of land;

$235,000 for renovating a campus building for classrooms, offices, and laboratories;

$1,200,000 for construction of an out-patient/ambulatory care facility;

$250,000 for a temporary out-patient facility;

$12,974,400 for construction of a Basic Medical Science Building;

$832,000 for salaries and operating expenses in 1975-76;

$778,000 for salaries and operating expenses in 1976-77;

$250,000 for 1975-76 and $325,000 for 1976-77 to implement the plan to increase the numbers of disadvantaged and minority students;

$360,278 for 1975-76 and $428,337 for the library budget;

$19,000,000 for a teaching hospital adjacent to the new PCMH.

The cover letter to Dr. Leo Jenkins said the "cost estimates are realistic and can be confirmed." It also noted that, as an alternative, the old county hospital might be purchased and renovated for no more than $5,000,000. [41]

The Panel of Medical Consultants had estimated that, conservatively, $66,806,000 would be needed for a new school during 1975-1982, of which $25,806,000 were for operating cost and $40 million for capital expenditures. It had calculated operating cost by taking an estimated cost per student and multiplying it by the anticipated number of students.

Dr. Monroe made the further point in his letter that the faculty group's comments should be considered in the context of their feeling that they had been unjustly appraised both by the panel of consultants and by the LCME survey team (on whose findings the panel depended heavily). They were taking an opportunity they had not had previously, to correct errors and misrepresentations before these had been disseminated by the press. [42]

The sharp contrast between the two sets of speculative figures was, of course, intended. The ECU faculty's total of $36,217,778 for both operating cost and capital expenditures, falling below the Bennett Committee's $40,000,000 for capital expenditures alone, could hardly have convinced anyone even mildly skeptical. It did have the virtue of being based on actual figures from the short operating history of the school, where the consultants' numbers were the result of purely theoretical calculation.

---

[1] Monroe interview, January 3, 1992.

[2] *Greenville Daily Reflector* , August 10, 1973; ECU Medical School Files, Bennett Committee folder for full text of Jenkins's speech to the panel.

[3] *Greenville Daily Reflector,* August 10, 1973.

[4] Letter from Edwin W. Monroe to William A. Dees, January 29, 1973, ECU Medical School Files, folder "EWM Correspondence."

[5] Jenkins Archives, letters from Edwin W. Monroe to William A. Dees March 6, 1973 and March 14, 1973.

[6] *Greenville Daily Reflector* , April 16, 1973

[7] *Raleigh News & Observer,* April 22, 1973

[8] *Greensboro Daily News*, April 17, 1973; see also Bratton, p. 415; *Raleigh News & Observer,* January 25, 1974, February 10, 11, 1974.

[9] *Greenville Daily Reflector* , Thursday, April 19, 73

[10] *Raleigh News & Observer,* April 22, 1973

[11] *Greensboro Daily News,* April 22, 1973

[12] *Greensboro Daily News,* April 1, 1973.

[13] *Winston-Salem Journal,* April 26, 1973.

[14] *Greenville Daily Reflector* , April 13, 1973

[15] *Greenville Daily Reflector* , July 16, 1973.

[16] Letter from William C. Friday to Archie K. Davis, July 17, 1973, William C. Friday Papers, Subgroup 1, Series 1, "Medical Education, July-Sept. 1973;" Friday's comment is quoted in Link, p. 431, note 24.

[17] Letter from William C. Friday to Senator Hamilton Horton, William C. Friday Papers, "Medical Education, July-Sept. 1973."

[18] Winston-Salem Journal, June 1, 1973

[19] Letter of John M. Uribe to Ivan L. Bennett, Jr., M.D., August 20, 1973, in ECU School of Medicine Files, Folder "Bennett Committee."

[20] Link, p. 230.

[21] Link, pp. 230-1; Letter from Dr. Wallace Wooles to Dr. Jules I. Levine, September 5, 1973, ECU School of Medicine Files, Folder "Report of the Panel of Medical Consultants Committee".

[22] Link, p. 231; Letter from Dr. Ivan Bennett to Dr. Wallace Wooles, September 13, 1973, ECU School of Medicine Files, Folder "Report of the Panel of Medical Consultants."

[23] ECU School of Medicine Files, Folder "Report of the Panel of Medical Consultants".

[24] *Greensboro Daily News*, (also in *Charlotte Observer, Raleigh News & Observer*), April 5, 1973.

[25] *Raleigh News & Observer*, May 1, 1973.

[26] *North Carolina Biblical Recorder*, May 12, 1973.

[27] *Salisbury Post*, June 2, 1973.

[28] Interview of Dr. Donald W. Barnes, January 15, 1992.

[29] *Greenville Daily Reflector* , January 13, 1974.

[30] Barnes interview.

[31] Chapel Hill *Weekly*, 23 July 23, 1973

[32] *A Statewide Plan for Medical Education in North Carolina*, Report of the Panel of Medical Consultants to the Board of Governors of the University of North Carolina, Chapel Hill. Sept. 21, 1973.

[33] *Statewide Plan*, p. 48, (italics in original).

[34] *Greensboro Record*, September 20, 1973.

[35] *Raleigh News & Observer*, September 28, 1973

[36] *Greensboro Record*, September 20, 1973.

[37] *Greensboro Record*, September 20, 1973.

[38] Link, pp. 232-233; *Greensboro Daily News*, September 28, 1973.

[39] *Greensboro Daily News*, September 28, 1973.

[40] "North Carolina is not in the midst of a health crisis," presented to ECU Board of Trustees, October 24, 1974, ECU School of Medicine Files, Folder "ECU re SOM -2."

[41] *A Plan for Medical Education at East Carolina University*, Greenville, October 1974. ECU School of Medicine Files, Folder "ECU re SOM -2."The document presented to the Trustees was subsequently printed, in a slightly augmented version, as *A Plan for the Expansion of Medical Education at the School of Medicine East Carolina University*, Prepared by the Faculty, October 1974. Two copies in ECU School of Medicine Files, Folder "ECU *re* SOM - 2."

[42] Cover letter to *Plan*.

Chapter 10
Fallout from The Bennett Committee

When the ECU Board of Trustees met on October 23, 1973, Dr. Ed Monroe told the members that the medical school issue was still unresolved, since the Board of Governors had not yet produced a definite proposal. He suggested that the trustees study all the alternatives before making their recommendation. He said the documents he had given to the trustees did not represent a policy action, but constituted an in-house study. He felt that the study should not be published, because it could be misinterpreted. The trustees accepted the report from the ECU medical faculty for information only, and agreed not to make it public. They also agreed to postpone making their own proposal until after the UNC Board of Governors had made a recommendation about medical education facilities in the state.[1]

A few days later, Dr. Wallace Wooles appeared before a joint meeting of the Medical Manpower Study Commission and the legislative subcommittee on health manpower training and education, and said that the expansion of residency training recommended by the consultants' panel to the Board of Governors was not inconsistent with plans to expand ECU's medical school to four years. He made the point that it was impossible to insure that an adequate number of doctors were trained in the state for an expanded residency program, without such an expansion. He found it "comforting" to hear that the medical consultants had recommended using community hospitals for training, since ECU was completely dedicated to that concept. The future of medical education in North Carolina depended on using county hospitals and practicing physicians to supplement the teaching hospitals.

He also said that more than 2,356 hospital beds were located within forty miles of Greenville. There were nearly 600 in the city itself, between the new 370-bed hospital and the old 200-bed hospital, which would be empty when the new one was completed. The older one could be used as a teaching hospital for the proposed medical school.

The inability of the UNC medical school to absorb more than about twenty first-year students into its second-year class limited expansion of the one-year school. ECU intended to expand into a second year program as soon as possible, and could begin to expand into a four-year, degree-granting institution by 1978-9.[2]

House Speaker James Ramsey announced on October 31 that he

had scheduled a briefing on medical education for November 16-17, the last weekend before the General Assembly began its session. All legislators were invited to the meeting. The dates fell on one of the only two weekends in November when Dr. Ivan Bennett would be available. Ramsey said that Bennett had accepted the invitation to brief the legislators on the committee's report.

Ramsey also said he had asked the Fiscal Research Division of the General Assembly to assemble cost figures on the various alternatives that had been proposed. He said he hoped, too, that the Medical Manpower Study Commission could have a report ready for the briefing. The Commission and a legislative subcommittee with which it had been working had finished holding public hearings and planned to meet November 13 to work on recommendations to be presented in the upcoming session.[3]

One member of the House of Representatives, Dr. John R. Gamble, Jr., wrote to Speaker Ramsey objecting to his issuing an invitation to a member of the panel of consultants. Representative Gamble felt that the presentation would be biased against providing additional physicians in North Carolina, and would give the opponents of that position an unfair advantage with the legislature. The proponents would demand equal publicity and time, and he thought that trying to give the two sides equal publicity and time could lead to nothing but complications.[4]

On November 9, Ramsey announced that he had decided to postpone indefinitely the legislative briefing, because the Fiscal Research Division could not get accurate figures together soon enough. Also, the Medical Manpower Commission would not have its report ready by the time scheduled for the meeting, and he wanted to have the results of their study for the briefing.[5]

Ramsey told an Associated Press reporter on November 12 that he expected health care legislation to be a major issue in the 1974 General Assembly, and that whatever action was taken would affect the state for at least the next ten years. He said he had not made up his mind on the question of ECU's four-year medical school, but believed it would come up in the 1974 session. He said he was seeking to get information on what it would cost to build a four-year medical school at ECU, what the medical consultant's alternative would cost, and what it was costing to educate a doctor at the medical school at UNC from his admission to his graduation.

He said he had returned to his idea of holding a briefing on medical education for legislators, and was making plans to hold it in Raleigh on December 6 or December 7, if the cost figures could be ready by then. Dr. Bennett had only two possible dates for November, but might be able to attend a December briefing. Ramsey planned for lawmakers to hear from the Medical Manpower Commission and review the consultants' recommendations. He commented that North Carolina needs more general practitioners, more clinical facilities, and some way to keep doctors in the state after they graduate.[6]

The next morning the Medical Manpower Study Commission met together with the Senate health subcommittee to discuss its final report. Members of the group strongly indicated that expansion of the ECU medical school program would be among the solutions it would propose. They also favored establishing a statewide network of AHECs.[7]

President Friday presented to the Board of Governors at their meeting on November 16, a proposal entitled *Recommended Actions Consistent With the Report of the Panel of Medical Consultants.* He classified the panel's eleven recommendations into four categories, to meet which he proposed four actions.   Action 1 presented a $29,679,000 expenditure during 1974-1975 to expand clinical education for postgraduate medical students and other health professions through a statewide network of AHEC's. From these funds, also, there would be a continuing census of medical personnel and monitoring of medical education programs. His program included establishment of nine Area Health Education Centers (AHEC) about the state, with 250-300 new primary care residencies and clinical clerkships for undergraduate medical students. UNC School of Medicine would operate the AHECs, to be established by 1980, assigning full-time clinical faculty to the community hospital centers.

The pilot AHECs already started on a small scale in five areas, using federal funds, would be expanded. These were at Charlotte Memorial Hospital; St. Joseph's Hospital in Asheville; New Hanover Memorial in Wilmington; Wake Memorial in Raleigh; and a single program (Area L) at Edgecombe General Hospital in Tarboro, Halifax Memorial in Roanoke Rapids, Wilson Memorial in Wilson, and Nash General in Rocky Mount, which together made up a northeastern regional center. New AHECs were proposed for Fayetteville, Greenville, the northwest region of the state, and at Moses Cone Hospital in Greensboro. About $26 million would be invested in capital improvements, and about $5 million in operating funds.

Each AHEC would offer clinical instruction for third and fourth year undergraduate medical students; residencies in primary care, including family medicine, internal medicine, and pediatrics; and training for allied health professions such as dentistry, nursing, pharmacy and public health. President Friday estimated operating cost of the AHECs would be $4,680,000 in 1974-1975 and would rise to $14,181,000 by 1979-1980 when all nine centers were operational. Three hundred residency positions would eventually be offered by the AHECs.

Other recommendations of the consultants could be implemented without additions to already appropriated or requested funds. One proposal Friday rejected was to pay Duke and Bowman Gray annually an amount equal to that received by UNC-CH from the state for each resident. He noted that there was already an agreement to pay the other schools $5,000 for each North Carolina student enrolled. He and officials at Duke and Bowman Gray had discussed the matter, he said, and had agreed that the present rate of funding should continue through 1974-75. The two schools had agreed to increase NC student enrollment from fifty-four to sixty-five in 1976-77, so he recommended a $7,000 "capitation grant" for each NC student, beginning in 1975-76.

Friday's Recommended Action 2 concerned the one-year program at East Carolina University, state assistance for North Carolina students enrolled in Duke and Bowman Gray medical schools, and continuation of the contract with Meharry Medical College. It also included programs to recruit and counsel minority students for premedical education, and to provide scholarships for financially disadvantaged undergraduate medical students.

President Friday advised the Board to continue the ECU medical program, but under the supervision of Dr. William Cromartie, associate dean for clinical sciences and professor of medicine at UNC-CH School of Medicine. Cromartie would work toward UNC control of admissions to the ECU school, as well as its budget, curriculum, student examinations, and recruitment and promotion of faculty. Friday's recommendation would formalize the arrangement that had been established under the joint committee, which Dr. Cromartie had already begun carrying out in June 1973. Included in Friday's recommendations was $277,000 to be added to $125,000 already allocated to the one-year program at ECU. The funds would be used to appoint four additional basic science faculty members by the basic science departments in the School of Medicine in Chapel Hill to teach in Greenville, additional support staff, supplies, and equipment, and for improving medical library holdings, and purchasing trailers for laboratory and office space.

The LCME had requested a progress report on the ECU program by January 1, 1974, and Friday proposed keeping the class size to twenty pending their reassessment of the program. The medical school at UNC would begin immediately planning, under the direction of the President's office, the future of the ECU program, in coordination with the residency and other clinical education programs in the Greenville area. When the present program had been accredited, Friday said, he would submit plans to the Board of Governors for expanding the one-year program, adding a second-year program, or other alternatives for strengthening the present one-year program at ECU. He allocated $50,000 for the planning effort.

He recommended awarding fifteen scholarships to financially disadvantaged medical students, which would cost $90,000. The undergraduate medical scholarships for financially disadvantaged students would go mainly to black students enrolled in accredited North Carolina medical schools. These scholarships would carry a $4,000 annual stipend and pay all tuition and academic fees. Friday estimated that the scholarship program would cost $90,000 during 1974-1975.

Recommended Action 3 required no additional funding, and was aimed at recruiting more physicians, improving retention, and improving distribution of physicians. It continued a program begun in 1945, and included both medicine and other health professions. It provided incentive loans for medical students who were residents of the state and attended a state-supported school. The loans were to be repaid with interest, unless the recipients agreed to practice in an approved small community in the state, a state health facility, or a state or local public health department. They had to practice one calendar year for each academic year for which a loan was received.

The Division of Education and Research in Community Medical Care at UNC-CH had begun in July, 1973, a pilot program to identify potential candidates among residents training in other states for North Carolina communities that need to recruit doctors. Friday proposed to continue this program, with the UNC School of Medicine providing technical support.

Finally, this Action proposed modifying the citizenship requirement for licensing foreign medical graduates to practice in NC.

The panel of consultants had recommended that the Board of Governors set up a committee to supervise University medical and other health professional programs, including AHECs and coordination of joint efforts with the state's private medical schools. Recommended Action 4 endorsed the steps already taken by the Board in enlarging its Committee on Educational Planning Policies, and Programs. In addition, it proposed continuing for two years the assignment of responsibility for all programs of medical education to the UNC-Chapel Hill School of Medicine. The Dean of the medical school was to report to the Vice Chancellor for Health Sciences and the UNC Chancellor with regard to activities at the Chapel Hill campus, and to continue his direct responsibility to the President for the medical education program at ECU and elsewhere outside Chapel Hill.[8]

With President Friday's proposal, conflict again erupted on the Board of Governors. A motion was made by W. Earl Britt, board member from Pembroke State University, to approve the recommendations. David Whichard, editor of the *Greenville Daily Reflector*, who was a long-time ECU protagonist, in an amendment to Britt's motion, suggested adding $25 million to upgrade the ECU medical program to a four-year freestanding medical school. The Board rejected the amendment. It also rejected a motion by Reginald McCoy of Laurinburg to present a minority report to the legislature favoring ECU. On a final vote, the original motion was passed. The Board of Governors meeting ended without any resolution of the conflicts within it.

ECU Chancellor Leo Jenkins said from Greenville after the meeting that he was disappointed in the decision, although he immediately endorsed the AHEC portion of President Friday's proposed budget.[9] He said that the missing piece in the comprehensive medical program was a degree-granting school at ECU. The places it would provide for North Carolina students in medical schools were needed to fill the proposed residency slots.[10]

With the rejection of attempts to amend its budget proposal to include more funds for the ECU medical school, the UNC Board of Governors shifted the dispute over expansion of the ECU school to the General Assembly. On November 19, the *Charlotte Observer* reported that a legislative study commission's report was prepared to recommend a two-year medical program at ECU. The newspaper reported also that Representative Jay Huskins of Statesville, co-chairman of the Joint Medical Manpower Study Commission of the General Assembly had said he thought the Commission's report was headed toward endorsement of another full-fledged medical school in the state. The final report, which he was writing, would be adopted by the full commission at a later date.[11]

The Advisory Budget Commission met in executive session on the last day of November to finish most of its work on the budget to be presented to the General Assembly in the new session. The commission approved $25 million of the $30 million medical education budget submitted by the UNC Board of Governors. It also voted to add $7.5 million to the $7.5 million reserve fund previously established to build a second medical school, if and when there was a decision to build such a school.[12]

UNC President William C. Friday said after the Budget Commission's meeting that he would ask the General Assembly to restore the $5 million they had cut from the university's budget request for medical education. The deletions included funds for the northwestern AHEC, and part of the funds for the Greenville AHEC. Friday said that all the elements of the package he submitted were essential to make the program work.

ECU partisans supported the Budget Commission's medical education budget. Chancellor Leo Jenkins and pro-ECU members of the Board of Governors denounced only the failure of the plan to include definite proposals for expanding or enlarging ECU's medical school.

The Commission's action appeared to be a slap in the face of the Board of Governors. The normal procedure under the 1972 legislation establishing the Consolidated University would have been to approve a lump sum appropriation, leaving its allocation to the Board of Governors. By itemizing the deletions, the Commission took back authority it had delegated to the Board.[13]

Representative Horton Rountree announced that House Speaker James Ramsey and Senate president *pro tem* Gordon Allen had invited members of the General Assembly to a special meeting with the UNC Board of Governors. The meeting was to run from one o'clock in the afternoon to about five in Chapel Hill on December 7. The first two hours would be given to the Board of Governors to explain the panel report and the Board's recommendations, then thirty minutes would be allotted for a minority report from board members Reginald McCoy and David Whichard. Half-hour segments had been designated to present the estimated cost of implementing the panel's recommendations, to explain cost estimates for a medical school at ECU, and present a cost analysis of medical education at the UNC School of Medicine. He said the special meeting had been called without consulting other members of the General Assembly. In particular, the special commission on medical manpower and the joint subcommittee on health had not been consulted.

Rountree observed, "It looks like to me it's giving the Board of Governors two hours in which to further press for support for the panel report . . ." He said he found it interesting that the Board of Governors were requiring East Carolina University to be specific as to the cost per square foot of its basic science building, the exact number of teaching positions, and the cost of equipment, while the University of North Carolina School of Medicine could ask for $29 million without specifying in detail how it would be used. He thought that what it would cost to implement this panel report was more important than the Board's explanation and recommendations, and that these questions should be answered at the meeting.[14]

The legislators met as Representative Ramsey and Senator Allen had arranged and heard the Board of Governors' review of the various medical education alternatives that had been proposed. Most of the material had been reported earlier, but had not been brought together at a single hearing. Both before and during the session, most of the legislators admitted privately that they have already made up their minds. One legislator told Senator Allen, as he was talking to a reporter during a break, that after hearing Dr. Ivan Bennett he was more than ever convinced a new four-year degree-granting school was needed.

In summarizing the recommendations of the consultants' panel of which he was chairman, Dr. Bennett stated emphatically that a four-year medical school was not an alternative to their proposed plan. "It is premature because it is not a viable alternative at this time. The capability for it does not now exist in this state," he said. He maintained that what was holding back expansion of enrollment at the three existing medical schools was a shortage of clinical teaching facilities, and the state's best approach to the doctor shortage would be to set up a series of AHECs about the state. Doctors who took their residencies at the hospitals associated with these centers would tend to practice in the same locations. By providing clinical facilities for undergraduate medical training and allowing the schools to increase enrollment, the Centers would provide 300 residencies that should lead to more doctors setting up their practices in the state.

At the meeting, William Dees, UNC Board of Governors' chairman, urged legislators to accept the Board's recommendations. He reminded them that the General Assembly had made it a main principle of their reorganization of higher education in the state that decisions should be based on the best informed professional judgment available. He said that the Board's plan embodied just that. The five-member panel had been chosen after consultation with all parties in the medical school controversy, with two of the consultants (one of whom resigned early in the year without being replaced) recommended by ECU-SOM officials, and a third by a Greenville doctor then on the Board of Governors.[15]

David Whichard and Reginald McCoy appeared before the legislative briefing, and presented the minority position of the eight dissident members of the UNC Board of Governors. Later, to insure that not only those who attended the briefing but all members of the General Assembly heard the minority viewpoint, they sent to the members of the General Assembly copies of the minority statement, signed by Clark S. Brown of Winston-Salem, Wallace N. Hyde of Asheville, Lewis T. Randolph of Washington, W. W. Taylor, Jr., of Raleigh, Rev. Dr. E. B. Turner of Lumberton, George M. Wood of Camden, and by McCoy and Whichard. Copies of remarks that Reginald McCoy had made at the briefing were also sent.

In his statement to the legislative forum, McCoy said, "No matter how many AHEC programs we start in North Carolina, we are not going to have enough doctors interested in going into primary care and staying in it until we can produce them through our educational system." He also said that he and the other Board members in the minority group were completely convinced that the doctor shortage would not be solved until North Carolina was producing more doctors in its medical schools.

He said that the Board minority wanted the ECU school expanded to two years immediately and then to four years when new buildings were finished. The school would admit only North Carolina students, with a fair proportion from minorities.

In the minority report the opponents of the recommendations implementing the Bennett Report recognized that some of the report's content and recommendations were valuable. However, they were disturbed by the statement that North Carolina was not undergoing a health crisis, and categorically rejected it. They commented that one of the consultants, Dr. Lloyd C. Elam of Meharry University, seemed to concur with them, in a recently published statement that the lack of sufficient manpower was the major limitation on adequate health care in the U.S. The Board dissidents contended that the health crisis in the state could be ameliorated only by producing more physicians. Expanding the school at ECU was the best way to deal with the deficiency.[16]

They pointed out that arguments put forward against the ECU expansion were the same ones heard in 1946 when there was a move to make UNC's medical school in Chapel Hill into a four-year school. For example, the deans of Bowman Gray and Duke medical schools had opposed the expansion. Two-thirds of the members of the North Carolina Medical Society had opposed the expansion. One opponent of the four-year school, Dr. W. S. Rankin of Charlotte, had said that the shortage was a matter of distribution rather than producing more doctors. In the summer of 1946, in a statement echoing the report of the Bennett Committee, the *Raleigh News & Observer* had said, "There is no evidence to support the conclusion that another school of medicine would add a single physician to the number now practicing in the State."

The minority report proposed amending Friday's report to the Board of Governors by deleting four pages of recommendations (Recommended Action 2-A) and substituting (1) authorization for a degree-granting school of medicine at ECU; (2) funding the upgrade of the one-year program to two years, as a step toward the four-year medical school; (3) continuing the UNC-Chapel Hill and ECU cooperation and collaboration on the one-year program while beginning to plan immediately for the two-year program, as well as setting up primary care residencies. Rural clinics staffed by physician extenders such as nurse practitioners and physician assistants would increase the demand for physicians rather than lessening it.[17] In time for the briefing, the Legislative Services Commission staff had furnished Speaker Ramsey and Senator Allen with cost figures on the AHEC program and on the four-year medical school. They estimated that the AHEC program would cost $4.65 million in 1974-75 (which agreed with President Friday's figures), to rise to $14.85 million in 1979-80 with nine centers. The staff confirmed Friday's estimate of a $25 million non-recurring capital expenditure at the community hospitals where AHECs were established.[18]

Expanding the ECU school would require a capital expenditure of $27,344,000 for land and constructing a medical science building, health science library and ambulatory patient care building. Another $500,000 would be needed for temporary buildings for expanded programs until the permanent construction was done, Mercer Doty, director of Legislative Fiscal Research estimated. If a teaching hospital was needed, this would cost about $19 million for a new facility, or about $5 million to purchase and renovate the old Pitt County Hospital, he said. Operating cost for 1974-5 of an expanded ECU school would add $3,244,902 to what had already been budgeted, and $8,929,759 more would be needed by 1979-80 for 400 students.[19]

Speaker Ramsey (who came from Person County, graduated from Roxboro High School, and attended UNC-CH for his undergraduate and law degrees) appeared on WNCT's program "Carolina Today" in Greenville on December 12. He said he favored expanding the medical school at ECU and that he felt that the 1974 General assembly would authorize the schools expansion to at least a two-year program

He said that most of the policy of the General Assembly was controlled by the budget, and appropriations for health care would be a part of the budget that the 1974 session had to consider. He said the General Assembly would also approve additional money to expand the Area Health Education Center programs and mental health services.

Ramsey believed that the only way to get more doctors was to educate more medical students. Everything needed for a four-year school at ECU would be provided by funding a second year program and funding the Area Health Education Center, he said.

When the television interviewer asked him about a four-year medical school at ECU, Ramsey said, "I would not be surprised if this General Assembly authorizes a degree granting program for general practitioners." Expansion for the Greenville school would take place over a period of several years. He also said that he thought the General Assembly had to keep the program under the Board of Governors. He was opposed to the suggestions that had been made to take medical education out from the board's jurisdiction or to create a special commission. "I would personally be opposed to this. I think we've got to keep it under one umbrella," he concluded.[20]

The Joint Medical Manpower Study Commission approved unanimously a report recommending expansion of the ECU medical school from one year to two years, and eventually to a four-year degree-granting institution. The report said that if it was to survive, the UNC Board of Governors had to recognize that the University of North Carolina consisted of 16 campuses, some big and some little. The report also rebuked the "medical establishment" for furnishing biased opinions about the feasibility of a medical school at ECU. "I'm sure that they're in collusion with Chapel Hill right now," Representative J. P. Huskins, Co-Chairman of the Commission told its members.[21]

UNC President William C. Friday responded on December 15 to the implication of the report of the Medical Manpower Study Commission that the Board of Governors has shown favoritism to the Chapel Hill campus. He said, "This is the first time in my experience that either the Board of Governors or my administration has been accused of favoritism. No one has come to me with evidence of these charges, and I have not been presented any evidence of this favoritism. As far as I know, the Board has always considered all 16 institutions of the UNC system impartially, and I myself have always tried to be fair in my considerations of the various institutions."

He considered that the recommendation of the commission that the ECU medical program be expanded immediately in effect asked the General Assembly to take over the operation of the higher education system, which was the function of the Board of Governors. He said that the Board's proposal differed from the Budget Commission report on nothing but what the next step for ECU should be. He said that Dean Christopher Fordham was already working on expanding the ECU program, and determining how fast the expansion should go, in what direction. The question was how to move from the present situation. There were only two possibilities: "Either the Board of Governors will deal with the ECU program in the same way it always does when it goes about expanding an existing program, or the General Assembly will pass bills to effect the expansion."

Responding to the Commission's statements on accreditation, Friday said he was bound to follow the recommendations of the LCME in handling the ECU program until March, when the accreditation status of the school would be determined by an evaluation of the steps taken to upgrade the school. He said that Commission's support of the AHEC plan proposed by the Board of Governors was reassuring.[22]

Representative J. P. Huskins, in a telephone interview from his Statesville office, told the *Greensboro Daily News* he had received more favorable reaction than unfavorable to the Medical Manpower Study Commission's report since it had been released. He thought the report, of which he was principal author, was a compromise that would be acceptable to the General Assembly, including supporters of the ECU medical school. He considered it a compromise because it did not go so far as to endorse a new four-year school at ECU, but went beyond the UNC Board of Governors' recommendation to hold the school at its present one-year level for another year while attempting to assess its future.

Huskins said that the recommendations in the report, if implemented, would eventually give North Carolina another medical school. The third and fourth years could be added at ECU once the AHEC system had made clinical training available for its students.[23]

UNC President William C. Friday on December 19 directed a report to the LCME on the steps taken since the previous April "to assure the quality of the medical education program at East Carolina University." In the report, Friday noted that in June he had directed Dean Fordham of the UNC medical school to assume full authority for the one-year program at ECU. Fordham had then appointed Dr. William C. Cromartie, UNC associate dean for clinical sciences, as director of the ECU program. The report said Cromartie had worked with ECU officials and faculty to improve the school's curriculum, admissions, examination, and promotion process, faculty selection, and planning and budgeting, and had established committees of UNC and ECU medical school faculty members for each major course in the curriculum. The report described fund allocations by the UNC Board of Governors for improvement of the ECU school, including $227,000 allocated in the medical education plan approved by the Board in November.[24]

An ad hoc committee of the UNC-Chapel Hill Medical faculty, working under Dr. Cromartie as project director, had begun a "comprehensive planning study to examine sound alternatives for the future of the medical education program at ECU." Cromartie had started discussions on the Greenville campus and had brought in Dr. Steven Beering, Associate Dean of the Indiana School of Medicine, for two days as a consultant. With another UNC faculty member, Dr. Cromartie had visited Florida State University in Tallahassee, and a second consultant, from the University of Washington School of Medicine, had been scheduled to visit East Carolina. Glenn Wilson, director of the state AHECs, was working with Dr. Cromartie in studying possible clinical teaching in the Greenville area, patient referral patterns, and the interest of the Pitt County Memorial Hospital staff in a joint clinical education program with ECU. The LCME was expected to act on President Friday's report in late March, 1974.[25]

Following the Board's decision to accept the Bennett Committee's recommendations, the UNC School of Medicine proceeded to implement the charge of planning for development of an overall design for medical education in the state. In December, Dr. William Cromartie's responsibilities at ECU were expanded to include studying the feasibility of adding a second year to the medical program. In an interview by a *Greenville Daily Reflector* staff writer, he was asked when he would report his recommendations. He said "I can assure it will be as soon as possible, in terms with good planning." He also said that the ECU medical students of the previous year appeared to be doing well at Carolina . "There's no reason why they shouldn't. Med students are so carefully picked that it's rare for one to have academic problems."

Dr. Cromartie discussed the arrangements that had been worked out for bringing UNC faculty to ECU to teach for one to three days at a time. Most of the teaching was being done by the ECU faculty, and the need to bring in others did not reflect in any way on the quality of the ECU faculty. He explained, "This is a small faculty, but it is a good one. The problem is one of numbers. It's just impossible for a small number of people to cover a curriculum the way modern medical education demands. Any good medical school is always seeking more faculty as the complexity of medical science increases. We'll be adding on more faculty as we can get the money appropriated. We'll be recruiting from the national and international pool of medical educators." [26]

[1] *Raleigh News & Observer* , October 24, 1973.

[2] *Raleigh News & Observer* , October 26, 1973.

[3] *Greensboro Daily News*, November 1, 1973

[4] Letter from John R. Gamble., Jr., M. D. to Speaker James E. Ramsey, October 30, 1973, in ECU School of Medicine Files, Folder "Huskins-MMPC 2."

[5] *Greensboro Daily News*, November 10, 1973.

[6] *Greenville Daily Reflector*, November 12, 1973.

[7] *Fayetteville Observer*, November 14, 1973.

[8] Recommended Actions Consistent with the Report of the Panel of Medical Consultants on *A Statewide Plan for Medical Education in North Carolina*, Report of the President to the Board of Governors, November 16, 1973, ECU School of Medicine Files, Folder "Bennett Committee;" also in William C. Friday Files, Subgroup 1, Series 1, "Medical Education, Nov. 1974."

[9] *Charlotte News*, November 17, 1973.

[10] *Kinston Free Press*, November 17, 1973.

[11] *Durham Sun*, November 19, 1973.

[12] *Chapel Hill Newspaper*, December 2, 1973.

[13] *Statesville Record and Landmark*, December 1, 1973.

[14] *Greenville Daily Reflector*, December 6, 1973.

[15] *Greensboro Daily News*, December 8, 1973.

[16] Link, p. 233; *A Minority Report from the Board of Governors to the Members of the General Assembly*, December 7, 1973, with covering letter from David J. Whichard II, December 13, 1973, in ECU Medical School Files, Folder "Bennett Committee."

[17] *Minority Report*.

[18] *Greensboro Daily News*, December 8, 1973.

[19] *Greensboro Daily News*, December 8, 1973.

[20] *Greenville Daily Reflector*, December 12, 1973.

[21] *Hickory Daily Record*, December 13, 1973.

[22] *Chapel Hill Newspaper*, December 16, 1973.

[23] *Greensboro Daily News*, December 19, 1973.

[24] Letter from William C. Friday to Dr. Marjorie P. Wilson, December 19, 1973, ECU School of Medicine Files, Folder "Liaison Committee on Medical Education."

[25] *Durham Herald*, December 22, 1973.

[26] *Greenville Daily Reflector*, January 13, 1974.

Chapter 11
The Medical Manpower Commission

In early 1973, after the Jordan Committee had reported to the Board of Governors and while the Bennett Committee was beginning its inquiry, supporters of both sides of the ECU medical school question continued to pursue support from community leaders, chambers of commerce, and other civic groups. On January 23, Dr. Robert Thurber, professor and chairman of the Department of Physiology at ECU School of Medicine, gave a talk on the need for a four-year medical school to the combined Rotary and Kiwanis clubs, at the Holiday Inn in Jacksonville, NC.[1] UNC President William C. Friday told the Charlotte Rotary Club on the same day that legislative interference or political meddling at this time could weaken the structure of the sixteen-campus university system.[2] And that evening, in Chapel Hill, Mayor Howard Lee endorsed the idea of the two-year school in Greenville in a speech to a workshop on the UNC campus, sponsored by the Health Careers Organization, a group composed of disadvantaged and minority students at UNC studying for health careers.

ECU Vice Chancellor For External Affairs John A. Lang, Jr., a Major General in the U. S. Air Force Reserve, told the Rocky Mount Rotary at its February 19 luncheon meeting that the school of medicine at ECU was ready to expand to a free-standing degree-granting school. Lang said: "We feel at East Carolina that what our state needs is a considerable new crop of doctors who are trained and motivated toward community practice in rural areas, and we believe that our situation particularly lends itself to the development and training of the type of general practitioner that every section of the state now requires." [3]

Dr. David Citron, president of Mecklenburg County Medical Society, said on February 22 that a medical school proposed by legislators to be located at UNC-Charlotte was not needed here, and would weaken existing medical programs in the state. There was speculation that eastern legislators might be trying to gain support for expanding the ECU medical school by proposing to build one in Charlotte, the same kind of gambit used when ECU sought regional university status in 1967. To gain support for their bill at that time, it was said, they included Western Carolina University, Appalachian State University, North Carolina Central University and North Carolina A & T State University.[4]

Representative Horton Rountree said there was no such bill, and he did not know who put the rumors out. Senator J. J. Harrington of Bertie County said that if there were such a bill he knew nothing about it. He added, "And I know it wouldn't come from the university. I'm close enough to ECU to know that." [5]

At a coffee and donut breakfast in Greenville on February 23, sponsored by Dr. and Mrs. Ray Minges of Greenville, Mr. and Mrs. Jack Lewis of Farmville, and Mr. and Mrs. David Spier of Bethel, Attorney General Robert Morgan, chairman of ECU Board of Trustees said that four-year medical school supporters must go to the legislature for help in establishing the program.[6]

Supporters of the medical school and their opponents were lining up in the General Assembly. With broad backing in both houses Senator Livingston Stallings from Craven County and Senator James Garrison from Stanly County introduced a bill in the Senate, and Representative John Gamble of Lincoln County in the House, to set aside a $25 million reserve to create an additional degree-granting school of medicine besides the one at the University of North Carolina in Chapel Hill. Stallings said the bill was aimed at telling the UNC Board of Governors that "the legislature feels another medical school is needed."

The bill did not say specifically that the $25 million was to go to ECU, but Stallings commented that East Carolina was obviously the logical place. Leaving it open for other locations enabled ECU strategists to pick up support from a number of legislators who were not backers of the school in Greenville, but were concerned about the physician shortage in the state.

At that time, Representative Gamble, a physician, and Senator Garrison, both new in the legislature, had not been identified with ECU's campaign, but ECU legislative partisans were encouraging them to join their cause. More than thirty members in both houses had signed the bill just before it was introduced, including Democratic leaders in both chambers. The supporters apparently intended to impress the UNC Board of Governors and administration with the strength of support in the legislature for a second public medical school.

Legislative leaders predicted that the odds were good for setting up the $25 million medical school reserve, and that if it was set up, then ECU could be almost sure of getting its medical school. Stallings said that if the board of governors recommended against funding the medical school for which his bill reserved funds, then it would be "another ball game." He said also that he would support the approach recommended by Representative Gerald Arnold of Harnett

County, to set up a separate legislative study of the ECU medical school question, because that would indicate that the legislature was going to override the Board of Governors.[7]

On Thursday, April 12, Representative Arnold introduced the bill to set up the Medical Manpower Commission to review all the reports and documents pertaining to the state's need for medical manpower, in particular the findings of the consultant panel now working for the Board of Governors of UNC. The commission would present its report in January 1974, along with specific legislative proposals to solve the medical manpower problem.

Arnold said that there was an immediate need for additional doctors. The ECU medical school was a reality which did not appear when the legislature created the UNC Board of Governors. He advocated rejecting the consultants' report unless it provided guidance for setting up another medical school.

He commented on a speech proposing a rural health program which Governor Holshouser had given, which Gamble thought was merely an attempt to block establishment of the medical school. That plan would bring the state nothing but second class medical services when what was needed was the means to produce first class doctors.

Dr. Edwin W. Monroe observed of Representative Gamble's bill that it was designed to arrive at a unified approach to the state's health care needs. It proposed that the legislature would review not only the anticipated report from the Board of Governors' consultants, but also all reports and legislative actions related to medical manpower needs over the past few years. The commission set up under it would then recommend some course of action that would provide a comprehensive approach to the problem and not a piecemeal, partial attack. Previous experience had show that a disunified approach did not produce significant results.[8]

On May 23, 1973, the General Assembly ratified a resolution (House Joint Resolution 1133) implementing Representative Gamble's proposal, and establishing a joint Medical Manpower Study Commission (MMSC). Among the reports and documents pertaining to the medical manpower needs in the state that this Commission was to review were all earlier and proposed legislative actions. The Commission was to hold public hearings throughout the state, and to review the recommendations submitted to the Board of Governors by the panel of consultants.

The commission members were Senator J. J. "Monk" Harrington, Senator William D. Mills, Senator Wesley D. Webster, and Senator Vernon E. White. Representative J. P. Huskins, Representative Gerald Arnold, Representative J. R. Gamble, Jr., and Representative John J. Hunt. Five of the eight members (Arnold, Gamble, Harrington, Mills, and White) had previously expressed their support of the ECU medical program, and Senator Harrington of Bertie County had backed it as early as 1965. Representative Huskins was moving from a position of mild opposition or neutrality toward one of support for the medical school.

UNC President Friday's hopes that the independent panel of consultants would take the issue of the medical school in Greenville out of politics were to be splintered by the Commission's recommendations that were made public in December 1973 and reported to the General Assembly in January 1974. However, there could have been no surprise in them.

In May, Representative Gamble, at the meeting of the medical consultants attended by House Speaker James Ramsey, Representatives Carl Stewart and Liston Ramsey, and to which Senator Ralph Scott declined the invitation, had presented a statement of the results of his own comparison of North Carolina and other southeastern states with regard to medical education. Then, on June 8, Gamble made a less heavily documented but more passionate statement at the Board of Governors' meeting in which he explained at length that there were not enough physicians in North Carolina to provide for the citizens' health care, that it would not be enough to expand the existing schools, the problem could not be solved by use of paramedical personnel, and that the state could afford to fund a fourth medical school without diminishing support for the three already existing. Gamble was not speaking for the Commission, but apart from his omission of any reference to the AHECs his statement paralleled the conclusions they finally reached.

The Commission held an organizational meeting on July 27 to arrange for a secretary and research assistance as needed. It also considered locations to hold hearings throughout the state and decided to meet regularly each Thursday. Representative J. P. Huskins and Senator Billy Mills were elected co-chairmen, and Representative Gamble vice-chairman.[9]

The Commission held nine two-day hearings in Waynesville, Wilkesboro, Asheboro, Shelby, Williamston, Lumberton, and Raleigh. The meetings were held on consecutive Thursdays and Fridays during September and October, with extensive publicity preceding each, and specific invitations to mayors, city councilmen, county commissioners, physicians, civic groups, labor unions, and other interested people.

On August 10, after meeting in the morning in the Legislative Building, the Commission adjourned to reconvene in the afternoon and meet with the panel of medical consultants. At the meeting on August 30, the Commission members were joined by Senator Kenneth Royall, Jr., Chairman of the Senate Committee on Public Health and Co-Chairman of the Joint Health Committees of the General Assembly, and Senator John T. Henley, Co-Chairmen of Health Subcommittee #3, which dealt with facilities and services. The Joint Health Committees had already heard from sixteen people, including deans of medical schools, and the two groups had been largely duplicating one another's efforts.

It was agreed that Health Subcommittee #3 and the MMSC would hold joint sessions when this was suitable, and separate sessions when it was considered advisable. They would join in preparing a single report for the Health Committee. (Separate but coordinated reports were, in the end, submitted to the General Assembly). When the discussion moved from how the committees might cooperate to the substantive issue of the medical care crisis, the group decided that a cost-effectiveness study would be made to establish whether the UNC medical school had reached a point of diminishing returns in Chapel Hill.

The Commission's staff, the members' office staffs, and researchers recruited from the Legislative Services Office gathered information from many sources, literature searches, correspondence with medical programs in other states, the Association of American Medical colleges, and combing through federal government documents and state records. There were studies of the cost of implementing the Bennett Committee recommendations, of expanding ECU to a degree-granting four year medical school, of the cost per student at the Chapel Hill medical school, of physician/population ratios and medical student/population ratios in North Carolina and in the nation, and of patients seen in emergency rooms.

On October 16, a meeting was devoted to evaluating the report of the Panel of Medical Consultants to the UNC Board of Governors. President William Friday attended this meeting, by invitation, to talk about the report and answer questions of the MMSC and Health Subcommittee members.

At the October 25 meeting, a group of six physicians and medical educators were invited to attend. Included were Dr. William W. Hedrick, who was in Family Practice in Raleigh, Dr. James G. Jones, President of the North Carolina Academy of Family Physicians, Dr.

Robert Smith, Director of the Department of Family Practice at the UNC School of Medicine, Dr. Charles Harper, Director of Community Health Services in the School of Public Health at UNC, Dr. Edwin W. Monroe, and Dr. Wallace R. Wooles. The inclination of the doctors who spoke at the meeting was mainly in favor of training more family physicians, and most of them leaned fairly definitely toward the expansion of the program in Greenville. The comments made by Dr. Wooles were reported in the newspapers. He said that the expansion of residency training recommended by the consultants' panel to the Board of Governors was quite compatible with ECU's plans, since an expanded residency program would require that more doctors should be trained in the state. He also said that medical education in North Carolina depended on using county hospitals to supplement teaching hospitals, and physicians already in practice to serve as preceptors.[10]

Dr. Hedrick stated that only ten percent of the 2500 doctors who graduated between 1957 and 1968 went into family practice in North Carolina. Dr. Jones added that over-specialization had to be countered by better distribution of family physicians. Nurse-practitioners and physician assistants could not provide the quality of medical care that was needed. He cited the AMA's recommendation that fifty percent of all graduates of medical schools should become primary care physicians.

The overwhelming majority of those who spoke at the nine public hearings held in western, eastern, and piedmont North Carolina spoke in favor of expanding medical care facilities in the state. Laypersons were virtually unanimous in their support of greater spending by the legislature to achieve this, and attributed the problem to a shortage of doctors. Medical professionals gave qualified support to more spending, but some of them favored the expansion of existing facilities and others favored a new medical school. The general public was ahead of the medical profession in its willingness to pay whatever was necessary to make health care more accessible. Virtually no one was heard to dispute the fact that obtaining medical care was a growing problem in North Carolina.

The Medical Manpower Study Commission met in joint session with Senate Health Subcommittee #3 on November 13 to discuss its final report. Members of the group strongly indicated that among the solutions it would propose would be expansion of the ECU medical school program, and that they also favored establishing AHECs. During the meeting, Representative Horton Rountree and Senator Kenneth Royall, longtime supporters of the four-year program at

ECU, agreed with the proposed solution. Co-chairman J. P. Huskins said that he favored expansion of the ECU one-year program, and no other legislators disagreed with him. "The logical, sensible approach would be to go to a first and second year program at East Carolina as soon as we can do it. We should make available to ECU enough money to employ decent faculty and to launch a second year. I think that will produce more doctors at less cost than any other program recommended," Huskins said. The Commission also recommended restrictions on funds given by the state to Duke and Bowman Gray to support NC students, including having state-subsidized medical students guarantee to practice in NC.[11]

On November 30, in an open letter to James Shumaker, the editor of the *Chapel Hill Newspaper*, commenting on an editorial in that paper on the ECU medical school proposal, Jay Huskins said that opinion is less useful than understanding based on study of available information when it comes to solving problems. He said that he had been chairman of the Board of Higher Education committee that recommended that rather than a two-year medical school at ECU, a first- and fourth-year school should be established. The 1971 legislature approved the recommendation and started the first-year program, but nothing had been done about the fourth year.

Huskins said he had agreed it would be more economical to expand the existing medical schools than it would be to start a new one, but had changed his mind on closer examination. About $20 million had already been appropriated for capital improvements at UNC-CH, and about $2 million a year, soon to be increased to $3 million, for only a small increase in the admission of North Carolina students to medical schools. ECU was only asking for $10.5 million in capital and $3.5 in operating funds to expand to a two-year program which the legislature had authorized in 1965.

The Board of Higher Education committee had recommended the first- and fourth-year approach, with the class limited to twenty because of the shortage of clinical teaching facilities. The committee had suggested that local hospitals be used for clinical training, an idea that the AHEC program was carrying out.

Huskins said he thought that since the Board of Governors wants to locate an AHEC in Greenville, it made sense to add the second year there so that students could go directly from the ECU campus to AHEC, rather than continue to "shuffle between the two campuses and the clinical training centers." Competent authorities had suggested that medical training could be done as cheaply at Greenville as anywhere in the state.

No further studies were needed, since no less than eight had already been done since 1965, some in great depth and at great expense. "If we study this problem much longer, the people of North Carolina are going to begin studying us," Huskins said.[12]

On December 13, it was reported that the Joint Medical Manpower Study Commission had unanimously approved recommending expansion of the ECU medical school from one year to two years, and eventually to a four-year degree-granting institution. The report said that if the UNC Board of Governors was to survive it must "recognize that the University of North Carolina consists of 16 campuses, big and little." The report also rebuked the medical establishment for furnishing biased opinions about the feasibility of a medical school at ECU. Representative J. P. Huskins, it was said, told commission members, "I'm sure that they're in collusion with Chapel Hill right now." Huskins, as a co-chairman of the Commission, drafted its report.

The report supported the AHEC centers proposed by the Board of Governors, but said that the Board discriminated in not assigning an AHEC to Greenville, and suggested that this be changed. It also suggested withholding the $10 million requested by Governor James Holshouser for expanding community health clinics in rural areas during the next fiscal year, pending evaluation of the effectiveness of present clinics. It said that the costs of starting a medical school had been grossly exaggerated, and estimated ECU would need $11.5 million in the fiscal year 1975-76 to begin its two-year program, expanding from twenty to forty students in each class. The plan would use the $7.5 million medical school reserve fund set aside in 1973.

According to the report, the ECU School of Medicine should concentrate exclusively on primary care and would admit only North Carolina residents. State support to Duke, Bowman Gray, and Meharry should remain at present levels.[13]

About accreditation, the MMSC report, after a detailed review of the various kinds of curricula at accredited medical schools, said, "We have cited these examples in great detail to emphasize that there are many roads leading to the M.D. degree. It is not unusual for medical schools in other areas to break out of the traditional straitjacket and still attain accreditation. It ought to be possible to do it in North Carolina." [14] The report also quoted the 1973 LCME findings that the problem of accreditation belonged to UNC-Chapel Hill only, so that no problem of accreditation existed for the ECU program, until a free-standing school was established. Accordingly, much that the consultants' report said about accreditation was "gratuitous, if not out of place." [15]

As was mentioned earlier, President Friday objected strenuously to the implications of favoritism in the report. He had never seen any evidence of favoritism, he said, by the Board of Governors or his administration. He also said that the MMPC recommended, in effect, that the General Assembly should take over the operation of the higher education system, which was the function of the Board of Governors. [16]

In January, 1974, as House Joint Resolution 1133 had specified, the Medical Manpower Study Commission presented its report to the General Assembly. Most of its content had already been publicized. Its attack on the contributions that representatives of the medical profession had made to the Board of Higher Education and legislative committees, and on the findings of the Panel of Consultants was even more scathing than the newspapers had reported. For example, it said that the cost estimates that had been provided for medical school startup costs were biased and misleading. It cited data from eleven of twenty new medical schools, from a lecture to the American Association of Medical Colleges by Dr. Cheves McC. Smythe, and from the AAMC itself, that were strongly at variance with what had been previously furnished. After reviewing the panel's projection of costs for expanding the medical education program at ECU, the report said, "Such distortions in the handling of raw data raise serious doubts about some of the other conclusions reached by the panel."

The panel of medical consultants had spent the first ninety pages of its report to the Board of Governors, the MMSC commented, in attempting to establish the proposition that "North Carolina is not in the midst of a health crisis." The MMSC report, in a clear political voice, made this comparison: "Now, to tell a sick man he cannot find a doctor because of maldistribution is like telling a hungry man there is a lot of rice in China. Neither answer speaks to the problem." It went on to state the Commission's conclusion from the experiences of its member, from the public hearings, from statistics on emergency room crowding in the state, and from the length of time it took patients to see a doctor, "that access to medical care is not only inequitably distributed in North Carolina, but seriously limited. And, if this state of affairs is not to continue into the 1980's and 1990's, it is now time to begin doing something about it."

The Commission's conclusions on the ECU medical school were diametrically opposed to those of the Bennett Committee. The group found that North Carolina must have more doctors and paramedical personnel, and should attack the shortage by training more medical students. The problem of uneven distribution should be addressed. Health delivery organizations such as community clinics and out-patient centers should be increased and made more effective, but with care not to set up a two-track system. Financial barriers to health care should be removed. A system of regular evaluation of practices should be instituted. The Commission recommended:

1. The legislature should approve and fund the Board of Governors' proposal for a network of AHECs.
2. An appropriate level of support of Duke, Bowman Gray and Meharry Medical Schools should be continued.
3. The ECU medical education program should be expanded to two years, and the class size increased from twenty to forty as soon as possible.
4. The legislature should appropriate funds for a basic science facility at ECU, and the school's operating budget increased "to provide for adequate staffing and enrichment of faculty."
5. More funding for community health clinics should be withheld until evaluation of those already in place, and a discussion whether county health departments could not be staffed and funded to do the same job.
6. The Area Health Education Center proposed for Greenville should be given high priority, to serve not only the Greenville area but northeastern North Carolina.
7. The expanded ECU program should continue to operate under UNC supervision while continuing actively to seek independent accreditation.
8. Only NC residents should be accepted to the ECU program, and it should be confined to producing primary care and family physicians.
9. Funds should be released from the $7.5 million reserve as needed to expand the ECU program.[17]

[1] *Jacksonville Daily News*, January 24, 1973

[2] *Charlotte Observer*, January 25, 1973

[3] *Rocky Mount Evening Telegram*, February 20, 1973.

[4] *Charlotte News*, February 22, 1973.

[5] *Raleigh News & Observer*, February 24, 1973.

[6] *Greenville Daily Reflector*, February 23, 1973.

[7] *Winston-Salem Journal*, April 12, 1973.

[8] *Greenville Daily Reflector*, April 13, 1973.

[9] The account of the MMSC's activities is based on the correspondence and minutes of the Commission, in ECU School of Medicine Files, Folders "Medical Manpower Study Commission."

[10] *Raleigh News & Observer*, October 26, 1973.

[11] *Fayetteville Observer*, November 14, 1973.

[12] *Statesville Record and Landmark*, November 30, 1973; letter from L. F. "Bud" Amburn of Edenton, in 1973 President of Albemarle Area Development Association, and Huskins's brother-in-law, to an unidentified ECU supporter, in ECU School of Medicine Files, Folder "Edwin W. Monroe."

[13] *Hickory Daily Record*, December 13, 1973; *Report of the Medical Manpower Study Commission to the General Assembly of North Carolina, 1974*, January 16, 1974, in ECU School of Medicine Files, Folders "MMSC."

[14] *Report of the MMSC*, p. 21.

[15] *Report*, p. 27.

[16] *Chapel Hill Newspaper*, December 16, 1973.

[17] *Report*, pp. 46-47.

Chapter 12
Into the Legislature

It was not predetermined that the General Assembly would prefer the findings of a group of its own members over those of the panel of outside medical experts. However, the Medical Manpower Commission, after its hearings across the state, was very persuasive when it concluded that the public was ahead of the medical profession in supporting better availability of medical care, however much it might cost. This conclusion threw the issue right back into the political arena. President Friday's efforts to turn the decision into an administrative or educational one had little chance to succeed when the 1974 legislature was left to make a decision between a popular position and one proposed by a panel of experts, however illustrious, from outside the state.

A bill to expand the medical school at ECU in the next year from one to two years and double enrollment from twenty to forty in the 1975-76 school year was drafted in a closed session of a joint committee of House and Senate leaders, chaired by Representative J. P. Huskins. Huskins explained that the committee members closed the meeting because they wished to be able to discuss freely the legislation's possible impact on the medical school issues' opposing factions, and devise a bill that was not "abrasive." The members of the committee, which was made up of members of the medical manpower subcommittees of the two houses and of members of the Medical Manpower Study Commission, said that their bill would be based on the report of that Commission. Democratic legislative leaders said that most of the legislators had made up their minds about the ECU school a long time ago.[1]

The dissatisfaction at ECU with the Bennett Committee caused further protests. UNC supporters claimed that it would irrevocably weaken the Board of Governors for the legislature to go against the Board's recommendations. ECU supporters countered that the Board's position was biased against ECU. They continued to argue that the shortage of physicians, especially in rural areas, made increasing medical education facilities urgent.

The Board of Governors met on Friday, January 11, 1974, and voted to fight actively against the proposal of the legislature's medical manpower subcommittee to expand the ECU medical program. William Johnson, who moved that the Board should act, said its position has been misconstrued and misinterpreted, and that the

Board was being maligned in many areas. No matter what plan might be adopted, he thought it should be based on the best information available.

David Whichard II of Greenville interjected that there were other valid views besides the Board's position, in the medical profession, legislature, and among citizens. He said it was a mistake to insist that all other voices be ignored.

The Board instructed Chairman Dees to take the facts behind the Board's actions to the General Assembly, the news media, and the people of the state. He should clarify the Board's position on the expansion issue, which had been misinterpreted, as had the facts about the state's need for more doctors and about how much it would cost to provide them.[2]

Dees, in an interview after the Board meeting, said he would ask to appear before the joint legislative committee that was considering the bill to expand ECU's medical program. He said that the Board had not "refuted anything in Raleigh." One allegation that had irritated him immensely was the charge that the consultant's report was stacked against ECU. If the report was biased in any way, he said, it was in ECU's favor, because three of the five consultants were picked by ECU administrators.[3] As was pointed out before, only two of the five were, and one of them resigned soon after the committee began its work. This member, Dr. Robert S. Stone, was not replaced. The third choice to which Dees referred was made, not by the East Carolina administration, but by a Greenville physician, Dr. Andrew Best. He proposed the Dean of his alma mater, the Meharry School of Medicine, Dr. Lloyd C. Elam.

Dees said one clear misinterpretation had been of the Board's position on an AHEC for Greenville. He said that not until that week had Pitt County Memorial Hospital and ECU administrators agreed to have an AHEC located there, although negotiations had been under way since 1966. Dr. Jack W. Wilkerson, chairman of the medical education liaison committee of Pitt County Memorial Hospital, and a member of the Hospital's Board of Trustees, said that Dees was in error when he said the PCMH was reluctant to join the AHEC program. Wilkerson said that the hospital had not been given time to plan for participating, and would not go into it without adequate study. He emphasized that the hospital has recently joined with the ECU School of Medicine in an AHEC program for nurses and allied health personnel.

Reginald McCoy said after the meeting that he and Whichard, who submitted a minority board report on medical education to the legislature, would continue to support the ECU position.

Representative Horton Rountree, Democrat from Pitt County, and a longtime supporter of ECU, explained to a reporter who called him after the Board meeting that the 1975 date for expansion of the ECU medical program was selected in the bill to be proposed because there had to be time to organize the program, hire faculty, and complete necessary construction. The committee had considered 1974, but rejected it as impractical.[4]

In his 1974 Legislative and Budget Message, Governor James E. Holshouser spoke in support of the AHEC system across the state. He said that under plans already being put into effect, the number of medical students would more than double before 1984. It was true that there were not enough doctors in the state, particularly family doctors, doctors practicing in the primary care fields. Still, the key to increasing the number of physicians in the state centered in residency programs, since the location of residencies most influenced a physician's choice of where to practice.

A major part of the problem, that of distribution, was one not specific to North Carolina. Some cities had an adequate doctor-patient ratio, while others, and many rural areas, did not. Spreading medical education across the state by expanding the AHEC system would bring doctors and other health personnel to numerous locations. Medical education would not be concentrated almost totally in Winston-Salem, Durham, and Chapel Hill.

Governor Holshouser said the problem was not just one of health care delivery, but also one of medical education within the university system. He did not specifically mention ECU nor the UNC Board of Governors' decision against a four-year school in Greenville. But he urged the General Assembly to keep faith with the university system, just when the young Board was starting to show its sense of accountability and to take responsibility for its decisions.[5] Democratic leaders in the legislature replied that the final responsibility rested with the General Assembly to decide one way or the other on expansion.

Dean Christopher Fordham urged the legislature again not to approve expanding the ECU program. The UNC medical school would find it difficult to find space for any more that the 20 students being taken as transfers.

The 1974 General Assembly was a trial run for annual rather than biennial meetings. At the opening of the session on January 16, there were about the same number of supporters on each side of the ECU medical school issue. In the house, UNC was thought to be slightly ahead, though forty-two legislators signed a statement calling for immediate expansion of the ECU program.[6] It was not promising for UNC that the sponsors of the declaration were James Garrison, an influential senator and ECU medical school supporter from Stanly County, and Representative J. P. Huskins, the respected co-chairman of the Medical Manpower Study Commission.

The medical school at East Carolina was supported by the Democratic Party leadership, and by most of the Democratic members of the legislature. In April 1974, there were sixty-four House supporters of enlarging the program at ECU, of which fifty-eight were Democrats; thirty-four out of fifty Republicans championed UNC.[7] Governor Holshouser was a Republican, but the Democrats were still in the majority in the legislature, and Lieutenant Governor James B. Hunt was the leader of the Democratic Party. He had supported the ECU program actively in his 1972 campaign for the lieutenant governorship. His advocacy for improved health care was central to his platform. He had been active in setting up the Medical Manpower Commission to review the Bennett Committee's findings and gather its own data on health care. He had asserted that health care took priority over the higher education system centered at UNC. In March, 1973, he had come out in favor of putting $25 million aside for expansion of medical schools in the state. He said that the final word on the proposal from ECU would be the legislature's, and that to get more family doctors a new school was necessary. He thought the ECU proposal was favored by legislators because it came from the grassroots and not merely from East Carolina University.

On Tuesday, January 22, Representative Huskins and Senator William Mills of Onslow County prepared to introduce identical bills in the House and Senate calling for expansion of the medical school at ECU to a two-year school increasing class size to forty, and allocating $14 million for construction of a basic science building. Huskins said there were thirty-nine or forty signatures of cosponsors, "including four or five Republicans," on the proposal.

ECU supporters had suggested that it would be better to have someone not from the east introduce the legislation in the Senate. Senator James Garrison of Stanly County had agreed to do so, saying, "We felt I should do this because I'm from the Piedmont and we want to get support from all over the state. It was something we all agreed with."[8] Introduction of the bill was deferred, but it was introduced on Friday, January 24. Senator Garrison had guarded against having anybody else sign it, but without his knowing it, Senator Livingston Stallings from New Bern had slipped in and signed the bill.

Garrison got up and said, "Mr. President, I have a bill to send forward," and Stallings went and put his arm around him, and said,
"We...." The ECU supporters, who had worked so hard to make sure
the bill came from outside the east, were embarrassed, but fortunately for them, Senator Stallings's intervention did no harm.[9]

That day, Representative John Stevens of Buncombe County, a
supporter of the UNC Board of Governors, said that he believed that
the House, in spite of being nearly evenly divided, would support the
UNC position. It was generally agreed among House members that it
was too close to call, but that the Board had been gaining support.

In the Senate, only nineteen members had cosponsored Senator
Garrison's bill, even though ECU supporters had worked hard to gain
support. Senator Monk Harrington of Bertie County admitted, "We
still need to pick up a few marbles."[10] He could not have anticipated
the split that was to come between Republican members of the legislature.

House Speaker James Ramsey asked Senator Ralph Scott and
Representative Carl Stewart to arrange a private meeting of ECU and
UNC administrators, members of the Board of Governors, and pivotal
legislators. Ramsey said the meeting was to give the legislators an
opportunity to ask for information they might not already have, and
an equal number of legislators on each side of the ECU issue, from
the House and the Senate, had been invited. A compromise to be
proposed, supported by ECU backers, would insure expanding the
ECU program, closely supervised by the UNC Board. It would also
give priority to developing the nine AHECs.[11]

On January 23, Dr. Edwin Monroe told a *Greenville Daily Reflec-
tor* reporter, "We have been invited to Raleigh to discuss a compro-
mise on expansion of our School of Medicine. Dr. Jenkins, Dr.
Wooles, and Dave Whichard, a member of the Higher [Education]
Board, will be there. I really can't imagine what will be talked about.
As I see it, the bill introduced yesterday was a compromise, so I can't
see how we can compromise further." Senator Vernon White and
Representative Horton Rountree had also been invited to attend.
Rountree said that he believed there would be about eight senators
present at the meeting, two of whom were opposed to the ECU
school. House members would be five for and five against.[12]

On Wednesday, January 23, Senator Ralph Scott commented on
the planned meeting. He said it was an attempt to work out a compromise on the medical education controversy, and avoid floor fights
in the General Assembly. He thought that the compromise would be
acceptable to the Board, but was not sure about agreement from

ECU supporters. He was going to offer a proposal that would try to reassure ECU proponents who did not trust the Board of Governors, by giving them some guarantee that the medical school at ECU would eventually be expanded, but leave the Board its prerogative to decide when the expansion would occur. There would be no dates specified in legislation or appropriations enacted during the current session of the General Assembly.[13]

On Friday evening, January 25, they met at the College Inn in Raleigh to discuss the ECU medical school question. Of the UNC administration, President William Friday, Dean Christopher Fordham, and Board of Governors Chairman William A. Dees were invited, and from ECU, Chancellor Leo Jenkins, Dean Wallace Wooles, and Dr. Edwin Monroe. Four or five UNC Board members and twenty legislators, ten selected by Scott and ten by Stewart, including Representative Horton Rountree and Senator Vernon White, were also asked to attend. Altogether, thirty-eight people were invited. Forty-five or more attended, prompting Senator Scott to remark, "This meeting has gotten so large that we wonder whether we can accomplish anything tonight. We'll have to go to Carter Stadium if we keep this up." [14]

Both ECU and UNC supporters had commented publicly that they saw little chance of any compromise between their respective positions. Dr. Monroe's comments have been quoted. On Monday, January 21, Dr. Christopher Fordham had told the N. C. Memorial Hospital Board of Directors that expanding the ECU school's class size would cause serious space shortages in the clinical facilities for UNC medical students. He also mentioned the lack of a strong basic science program at ECU and the impossibility of having medical students trained at Pitt County Memorial Hospital before 1977 when the new hospital was completed. Earlier, he had told the Mecklenburg County Medical Society that "expansion of the ECU program to two years is not a compromise..., it is a possible educational tragedy," which would not help solve any of the state's health care problems, including that of the maldistribution of doctors.[15]

Speaker James Ramsey described the meeting he had suggested as an opportunity for legislators to get information that they might not already have. He said, "We are reaching a point of no return. This is an area that we ought to explore more. There might be something that comes forward in the confrontation." [16]

Senator Scott said, "We want to get something that both sides can accept without having a bloodletting." The purpose of the gathering was to get the "ECU and the UNC people to agree to something we can go with. The trouble is that the ECU people don't trust the Board of Governors to agree to do something that they are talking about. We want the Board to agree to enough so that everyone will be certain that it will be carried out."[17]

The compromise proposal that was discussed at the meeting provided for adding a second year of instruction at ECU, but under the close supervision of the UNC Board. It would also guarantee the construction of nine AHEC centers, giving them priority over the ECU expansion. Senator Scott said he thought that ECU would accept the compromise if they were assured their program would be protected. UNC would be foolish if they did not accept it. "The power is here in the legislature. It's the legislature that gives out the money." Neither side acted as he thought they would.

After the meeting, Representative Carl Stewart said that no agreement had been reached that would make it possible to avoid a confrontation in the General Assembly, but that he thought the group was getting nearer to an answer. They had agreed to meet again at an unspecified later date, inviting a member of the LCME to attend.

Senator Ralph Scott and Representative Carl Stewart continued discussions with President William Friday and other members of the UNC administration, who were still trying to block Chancellor Jenkins's expansionist plans.[18] On February 5, Scott and Stewart proposed a plan under which ECU would add the second year of instruction as soon as they could manage, but the UNC Board of Governors would exercise control. It was essentially the "compromise" that had been offered and rejected at the College Inn meeting. Expectably, Friday declined to endorse it, and it became clear to Scott and Stewart that UNC would not accept specific target dates for expanding the ECU program. A compromise offered by Representative Herbert L. Hyde, which skirted the question of expanding the ECU medical school, aroused little interest, even among UNC supporters.[19]

In 1973, Representative Larry Eagles of Edgecombe County had introduced a $50 million bond referendum to pay for a medical school at ECU. Eagles had said then that more studies were unnecessary and that the people of eastern North Carolina had enough sense to know more doctors were needed and where the school ought to be. Eagles's act had come as a surprise to Dr. Leo Jenkins, and he had been against it. Early in February, 1974, House speaker James Ramsey and House majority leader Billy Watkins of Granville County, revived the Eagles proposal as a potential way out of the deadlock between ECU and UNC. However, both the General Administration and ECU rejected the bond issue, and on February 7 it was voted down in committee.[20] Nothing was left but to take the question to the legislature, and both parties marshaled their support.

On February 19, 1974, the Joint Appropriations Committee began public hearings on the ECU medical school proposal, with special attention to the minority report to the Board of Governors in the fall of 1973. On one side of the hearing chamber were President William Friday with his staff, and with the leadership of the Board of Governors, including Watts Hill, Victor Bryant, and others from the former UNC Board of Trustees, along with some of the pro-UNC members of the legislature. Opposite them were ECU supporters, somewhat fewer in number than those for UNC. They included Mutt McCoy, David Whichard and Dr. Andrew Best, with other members of the Board of Governors who backed ECU, representatives of the Farm Bureau, the State Grange, the Lions Club, the Jaycees, and other civic organizations whose members had been addressed by Leo Jenkins, Ed Monroe, and Wallace Wooles during 1971-1973. The mayors of many towns in eastern North Carolina were there, and some members of the medical profession, including Dr. Ernest Furgurson and Dr. Lenox Baker, who had recently retired from the faculty of Duke University School of Medicine. Dr. Ed Monroe on one side, and on the other President Friday, Dr. Raymond Dawson, and Felix Joyner orchestrated the presentations. Altogether, twenty-two persons spoke before the committee, supporting both sides of the issue.[21]

Representative J. P. Huskins made a memorable speech to the Committee. It was a capsule history of what had gone on in the campaign to set up a medical school at East Carolina University. The speech was more than a summary. In effect, it defined the parameters of the General Assembly's discussion of what was to be done about ECU's request.

He began, "I feel somewhat like the young man out on his first date. I know what I want to do. I just don't know where to start. Perhaps I had better start with a little story one of your co-chairmen told me.

"It was after one of the many conferences we had held in an effort to reach some compromise on the medical manpower dilemma when he came up to me and said he had been talking with a member of the Board of Governors and would tell me something funny if I would promise not to get angry. When I assured him I was getting too old for that, he continued, 'Well, we were talking and your name came up and he said, "And he's such a quiet little son of a bitch."

"Now, my problem for the next 15 or 20 minutes is how to dispel the first part of that image without confirming the second part."

He spoke for about twenty minutes, reviewing his experience with the question of the East Carolina School of Medicine, from his first encounter with it during his service on the Board of Higher Education, through the investigations of the Medical Manpower Commission—a period of nearly ten years of close involvement. He described how he had not at first been in favor of the school in Greenville. When it failed to win accreditation from the LCME by January 1, 1967, and the decision fell back to the Board of Higher Education, he had supported establishing what became the School of Allied Health Sciences at ECU, as a first step toward providing the foundation that ECU lacked for a medical school.

When the General Assembly gave ECU university status in 1967, and appropriated funds in 1969 for planning and developing a two-year medical curriculum, it made the program subject to approval by the BHE and accreditation by the AMA and the Association of American Medical Colleges. In the fall of 1970, ECU applied for approval of a two-year master of medical education program. The BHE considered the application, with its accompanying request for $13.5 million capital and operating funds for an initial class of twenty medical students. At the same time, UNC-Chapel Hill requested funds to enable it to enlarge the UNC Medical School's entering class, and proposed subsidizing Duke and Bowman Gray for each North Carolina student they accepted.

The BHE, after calling in its own consultants and visiting other states where innovative approaches were being taken to medical education, recommended against a two-year medical school at ECU. Huskins said that if he had possessed the information in 1970 that he had in 1974, he would not have gone along with the recommendation. He mentioned the misleading statements that two-year medical schools were not being accredited, including an LCME report that seemed to reinforce the contention. He mentioned the missing page from the 1970 LCME site visitors' report, which said that ECU had "the potential for developing a fully-accredited two-year school of basic medical sciences," and could look for provisional accreditation by the fall of 1972.

He reexamined the lack of accurate cost figures, which had made a rational decision impossible. It had been said that it would cost $100 million or more to start a new four-year medical school, but actual investigation had shown that the cost of a school of medicine varied not only from one state to another, but according to the goals of the school. Schools centered on research and on training paramedical personnel would cost much more than those whose mission was training more physicians. Some schools had been built during the past five years, he said, for $30 million or less, and the average had been $56 million.

He described how he, Dr. Cameron West and Lem Stokes of the Board of Higher Education staff had persuaded Governor Robert Scott that the two-year program at ECU, which he had strongly and publicly supported, was not practical. With Scott's agreement, the BHE had recommended successfully to the 1971 legislature that it fund enlarged classes at Chapel Hill, subsidize Duke and Bowman Gray, and authorize a first- and fourth-year program at ECU. First-year students were to transfer to UNC-CH for their second and third years, then return to Greenville for their fourth, clinical year. Governor Scott accepted their proposal because it kept the door open for future expansion at ECU.

As a member of the legislature and the new Board of Governors, Huskins said, he discovered that the cost of medical education was going up. The committee headed by Robert B. Jordan III that reported to the Board in December, 1972, recommended increasing the subsidies to Duke and Bowman Gray to about double what they had been. Besides the $3.5 million for remodeling MacNider Building to make expansion of the first year at Chapel Hill possible, the committee recommended $11.5 million for a new laboratory-office building. Instead of resolving the question of ECU expansion, the Jordan Committee had recommended calling in a panel of outside consultants.

The consultants were then appointed, under the chairmanship of Dr. Ivan Bennett. Meantime, while Huskins was chairman of the Board of Governors' budget committee, another $16 million was requested from the legislature, beyond the $12 million being asked for renovating and expanding Memorial Hospital. He was successful in the advocacy appropriate to his chairmanship, and the 1973 legislature appropriated over $28 million to expand medical education at Chapel Hill, and increased its commitment to Duke and Bowman Gray to about $3.5 million for the biennium.

In the summer of 1973, he continued, House Speaker James Ramsey asked him to serve with Senator William Mills as cochairman of the Study Commission authorized by the General Assembly to study the physician shortage in North Carolina, hold hearings, review published materials, including the Bennett Committee's report when it was issued, and to make recommendations to the legislature concerning how to solve the medical care dilemma.

That commission was made up equally of members from the eastern and western regions of the state, including a doctor, a dentist, a lawyer, a publisher, a banker, a manufacture, a merchant, and a farmer. In public hearings held all across the state, the study group heard from the people at large, none of whom had previously had a voice in plans being made for their health care needs. They had not been heard by the Jordan Committee, they had no voice on the Bennett Committee, nor in the formulation of the proposal presented by the Board of Governors. While the panel of outside experts were developing statistics to show that North Carolina was not experiencing a crisis in health care, the Health Manpower Commission learned that doctors are inequitably distributed in the state, that there was such a grave shortage of primary care physicians that many people already economically at risk were at a great disadvantage in seeking medical care.

They found that the citizens of the state were worn out with spending long hours in doctors' offices waiting to be seen, tired of having to resort to emergency rooms for primary care, and more and more alarmed to hear the refrain, "The doctor is not taking any new patients." They found that, more than anything else, the people were tired of hearing how happy they were with the arrangement. In actuality, of the fifty states, North Carolina was forty-third in doctors per capita, and forty-sixth in the proportion of medical students to population.

Once the Commission was convinced that there was a genuine crisis in medical care in the state, its members began to consider the various ways that had been suggested to solve the problem. They had received the proposal of the UNC Board of Governors, based on the Bennett Committee's recommendations, and a great body of data that the Commission's researchers had gathered from all across the United States. They found it puzzling that the Board had adopted the Bennett panels report within a week of its release, and prepared a proposal for medical education for the state to be presented to the legislature, without consulting either the Medical Manpower Study Commission or the Joint Committees on Health, who were at the time studying the problem at the General Assembly's direction. More disconcerting still was the fact that the Board, having prepared its proposal without consulting the legislature's study groups, was insisting that the legislature proceed in equally blissful disregard of alternatives, and fund the Board's request without challenging it.

The report of the Medical Manpower Study Commission, Huskins said, had taken account of the panel of experts and the Board of Governors in preparing its report. It had found that the experts' analysis of costs at ECU were so full of gross errors that they cast the entire report into doubt. Also, the Board of Governors' projections into the 1990s of the production of new physicians under its plan was far more optimistic than there was any basis for believing.

Above all, the Commission had found that when the Board of Governors and its panel of experts talked about "beefing-up" existing medical schools as the best way to go, "they were talking about money, not meat." When the legislature set up the two-year medical science program at ECU in 1969, the estimated cost for an entering class of forty students was $11 million in capital funds and $2.5 million in initial operating funds. Since 1969, the legislature had appropriated $44.8 million in capital funds to "beef-up" the Chapel Hill program. Further, the UNC-CH medical schools had received $10 million in state and federal funds for the AHEC, and was asking for $24.9 million more for that program. The total was $79.8 million either appropriated or requested for expanding the UNC-CH medical school from 100 entering students in 1970-71 to 160 by 1976-77, including ECU's twenty students. This did not include the UNC medical school's increased operating budgets, nor the Duke and Bowman Gray subsidies. If this was not enough, before there was an entering class of 160 the medical school in Chapel Hill would be back for additional funds to expand its physical plant to provide for its expanded enrollment. It had already asked for planning funds for that project.

Huskins then asked whether the Board of Higher Education and the General Assembly were perhaps wrong in 1970 when they decided to "beef-up" Chapel Hill, Duke, and Bowman Gray. He wondered whether there was still time to improve the situation and make a new beginning. He said that the members of the Medical Manpower Study Commission believed it was possible, that although statesmanship did not prevail in the first instance it still might. He went on to outline the proposals of the Commission and emphasize their foundation in the best evidence they could muster.

He proceeded to argue forcefully for the recommendations of the Commission, particularly expansion of the medical education program at ECU, concurrently with developing clinical training facilities in AHEC centers across the state. If a spirit of cooperation and good will could be generated, then the question of a four-year school at East Carolina would no longer be an issue. He concluded: "For ten years now the legislature has been holding a medical school carrot in front of East Carolina University; and every time ECU has reached for the carrot, somebody has hit it across the knuckles. This time ECU was too timid—or too experienced—to reach. The Medical Manpower Commission is doing it for them. And in suggesting that we at long last deliver the carrot, we are not trying to undercut the Board of Governors. We are trying merely to enlarge its vision." [22]

The speech is cited at length because it was so influential, and its terms came up again and again in the continuing debate. It convinced the legislators of Representative Huskins's grasp of the issues involved. It was effective because he had personally made the whole journey; he had gone from advocating expansion of existing medical schools and opposing the two-year program at ECU, to favoring the medical school. And it was obvious to his fellow legislators that the last step in changing his position had been brought about mostly by his Commission's inquiries throughout the state, looking at what was going on and listening to the people involved, and not just to arguments from the two parties to the contention.

At the February 19 hearing, the Rev. Coy Privette of Kannapolis, president of the Christian Action League, an influential Baptist organization set up to fight liquor-by-the-drink in North Carolina, spoke in favor of the ECU school. At a later hearing, he expanded his statement by adding that to reduce the physician shortage in the state, the ECU medical school should be expanded "to feed more family doctors into the pipeline." The General Assembly should make the decision, not the UNC board, who responsibility is higher education policy, not health care. The General Assembly is closer to the people, and elected to represent them, where the Board is appointed. He noted that twenty-one of the thirty-two Board of Governors members were UNC graduates, and asked, "Do you really believe that they would vote to expand a med school at ECU no matter how desperate the need?" [23]

On Monday night, February 25, Senator Scott, Representative Carl Stewart and leaders of the ECU partisans met in the office of Senator Thomas Strickland until midnight, and Representative Huskins, author of the original ECU bill, agreed to defer to the compromise Scott-Stewart bill. Strickland promised to push for an amendment nailing down the construction money for the medical school, and a second amendment instructing the governing board to work toward independent accreditation of the ECU school. Both were passed by the committee. [24]

The Republicans in the legislature, who had been reliable UNC

supporters in the past, were split by the dissension between the conservative branch of the party, led by Senator Jesse Helms, and the
moderate branch affiliated with Governor Holshouser. In February,
the Holshouser group had brought about the withdrawal of conservative state Senator Hamilton Horton from the U. S. Senate race by
pushing forward William E. Stevens of Caldwell County, a moderate,
to oppose him in the primary. Horton's friends in the legislator said
the Governor had led him to believe that he would remain neutral in
the Senate race. The ECU controversy gave the conservatives a con-
venient issue on which to retaliate against Holshouser. Phil Kirk, the
Governor's legislative liaison with the legislature, attempted on that
Monday night, February 25, to persuade lawmakers that Holshouser
had not broken his promise of neutrality, but had told Horton that
Stevens was a likely candidate.[25]

Also on Monday night, Holshouser met with GOP members of
the Appropriations Committee to explain his position, but was unable to rally effective support for it. Frank Rouse, who had been defeated by Holshouser's moderates in his bid to become state Republican chairman, joined in the lobbying against the Governor. Representative Stevens's vote was lost when he resigned from the House to
declare for the state Senate race. Altogether, Holshouser lost three to
five votes, depending on who was making the count, to East Carolina
supporters.[26]

On February 26, Senator Scott made a statement before the
Joint Committee. Scott described the three bills being sponsored by
legislators: (1) the "East Carolina Bill," or Huskins-Garrison bill,
proposing a medical school at Greenville to be built by a definite
time, (2) the "Board of Governors' Bill" proposed by Herbert L. Hyde,
which did not support building a medical school at Greenville, and
(3) the "Scott-Stewart Bill," which was a compromise, and called for
building the school, but without a definite time frame. He admitted
that his description was an oversimplification, since each bill contained other things than those he used to label it. Simplification was
needed, he thought.

Scott said that the process had not begun because ECU wanted
a medical school and the Board of Governors did not want them to
have it. Rather, it started because the people of North Carolina
wanted good health care and were not getting it, and wanted to be
able to find doctors when they needed them. The medical school in
the east was proposed as a possible solution to the problem, and it
was a commonsense solution, opposed only by so-called "experts".
The proposal went through channels, and when it reached the Board

of Governors, they would not go along with it.

The people turned to the General Assembly for help. This was not an attack on the Board, but a recognition that they had failed to respond to a public need. He said that Dr. Lenox Baker, the retired orthopedic surgeon from Duke, had recalled hearing opponents of Duke, Bowman Gray and UNC put out the same negative excuses. If they had been listened to, no medical schools at all would have been built. Senator Scott found it interesting that the very people who were supporting the Board on the present issue were those who had fought its creation in the first place.

It was equally interesting how not only the content but the rhetoric of Representative Huskins's eloquent statement was reappearing in the discussion.

The General Assembly, made up of the people's elected representatives, Scott said, was responsible for doing something about medical education. His own efforts had all been directed at trying to make this happen. All the meetings and discussions had been aimed at nothing else, and what he had been forced to conclude from them was that neither side was willing to compromise. However, he hoped that both sides in the ECU conflict would support the compromise measure, which although not perfect, was probably the best that could be had. He thought that if it was not passed, they might leave the session without a bill, and everyone would lose.[27]

When the Joint Appropriation Committee met on February 26, it was still closely divided on the ECU medical school issue in spite of the understanding that the key players had reached. The session of the committee went on for two and a half hours, with the committee room packed with committee members, other legislators, lobbyists, reporters, and visitors. By the end of the session, the air was hazy with cigar and cigarette smoke.

The committee voted by forty-nine to twenty-eight to send forward the Scott-Stewart compromise bill. By a single margin vote of forty to thirty-nine, the school's supporters managed to have the medical school funding included in the main appropriations bill, rather than in a separate bill. They felt that including their expansion funds in that bill increased their chances to succeed in their plans, since the budget bill, usually the last major bill approved by each session, would be difficult to amend on the floor.[28]

Section 46 of the bill provided, after quoting the report of the Medical Manpower Study Commission, that the Board of Governors should include in its operating budget for the 1975-76 fiscal year funds for expanding the medical education program at ECU to the second year and enlarging the class from twenty to forty as soon as possible, with concentration on training family care physicians and on recruitment of minority students. Fifteen million dollars were appropriated for a Basic Science facility at ECU. The UNC Medical School and the ECU Medical School were directed to work cooperatively together toward full accreditation of the expanded medical education program at East Carolina University, so that its graduates might transfer freely to the medical school in Chapel Hill.[29] Supporters of the UNC board's position promised that there would be floor battles when the budget was presented in each House, but the final version of the bill was ratified on April 8.[30]

While the Joint Appropriations Committee was debating and voting, elsewhere in Raleigh the trustees of the Christian Action League (CAL) were also debating and voting. During the hour-long discussion preceding the vote, Dr. Edwin Monroe of the ECU medical school and the Rev. Tommy J. Payne of Greenville, a trustee of the League, spoke in support of East Carolina. Payne said the university's expansion bid had been subjected to "damning editorials and scathing cartoons" in the newspapers. He said the existing medical schools did not enroll enough North Carolinians, and that at Board of Governors meetings no one had spoken for the people.

J. Marse Grant, editor of *The Biblical Recorder*, proposed a substitute motion to replace the recommendation of the CAL executive committee. The substitute recommended that the League commend the Joint Appropriations Committee of the General Assembly for its action on better medical care in North Carolina, and urged the legislature to approve this or a similar plan to assure more family physicians for the state. Speaking in favor of the substitute motion, Grant and Dr. A. L. Parker, pastor of Greensboro's Friendly Avenue Baptist Church and former Baptist State Convention president, noted that the motion did not back either the ECU proposal or that of the UNC Board of Governors. They said it was carefully worded to recommend that or a similar plan so legislators would understand that CAL supported the General Assembly in all efforts to get more and better medical care for all of North Carolina's citizens.

Some trustees said that CAL's two-week campaign in favor of the expansion had already influenced enough legislators to assure ECU of winning. The Reverend Coy Privette, CAL president, commented on the vote, "We got what we wanted."

The vote came after Dr. W. Perry Crouch, general secretary-treasurer of the Baptist State Convention, asked the trustees not to continue supporting ECU expansion, because the issue was debatable, and statistics quoted for and against it confusing. The Reverend Tom Freeman of Dunn, immediate past president of the Baptist State Convention, said that the League should not get involved in partisan politics. He said the League was in a strong position and should not alienate its friends. He was obliquely referring to the League's success in campaigning against a statewide liquor-by-the-drink referendum in the previous November's election.

Mrs. George D. Wilson of Fayetteville, a member of the UNC Board of Governors, spoke against CAL involvement in the controversy. She said partisans were using "suspicion and distrust, emotionalism and sectionalism to confuse the issue and work to the detriment of the people of North Carolina." She described the particulars of the Board of Governors' proposal for the trustees.[31]

The arguments favoring neutrality or the UNC position did not prevail. In the end, the trustees approved, with only one dissenting vote, a motion that commended the Joint Appropriations Committee for its action on medical care in North Carolina.

The decisions of the Joint Appropriations Committee and of the General Assembly were a defeat for William Friday, the General Administration, and the Board of Governors. However, it left undecided where control over the two-year program would lie. On March 8, the Board met and Chairman William Dees reported to them on the Joint Appropriations Committee's action. When the meeting was over, Dees stated that the Board would abide by whatever the General Assembly decided, would stop lobbying, and accept whatever the decision the legislature reached.[32]

The General Assembly approved on April 8 the general appropriations bill containing (in Section 46) the compromise provisions which Senator Scott and Representative Stewart had introduced. The Board of Governors was directed to include in its 1975-1976 operating budget funds for expansion of the ECU medical school's first year, to add a second year program emphasizing family care, and to make special efforts to encourage racial minorities for the medical program. A sum of $7,500,000 was appropriated, to be added to the $7,500,000 already in reserve, for the erection of a basic medical science building.[33]

President Friday raised the question whether there was any intent in the legislature's action concerning a four-year medical school at ECU. On May 23, Senator Scott wrote to him that there was no such intent, and "that the question of establishment of such a four-year institution will have to be resolved by future sessions of the General Assembly."[34]

After the Board of Governors capitulated and the legislature acted, President Friday called on Chancellor Jenkins for a proposal on how UNC and ECU could best work together to make the ECU program ready for accreditation. He accepted Jenkins's contention that the primary responsibility should be ECU's. UNC Chancellor Ferebee Taylor and Dean Christopher Fordham agreed with Chancellor Jenkins's proposal. On May 10, President Friday reported this to the Board of Governors. He assured the board that the Liaison Committee on Medical Education would approve the plan.[35] The Board authorized him to turn over to Dr. Jenkins the job of laying out a curriculum for a two-year program.[36] At this juncture, the Liaison Committee on Medical Education appeared on the stage again.

On April 12, 1974, Dr. Glen R. Leymaster, Secretary of the LCME, had written to tell President Friday that the committee had accepted, as information, the progress report on the ECU program he had submitted on December 17, 1973. Leymaster requested another progress report in a year. The committee approved the enlarged entering classes at UNC School of Medicine, including twenty students per class from the ECU program.[37]

Friday wrote to Dr. Leymaster on April 29, informing him of the General Assembly's actions concerning the ECU program. On May 15, he sent another letter to apprise the LCME of the Board of Governors action of May 10 authorizing him to assign to Chancellor Leo Jenkins responsibility for a two-year program at ECU aimed at obtaining accreditation. He wrote to Chancellor Jenkins on the same day, "I do not want a situation to arise in which objection is later made by LCME to our approach to the development of the program with all that could entail in the loss of time." [38]

The Liaison Committee had renewed UNC's accreditation in January, 1973, with a warning that the ECU situation was not acceptable. Failure to deal with it could threaten UNC's own accreditation.

On June 14, Dr. Leymaster informed President Friday that the Committee would not consider granting accreditation to the proposed free-standing two-year school whose students would be guaranteed acceptance at UNC-CH, because the school would not meet the LCME's criteria for basic medical science programs that had been adopted by the LCME and its two parent Associations in 1973. He enclosed a copy of those criteria, which dealt with two-year schools on the way to becoming four-year schools, and with two-year schools accredited as components of four-year schools.[39]

President Friday announced on the day of the Committee's reply that their ruling would not prevent going ahead to carry out the legislature's clearly stated purpose. He intended to proceed with planning the two-year program. To do this would require, of course, revising his agreement with Chancellor Jenkins about assigning responsibility to ECU and dissipating all of the considerable effort spent in negotiating that arrangement. Jenkins said publicly that he did not consider the LCME's action a setback for the ECU medical school's expansion. "The simple truth is that the proposal of the board of governors for a stand-alone two-year medical school is not possible according to national medical authorities," he said. "President Friday and I have therefore agreed to pursue the expansion with close cooperation of the medical school at Chapel Hill. I have no reason to believe we will not receive the full cooperation of all the people concerned with medical education in Chapel Hill, where I have today been assured of this by President Friday." [40]

On July 11, Friday met with the planning committee of the Board of Governors, on which UNC Board members David Whichard and Reginald McCoy still served, to discuss the altered situation. Chancellor Jenkins, Dean Christopher Fordham, and Drs. Edwin Monroe and Wallace Wooles were also invited to the meeting. [41] McCoy and Whichard voiced strong objections to the arrangement imposed by the LCME. Some committee members at the meeting said that a few individuals grew angry and used strong language. Whichard questioned Fordham, without obtaining a direct answer, about his many public statements that he thought the ECU school should be closed down and all state-supported medical education concentrated in Chapel Hill. [42] After the meeting, Friday characterized Fordham's remarks as candid rather than negative. [43]

The *Greensboro Daily News* reported on Saturday, July 13, that on the day of the planning committee meeting, ECU Chancellor Dr. Leo Jenkins had pleaded again with Friday to leave management of the program in ECU's hands. Friday passed Jenkins's request on to the LCME, but the committee declined to authorize it. [44]

At both the committee meeting on July 11 and the Board of Governors meeting on the following day, President Friday said that no action on his proposal was needed. At the Board meeting, he said, "The time has come to end the discussions and get down to work and obey the law. I want to make clear this is the way all work (on development) is to move forward. There is no other way to move." He noted that the accreditation committee had reiterated that everything done on the ECU medical school expansion must be under control from Chapel Hill, and said, "They are not telling us what to do, but saying that whatever is done must come from here. I will make that clear in a memo to the chancellors."

He had instructed Dean Christopher Fordham to appoint a person to work full-time on the ECU campus during the planning stages, to report to Fordham, who would in turn, report directly to Friday. He told the board that Dr. Fordham had to have full authority to act, and that he (Friday) intended to be ready to report to the 1975 General Assembly as required by the law. All future reports would deal exclusively with the progress being made.[45] Friday also told the board that Dean Fordham should have full authority in planning the expansion of the ECU medical school, since he would be completely responsible for it.[46]

---

[1] *Greensboro Daily News*, January 11, 1974.

[2] *Raleigh News & Observer*, January 12, 1974.

[3] *Greenville Daily Reflector*, January 11, 1974.

[4] *Raleigh News & Observer*, January 12, 1974.

[5] Governor James E. Holshouser, Jr., 1974 Legislative and Budget Message, North Carolina General Assembly, January 17, 1974, 12:00 Noon. Text in ECU School of Medicine Files, Legislation series, Folder "1974 Message to the General Assembly."

[6] Link, pp. 234-5; *Raleigh News & Observer*, February 3, 1974.

[7] Link, p. 235; *Raleigh News & Observer*, April 17, 1974

[8] *Greenville Daily Reflector*, January 23, 1974.

[9] Rountree interview, October 14, 1991.

[10] *Greenville Daily Reflector*, January 25, 1974.

[11] *Raleigh News & Observer*, January 23, 1974.

[12] *Greenville Daily Reflector*, January 23, 1974.

[13] *Greensboro Daily News*, January 24, 1974

[14] *Raleigh News & Observer*, January 24, 1974.

[15] *Greenville Daily Reflector*, January 23, 1974.

[16] *Raleigh News & Observer*, January 23, 1974.

[17] *Raleigh News & Observer*, January 23, 1974.

[18] *Greensboro Daily News*, February 6, 1974.

[19] *Raleigh News & Observer*, February 21, 1974.

[20] *Chapel Hill Newspaper*, February 6, 1974; *Charlotte News*, February 7, 1974.

[21] Monroe interview, January 3, 1992.

22 Text of speech in ECU School of Medicine Files, Folder "MMPC-2."

23 *Winston-Salem Journal*, February 22, 1974.

24 *Winston-Salem Journal*, February 27, 1974.

25 *Charlotte Observer*, February 27, 1974.

26 *Charlotte Observer*, February 27, 1974; Link, p. 237.

27 Statement by Senator Ralph Scott, February 26, 1974. Copy in ECU School of Medicine Files, Folder, "Scott-Stewart Bill."

28 Link, p. 237.

29 Chapter 1190, 1974 Session Laws.

30 *Chapel Hill Newspaper*, February 27, 1974; Chapter 1190, 1974 Session Laws, adopted on April 8, 1974.

31 *Greenville Daily Reflector*, February 26, 1974; Greensboro *Daily News*, February 27, 1974.

32 *Raleigh News & Observer*, March 9, 1974.

33 *Raleigh News & Observer*, April 6, 1974.

34 Letter of May 23, 1974 from Senator Ralph H. Scott (signed by both Scott and Representative Carl J. Stewart, Jr.) to President William Friday. Copy in ECU School of Medicine files, Folder "Scott-Stewart Bill, Feb.- 1974."

35 Letter of July 22, 1974 from Reginald F. McCoy to Mr. J. P. Huskins, in ECU School of Medicine Files, Folder "J. P. Huskins."

36 Link, p. 239.

37 Letter from Dr. Glen R. Leymaster to William Friday, April 12, 1974, in ECU School of Medicine Files, Folder, "Liaison Committee on Medical Education."

38 Letters from William Friday to Dr. Glen R. Leymaster, April 29 and May 10, 1974, and to Leo Jenkins, May 10, 1974, ECU School of Medicine Files, Folder "Accreditation—Med School."

39 Letter of June 14, 1974 from Dr. Glen R. Leymaster to Mr. William Friday, in ECU School of Medicine Files, Folder "Liaison Committee on Medical Education;" King, pp. 186-7

40 *Greensboro Daily News*, June 15, 1974.

41 McCoy letter of 22 July 74 to J. P. Huskins.

42 McCoy letter.

43 Link, p. 239.

44 *Greensboro Daily News*, July 13, 1974.

45 *Greensboro Daily News*, ibid.

46 *Chapel Hill Newspaper*, July 30, 1974.

Chapter 13
Launching a Two-Year School

On July 16, 1974, President Friday wrote to Chancellor Leo Jenkins, Chancellor Ferebee Taylor, and Dean Christopher Fordham III, assigning full responsibility for planning and carrying out the joint UNC-ECU program to Dean Fordham. He was to report directly to Friday. To comply with the strictures imposed by the Liaison Committee on Medical Education, the ECU medical school would be administered as a component of the Chapel Hill medical school. Dean Fordham was to appoint a full-time director for the East Carolina University School of Medicine, with a faculty position at UNC-CH.[1] Complete responsibility for financial dealings were assigned to the director, including for initiation of requests for funds from the $15 million provided by the 1974 General Assembly for a medical science building and expanding the medical education program.

Board of Governors member Reginald F. McCoy wrote to Representative J. H. Huskins that the memorandum to Jenkins and the others seemed to present a "much harder position" than the one Friday had presented to the planning committee and the Board. The memorandum practically removed Drs. Jenkins, Monroe, and Wooles from the scene, leaving a two-year school entirely administered by the UNC group being sent to Greenville.[2]

When the demands of the LCME and the arrangements laid out in the July 16 memorandum became known to ECU supporters, there was a new furor. Two members of the ECU Board of Trustees, Robert Morgan and Robert Jones, called on Chancellor Jenkins to oppose President Friday's decision. Jenkins tried to calm them, and proceeded to meet with Dean Fordham to begin talking about specific plans for the medical school expansion. A search committee was to be set up for a full-time director for the program.

The UNC Board of Governors discussed regulations to prevent chancellors or other university officials from publicly disagreeing with established board policies without prior consultation with the chairman of the board and the university president. Unidentified individuals charged that these regulations were a response to Chancellor Jenkins's going over the head of the board in seeking the General Assembly's approval of the medical school in Greenville. The board postponed making a decision on the new rules.[3]

On July 22, Dean Fordham met with Chancellor Jenkins to discuss administrative arrangements, including reassigning Dr. Wooles to other duties, and the relationship of the Director and the School of

Medicine to the Vice Chancellor for Health Affairs.

On July 25, Jenkins telephoned to warn Friday that their agreement was coming apart. Dr. Cromartie had asked for Dean Wallace Wooles to resign and return to his position in the Department of Pharmacology. The ECU school's faculty and members of the board of trustees were vigorously opposed to the action. Dean Fordham's log of the ECU planning effort noted that Dr. Jenkins had earlier agreed with Wooles's resigning, and was reversing his position in late July.[4]

Encouraged by President Friday, Fordham flew to Greenville the following day to confer with Cromartie and Jenkins. While they were riding from the airport, Jenkins said that he felt Dr. Wooles was resistant to reassignment, and was supported by Robert Morgan and other ECU trustees. He said that he did not feel he could move ahead against all the opposition, although he understood the need for Fordham and Cromartie to have their own contingent to work with them. At the office, Fordham urged Jenkins to proceed with the reassignment of Wooles.

They were joined, Dean Fordham reported, by Vice Chancellor Robert Holt, Vice Chancellor Edwin Monroe and Dean Wallace Wooles, who were still antagonistic, and unwilling to forget what had gone before. Monroe said that reassignment of Dean Wooles would be a mistake. Fordham characterized Monroe's manner as "more or less inquisitorial," with the others chiming in. Monroe informed him that he was committed to a four-year school.[5]

The same day, Dr. Monroe wrote to Chancellor Jenkins about things that had happened during July and that seemed to him to rearrange and disrupt the established administrative structure "without due process." He presented four points:

> 1. The July 16, 1974, memorandum from President Friday to Chancellor Jenkins, Chancellor Taylor, and Dean Fordham removed the School of Medicine from any jurisdiction by the Division of Health Affairs, by Vice Chancellor Holt, or by Chancellor Jenkins. In effect, it removed a statutorily authorized school from the administration and governance of East Carolina University with no prior consultation with the Chancellor or Board of Trustees of ECU.
>
> 2. The specific directives in the July 16 memorandum contain no direct or implied actions to indicate that they were in keeping with the language of Section 46 of the 1974 Appropriations Act.

3. He had serious reservations about the removal of Dr. Wallace Wooles as Dean of the ECU School of Medicine.

4. He was completely familiar with the 1973 accreditation report and with the guidelines adopted in that year by the Liaison Committee on Medical Education, dealing with accreditation of two-year programs. He agreed that Dean Fordham did have ultimate responsibility for the medical education program, but not that this requirement should justify the removal of the ECU School of Medicine from the administration of the University or the removal of Dean Wooles from his position.[6]

On Monday, July 29, Fordham, feeling that in spite of his efforts matters were at a standstill, met with Friday, Raymond Dawson, and Felix Joyner, and told them that he found Monroe and Wooles reluctant to make a new start and proceed with the planning effort.[7]

That same day, Representative Horton Rountree said to an Associated Press reporter in Raleigh that he believed that Dean Christopher Fordham would appoint Dr. William Cromartie, who had been UNC's liaison with the ECU faculty since April, 1973, as the director of the Greenville medical school. Representative Rountree was concerned that Dr. Fordham intended to push aside Dean Wallace Wooles and Dr. Edwin Monroe and replace them with a director from the UNC campus. Dr. Wooles would hold only his position as chairman of the pharmacology department, and Dr. Monroe would no longer be Vice Chancellor for Health Affairs, but be relegated to head of the Allied Health programs, not related directly to training doctors. Rountree said that ECU officials hoped that Wooles or Monroe would be appointed director. Reporters attempted unsuccessfully to reach Dr. Wooles for his reaction.[8] Rountree also said that UNC officials had taken it upon themselves to merge the ECU medical school completely with the one in Chapel Hill. He said that this was not the intent of the General Assembly, and that a lot of legislators were disturbed by President Friday's decision.

When he was questioned about Representative Rountree's predictions, Dean Fordham declined to discuss them specifically, allowing only that he and Dr. Jenkins had been discussing plans for the ECU program. He said that there had been no final decision about personnel.[9] President Friday also denied that he knew of any decision made by Fordham regarding personnel at ECU.[10]

On the same day, Robert L. "Roddy" Jones, chairman of the ECU board of trustees announced that he was asking the state attorney general for a ruling on the legal status of the ECU medical school. Jones confirmed Representative Rountree's statement that Drs. Wooles and Monroe were being pushed aside. He said, "I would like to know if the legislature intended for there to be a typical two-year medical school program at ECU or if the intent was to make ECU a component branch of the medical school at Chapel Hill." He added that the ECU administration was left by President Friday's assignment of authority with no responsibility for its medical school other than maintenance and custodial services.

On July 30, a small tempest blew up that later escaped its teapot and turned into something of a tornado. On that day, Dean Christopher Fordham received a letter from Dr. Sylvanus W. Nye, Professor and Chairman of the Department of Pathology at ECU, expressing his concerns about the organization and administration of the medical school. He asked for an immediate decision on several matters which were important to him in deciding whether to remain on the faculty or not. He said that he thought the school's objectives should be improving the first-year program, and developing a two-year program within the next two and a half years. Nye thought a master plan should be developed immediately, supported by President Friday, and presented to the Board of Governors and General Assembly in 1978. The plan would call for funding a university medical sciences center in Greenville, to award the M.D. Degree, and to be completed and accredited in the mid 1980's.

He asked for some guarantee that funds earned from pathology services would be used only for Department of Pathology purposes, that the majority of members appointed by Fordham and Cromartie to the committee to plan expansion of the school would be ECU faculty. He also asked for assurances that the Director to be appointed would not be able to discharge him from chairmanship of the Department of Pathology for five years after his appointment. Nye sought written approval to request bids for two additional trailers for pathology, a personnel budget, with authority to fill four positions besides his own, and that his annual salary should be raised by increasing the portion derived from service income.

Fordham replied to Dr. Nye immediately that he understood his need for clarification and commitment. Since a great deal more work had to be done on the planning effort before a resolution was possible, he suggested that Dr. Nye in the meantime work closely with Dr. Cromartie. Later (August 12), Fordham asked Dr. Cromartie to answer Dr. Nye's letter also, which he did. Cromartie suggested Nye proceed to fill the two faculty positions then open in the Pathology

Department, and talk with him about additional steps needed to plan for the teaching program in 1974-75. He scheduled a meeting during the week of August 19 to discuss Dr. Nye's views on developing a pathology department in implementation of Section 46, and other questions he had raised.[11]

Finally, also on Tuesday, July 30, Dean Christopher Fordham returned to Greenville for his third conference in ten days with Chancellor Leo Jenkins on the future of the medical school.[12] They met privately for two hours over lunch, with no reporters allowed, and Fordham asked Jenkins to give him a statement or memorandum indicating the cooperative nature of their effort and his support.[13]

At the end of their meeting, Dean Fordham announced to reporters that he was appointing Dr. William Cromartie acting director of the ECU medical education program. Cromartie would report directly to Fordham, with no responsibility to ECU administrators. The *Greensboro Daily News* reported that Fordham wanted Dr. Edwin Monroe to give up all control over the medical program, and direct only the Allied Health and Nursing Schools. It also said that Fordham did not concede that the 1974 legislative mandate meant that a traditional second year of medical training would be added. As he interpreted it, the second year could be used for advanced clinical training for students from the medical school at Chapel Hill or elsewhere. Fordham's only comment on the issue was that the legislative mandate called for "innovative thinking" about the second year program. After the meeting, it was also learned that Fordham had refused to allow ECU officials to use any of the $15 million allocated by the legislature for development of the school. He said that such a decision required planning, and that could not begin until jurisdictional differences were settled. ECU officials wanted to purchase land that had become available for a good price near the new PCMH and have an architect begin designing the new medical science building.[14]

Dr. Fordham refused to make any comment about what effect the appointment of Cromartie might have on the position of Dean Wallace Wooles. He said that Dr. Jenkins would make a statement about that later in the week. He also stated that he had still not selected a person as permanent medical director at ECU, as he had been instructed to do by President William Friday.[15]

Friday told the *Chapel Hill Newspaper* on Tuesday that Fordham would appoint a new director in accordance with the conditions established by the Liaison Committee on Medical Education, which had stipulated that UNC must have full authority over the ECU school.

"The accrediting people view the ECU program as a constituent of the UNC medical school," he said. He and Chancellor Jenkins had recently requested permission from the LCME for the ECU administration to be put in charge of planning the expansion of the school in Greenville, and had been turned down. "In rejecting Chancellor Jenkins' and my proposal, the Liaison Committee required me to report to them on Jan. 1, 1975, as to what we had done to implement the conclusions in their report of April, 1973," Friday commented.[16]

Early on Wednesday, July 31, Chancellor Jenkins telephoned President Friday to tell him about the friction he was experiencing with the ECU Board of Trustees. He had tried to pacify Chairman Robert Jones, but had not been able to dissuade him from writing to Attorney General Robert Morgan to complain about the interference from the Liaison Committee and about President Friday's memorandum of July 16. Jenkins protested again about the memorandum of July 16. He charged Friday with being dictatorial.[17]

Jenkins said he was very tired of the whole problem, urged Friday to rethink his memorandum, and asked that Wooles should be permitted to stay on as Dean of the medical school.[18] Then he became calmer, and agreed with Friday to try to pacify Wooles by giving him another appointment.[19]

President Friday said that he would approve Dr. Wooles's appointment as associate vice chancellor for health affairs as soon as Chancellor Jenkins submitted a formal request. Wooles would continue as chairman of the pharmacology department. No approval by the Board of Governors was required for the change in his status.[20]

Representative Horton Rountree told a Greenville *Daily Reflector* reporter on that same Wednesday morning that the renewed problems about the ECU medical school had led him to consider calling for a special session of the General Assembly. He said, "It appears to me that the Legislature has given Friday too much power and it further appears to me that what he has done is turn aside to what the General Assembly reviewed and turned down during the fall of 1973." Rountree thought that something must be done immediately if the president of the University of North Carolina system thought he could completely bypass the trustees of one of its constituent institutions on issues involving more than academic instruction and financing. He said, "The General Assembly should possibly look to a specific session if necessary to call a halt to this type of maneuvering."[21]

Senator Ralph Scott commented, "What I'm after is a medical school at East Carolina and I'm holding Bill Friday responsible for getting it in, and not in 10 years either." Scott and Representative Carl Stewart agreed that they would prefer not to comment on the present controversy until they have had more time to consult with those involved. On the question of a full-time director of the ECU program, Scott said, he did think that Fordham would have to appoint the person whom he though could do the best job.[22]

Fordham's office announced, also on Wednesday morning, that Dr. Cromartie had asked not to be considered for a permanent position. His appointment to last only until a full-time director was recruited.[23]

UNC Board Member and ECU champion David Whichard called Jenkins Wednesday morning, and in a half-hour conversation, which Jenkins described as "exceedingly abusive and profane," accused Jenkins of selling out to Chapel Hill.[24] In a statement he made the same day, UNC Dean Christopher Fordham commented, "I am deeply disturbed by the regional polarization which has resulted from this continuing conflict. I would like very much to attempt to move ahead on a basis of cooperation with the chancellor and his supporters." He also called on Jenkins to support expansion of the medical school "in good faith." [25]

On Thursday, August 1, Dr. Wallace Wooles resigned his position as dean of the ECU School of Medicine. He said, "It is not without regret that I submit this resignation. For four long and difficult years we have worked continually to develop and expand the medical school. I acknowledge with thanks the continued support of the ECU administration as we all have worked toward a common goal of providing increased numbers of physicians to help meet the needs of the people of North Carolina." [26]

As Chancellor Jenkins and President Friday had agreed, Wooles was appointed associate chancellor for health affairs, and retained his position as chairman of the Department of Pharmacology. As a tenured professor, his faculty position was already guaranteed. On Wooles's resignation as dean of the medical school, Dr. Dean Hayek was named acting assistant dean.

Fordham had called Jenkins on Thursday morning, August 1, about critical remarks attributed to Jenkins in a news article. He said that he planned to talk with Jenkins again, but he left Chapel Hill for a vacation without contacting him. On his car radio, late in the afternoon, Fordham heard Jenkins's statement about Wooles's resignation.[27]

The *Raleigh News and Observer* reported that sources inside ECU had said that the administration of the university never expected Wooles to remain permanently as medical school dean, a position that is almost always occupied by an M.D. However, it had been anticipated that he would remain in the job for some time longer, probably until the school was ready to become a four-year program. Dr. Wooles had not been hired as dean of a four-year medical school, and had no reason to expect that he would stay in the position when the school was upgraded.[28]

Chancellor Jenkins held a press conference to announce Dr. Wooles's new appointment, and to respond, without direct reference to them, to Fordham's allegations. He said, "I want to assure you that I, Dr. Monroe, and Dr. Wooles are doing everything possible to carry out the wishes of the General Assembly and the people of North Carolina, in close cooperation with Dean Fordham . . ."

Jenkins said that Dean Christopher Fordham had requested that the expansion of the medical school should be carried out with his own team, and that "In keeping with the great spirit of cooperation, Dean Wooles unselfishly has offered his resignation." At the press conference, Jenkins took the opportunity to rebuke the press for reporting statements that he was not cooperating with Dean Fordham, without reporting statements that said the opposite. He said that Fordham had been given the sole responsibility to develop the program at ECU with his team. This was understandable, happened often in the business, professional and academic worlds. This meant, of course, that Fordham and his representative, Dr. William Cromartie, were now in complete charge of the ECU school. He also said that he wanted to emphasize as strongly as possible that there would be a first rate medical program at East Carolina University in accordance with the directive from the state legislature. "We in North Carolina have the need, the money, the ability, and the desire to accomplish this," he said. "Any detractors may as well pack their bags and let us alone." [29]

Dr. Edwin W. Monroe observed later that when Dr. Cromartie took over, Chancellor Jenkins began to withdraw from the fray. He said, "Leo, at that point, was looking ahead to only 3 to 4 more years before he had to retire. He had become more and more aware of how Bill Friday operated as his boss. They were superficially pleasant and courteous and hated each other's guts. Leo was getting very antsy about challenging Bill Friday's authority. He had stopped going to the legislative building in '71, as soon as Friday took over as Chief of the new university system. He would, down in his home territory, make challenging kinds of comments, but none up in that arena in Chapel Hill. He waffled at every opportunity." [30]

Jenkins said he wanted to discuss next with Fordham and Friday the question of whether the ECU medical school's faculty would be considered faculty members of ECU or of UNC-Chapel Hill.[31] Friday, in a separate statement, said that Fordham and Jenkins had met "in a spirit of cooperation and good will and made substantial progress in resolving problems."[32]

Dr. Monroe, interviewed by telephone on Thursday night, August 1, declared that it had never crossed his mind to consider resigning. He said that there were two issues that might appear unimportant, but would have very important bearing on the question of integrating the medical program with nursing and allied health education. These issues were, first, the degree of control that UNC would exercise, and second, what the status would be of the faculty already recruited for the medical school. Dr. Monroe expressed concern about the nursing and allied health programs that would still remain under the jurisdiction of the ECU Division of Health Affairs, if UNC took complete control of the ECU program. He also felt considerable uncertainty about the appointment of professors.[33]

Mr. Robert Jones, chairman of the ECU Board of Trustees, had posed the first question to the state attorney general when he asked whether UNC would have complete authority over the medical school, or just oversee it. Would Chapel Hill control faculty appointments, admissions, curriculum, and planning? The second question was equally complex: Would the faculty at Greenville be given appointments on the UNC School of Medicine faculty? Would they be given joint appointments to the two schools? Dr. Leo Jenkins said that he wished to have the medical school teachers belong to the East Carolina University faculty. It was by no means definite that this would be the case.[34]

The seventeen full-time faculty members in the medical program at ECU, all of whom had come to Greenville expecting eventually to be part of a medical school in full operation, were becoming discouraged from the continuing uncertainty. The interference by UNC with their planning and teaching and their sense that the Chapel Hill administration was intent on preventing development of a first-class program at East Carolina made them increasingly resentful. Especially galling to the people at ECU was Fordham's refusal to release any of the $15 million that had been appropriated for the school's expansion.[35] Suitable land had became available for a basic science building, at a low price, but they believed he had blocked its purchase.

The UNC News Bureau said in a news release that Dean Fordham had asked Chancellor Jenkins to be more cooperative in planning the expansion of the ECU medical school, and that he felt he could not proceed with the planning effort unless Chancellor Jenkins and his constituencies would support the effort in good faith.[36]

The ECU administration and faculty's mistrust was not illfounded. President Friday had worked, albeit behind the scenes, against establishing an independent medical school in Greenville. His capitulation to the legislature's mandate and short interim of cooperation with Dr. Leo Jenkins had been brought to an end with the LCME's rejection of ECU's self-direction. Even as Fordham and Jenkins contentiously maneuvered to reach some accommodation, it was increasingly evident to both sides that the situation was not improving.

Fordham's suspicions of Jenkins and his staff were at least as deep as theirs of UNC. He believed that Jenkins was treacherous, and that to hope for open and honest discussion with him was naive and impractical. Fordham was particularly distrustful of ECU officials, especially of Dr. Edwin Monroe, whom he thought never let pass an opportunity to undermine attempts to bring the ECU program under control from Chapel Hill. In his log, he commented on a letter which Chancellor Jenkins had sent to President Friday near the first of August that an agreement Jenkins mentioned had not been made. He said that Jenkins had not had the courtesy to discuss the matter with him, and that it was "frank treachery." He thought Ed Monroe might have composed the letter.[37]

Supporters of ECU were disturbed by the actions President Friday had taken. An editorial in the *Goldsboro News-Argus* said, "In the minds of many supporters of the ECU medical school, there can be but one interpretation: Dr. Monroe and Dr. Wooles, both key men in the school's survival, have been shot out of the saddle. There is an inherent distrust of Chapel Hill by the most ardent supporters of ECU and its medical school. And among many at Chapel Hill and elsewhere, ECU traditionally has been regarded with a presumption of inferiority and that allocations for ECU's development have been at the expense of UNC at Chapel Hill. These two attitudes have never made for compatibility."[38]

Equally caustic remarks were made by newspapers on the other side. The editor of the *Fayetteville Observer* of August 1 wrote, "Chapel Hill is now taking over control of ECU's medical school, in accordance with the directive [of the LCME]. The first move will be to remove the top officials of ECU's medical school, reassign them to positions more in keeping with their qualifications, and bring in a set of qualified administrators.

"Predictably, ECU is squealing like a stuck hog. The chairman of ECU's Board of Trustees is asking Attorney General Robert Morgan, an ECU advocate of long standing, for a friendly opinion on the legal status of the new medical school, particularly as it pertains to Chapel Hill's authority. Rep. Horton Rountree of Pitt, ECU's No. 1 cat's paw in the Legislature, is agitating, giving the heavy implication that if something isn't done to stop the takeover beforehand, the 1975 General Assembly will be asked to intervene. Rountree is also ranting that he doesn't give a Continental about accreditation, which says more about Rountree than about medical education. ECU Chancellor Jenkins so far has limited himself to wearing that familiar Giaconda smile." [39]

The *Durham Morning Herald* of the next day commented, "If accreditation is meaningless to Rep. Rountree, it is far from that to the students who will attend the ECU school. If they are trained in a school that is not approved by national medical authorities, they cannot practice medicine outside of North Carolina. Even more significant, it will mean that the Greenville school does not measure up to nationally accepted standards for medical training.

"The establishment of a medical school at East Carolina was, in our judgment, a mistake. But that issue has been settled once and for all, and it would be folly for the State of North Carolina to permit that school to be a third-rate institution. It would be an insult and a disservice to the people in the East and to the taxpayers all over North Carolina.

"All the other issues have been settled in favor of supporters of a medical school at Greenville. The only question remaining is whether it will be an excellent school or a third-rate school, and that, of all things, should not even be an issue." [40]

The sanguine conclusion of the *Durham Morning Herald* was premature. There were still plenty of questions. Dean Wallace Wooles's withdrawal did little to clear the atmosphere of mistrust that still hung on between UNC and ECU. Fordham complained to President Friday and Dr. Raymond Dawson that it would be naive to expect any frank discussions with Leo Jenkins, who was deceitfully working against his efforts. He noted in his log his intention to write an expression of distress to Jenkins, describing his "continued carping, especially in the public media during the planning effort as destructive and uncooperative." [41] The letter was apparently not written.

He briefed President Friday and Dr. Dawson on what he saw as continuing efforts by Ed Monroe and others to undermine everything that UNC attempted to do. The efforts to hinder were "regrettable, but apparently unstoppable." [42]

On August 2, Lieutenant Governor James Hunt wrote to President Friday pressing him to make the ECU program independent. He contended that it had been the legislature's aim to have a four-year school set up in Greenville. The UNC administration had, he protested, been holding up progress and keeping ECU out of the planning.[43] Friday talked with Hunt three days later, and attempted to satisfy him that headway was being made at ECU. He showed Hunt a letter dated May 23, 1974, signed by Senator Ralph Scott and Representative Carl Stewart, stating that Senate Bill 1072, which was substituted in committee for the House bill (Bill 1549), had not expressed any intent about a four-year medical school. Senator Gordon P. Allen of Person County had proposed to the Joint Appropriations Committee amending the bill to include instructions to the Board of Governors to develop a four-year medical school, but his amendment had been voted down. Section 46 of the appropriation bill (Senate Bill 977) had included the language of the substitute bill, without Allen's amendment or the phrase "additional degree-granting school" from the House bill. Senator Scott concluded that the decision on the four-year school would have to be made by a future General Assembly.[44]

On Wednesday, August 7, Senator Scott, appearing in Greenville on the WNCT-TV "Carolina Today" program, said that the bill directing the expansion of the one-year ECU medical school had intended for the school eventually to become a four-year degree-granting school. He was concerned that responsible plans should be presented to the legislature. He also said that the only persons responsible for planning the expansion of the medical school were President William Friday and Chancellor Leo Jenkins. They were working together to develop a meaningful program.[45]

On August 15, Vice Chancellor Robert L. Holt responded to a request made by Dr. Cromartie during the first week of August, and identified six persons who should be consulted on administrative questions. These were Clifton G. Moore, Vice Chancellor for Business Affairs; Edwin W. Monroe, Vice Chancellor for Health Affairs; Wallace R. Wooles, Associate Vice Chancellor and Chairman, Department of Pharmacology; John M. Howell, Provost; J. D. Boyette, Dean of the Graduate School; and Vice Chancellor Robert Holt himself. This group began meeting weekly, and was furnished with weekly reports on the progress of planning by Dr. Cromartie from September to October 21. They made up an advisory committee for Dr. Dean Hayek, the acting assistant dean of the medical school, as well as for Dr. Cromartie. The committee made recommendations in writing regarding the use of existing space on the ECU campus for the medical program, selecting an architect, organization of the faculty and administration, joint programs between the medical and other university programs, and the health affairs library.

The search committee for the director of the ECU medical school was announced on August 16 by Dean Fordham's office. The committee had a majority of one from the UNC School of Medicine faculty: five members were from UNC, two members were on the ECU School of Medicine faculty, and two Greenville physicians were appointed. The UNC members were Dr. William Cromartie, Dr. Robert Crounse, Dr. Logan Irvin, Dr. Frederic Dahldorf, and committee chairman, Dr. Daniel T. Young, professor of medicine at Chapel Hill. Four Greenville appointees included private physicians Dr. Earl Trevathan and Dr. Andrew A. Best, and two members of the ECU medical school faculty, Dr. Evelyn McNeill, assistant professor of anatomy, and Dr. William H. Waugh, professor of medicine. The announcement also said that the committee had not yet begun meeting to start the process of selecting and interviewing candidates, and that no date had been set for its report to Dean Fordham. He would make the final choice from the list of candidates which the committee submitted to him.[46]

Robert Jones, chairman of the ECU board of trustees, met with UNC Vice President Raymond Dawson, UNC counsel Richard R. Robinson, and assistant attorney general Andrew Vanore to discuss his request for a ruling on the right of UNC to control ECU's expansion plans. He had become convinced that there would be no point in filing a lawsuit. On August 20, Jones announced that he had withdrawn his request to the Attorney General, because he had decided the General Assembly should decide the fate of the ECU medical program.[47]

Seven years before, in August, 1967, a number of interested people from Pitt County—physicians, business men, and the Board of Trustees of Pitt County Memorial Hospital—had decided to propose building a new hospital. Expanding the existing facilities was also discussed, but they decided that this was not the best approach. Dr. Edwin W. Monroe began at least as early as 1968 discussing with hospital officials the needs that ECU would have for clinical training facilities, starting with those for the various allied health programs, and what might be required for activities associated with the Regional Medical Program of North Carolina. Monroe, other members of East Carolina College and of the Regional Development Institute were active in the planning. Especially after January 1969, Monroe conferred regularly with the County Commissioners, the hospital's Board of Trustees, its medical staff, and with Charles P. Cardwell, Jr., of the Medical College of Virginia, about the projected expansion of the hospital. When, in November, 1970, a bond issue was passed, and definite building plans were formulated, the needs of the medical program at ECU were taken into account.

Glenn Wilson, associate dean of the UNC School of Medicine, had come to Chapel Hill in the spring of 1970, for the purpose of helping the University set up the Orange-Chatham Comprehensive Polio Health Center. He became also the director of the Division of Community Health Services in the Dean's office, which became the Area Health Education program, during 1970-74. In the spring of 1972, he talked with the medical staff of the Pitt County hospital about an affiliation with Chapel Hill. His purpose was to set up a family practice residency under an Area Health Education Center. A number of such centers had already been set up across the state. Under the AHEC residency arrangement, every patient in the hospital was to be made available for teaching, and there was to be no compensation to the local physicians for giving their time to this. At the same time, the residents would take some of the pressure off the medical staff. Wilson carefully investigated the facilities and staff available, and in April, submitted a specific proposal. The hospital staff, citing the lack of time to give his proposal adequate study, voted against it.[48]

On August 20, Dean Christopher Fordham announced that the UNC planning staff were evaluating clinical facilities in the Greenville area, to establish the best way to expand the ECU medical school. More than half of the medical courses past the first year would require facilities for clinical teaching, so that the eventual proposal for the two-year teaching program would depend in part on the availability of clinical facilities.[49] When he was asked about the lack of clinical facilities in Greenville, the dean answered that it was one of the key factors. He would say nothing more on the subject, and refused to discuss details of the program whose planning was under way.[50]

After meeting with UNC officials to discuss an affiliation agreement between Pitt County Memorial Hospital and the ECU medical school, Jack Richardson, administrator of the hospital, said that limited clinical facilities at the hospital might make it "a little awkward" to add a second-year program at ECU until the new hospital was completed in 1976. The UNC and ECU planners had been discussing the role that PCMH might play in the expanded program, Richardson said, and there had been discussions of developing a third- or fourth-year program utilizing clinical facilities at other hospitals in the area, rather than a program for a second year in Greenville. In late 1975 and 1976 when second-year medical students from ECU begin to utilize the hospital for clinical training, the situation might become crowded. It would not, however, be impossible to manage temporarily until the new hospital was completed in 1976.

There had also been discussions between the school planners and hospital medical staff concerning the part that the physicians would perform in teaching medical students, and Richardson commented that although details had not yet been worked out, there was considerable enthusiasm for it among the medical staff. He also said that the discussions between planners and hospital representatives had not had the animosity that had characterized those between ECU and UNC planners. He had found the planners very cooperative and reasonable, and said, "I hope we can get down to serious business." [51]

The day after Richardson made his comments, Representative Horton Rountree remarked, "I think that East Carolina University, before Chris Fordham took over, had already analyzed the clinical facilities in the area. All Fordham has to do is look back over what East Carolina University has already plowed the ground on, and he could find out about all different types and kinds of clinical service in Eastern North Carolina. It looks like a foot-dragging thing as far as I'm concerned." [52]

On August 6, there was a meeting between Drs. Cromartie, Holt, Monroe, and Wooles, and Mr. Cliff Moore, ECU Vice Chancellor for Business Affairs, regarding the contract made with pathologist Dr. Sylvanus Nye. Wooles agreed to review the agreement signed with Nye concerning compensation for pathology services he provided to Lenoir Memorial Hospital in Kinston.

At the time Nye had joined the ECU medical school faculty, Drs. Charles F. Gilbert and Robert L. West were under contract with PCMH to provide autopsy and other pathology services. They declined to withdraw from their contract, although they were asked to. To make a pathology program for the medical school possible, it was necessary to set up Dr. Sylvanus Nye in some arrangement that would provide the necessary materials and practical exposure necessary for teaching. An agreement was made for him to provide pathology services to Lenoir Memorial Hospital.[53] Dr. Wooles did not think that Dr. Nye had voided his agreement, although he had written to state he was canceling it.

On August 21, Dr. Cromartie followed up the meeting in a memorandum to Vice Chancellor Holt, asking a series of questions about the contract with Dr. Nye. He wished to know if it was appropriate for a full-time faculty member of the medical school to enter into such a contract, and if this arrangement was consistent with University and State personnel policy. Had the contract been approved by all appropriate University authorities? Was the contract in keeping with the University's fiscal policies?

Dr. Holt replied that he thought the questions had been answered at the August 6 meeting, but since Dr. Cromartie did not share this view, he would say the following: The contract was approved appropriately, and would not have been allowed if it had not been approved. It was in keeping with the University's fiscal policies, and all funds and expenditures under the contract were handled according to procedures approved by the State Auditor's Office.

The contract between Dr. Nye and the Lenoir Memorial Hospital was to provide pathology service, a necessary and valuable adjunct to the pathology department and the medical school. It was important for teaching purposes, extremely helpful in collection of teaching material in pathology, and a valuable adjunct to the development of a pathology department. It had provided clinical experience for three full-time pathology faculty the year before, and one of them had been paid solely by funds generated by the contract.

Vice Chancellor Holt considered that under the circumstances in which the medical school had to begin, the contract was an appropriate arrangement. Dr. Cromartie had been asked to suggest alternatives, but had not suggested ways either to improve the contract or write one more advantageous.

Dr. Sylvanus P. Nye formally submitted his resignation to Chancellor Jenkins on August 27, 1974. Before accepting the letter of resignation, Dr. Jenkins told Vice Chancellor Holt he would like an investigation of the reasons for the resignation.

On August 30, Dr. Monroe wrote to Jenkins that he was concerned about Dr. Nye's resignation, which was, however, not a surprise, since he had said in May he would resign if the administrative and organization problems regarding the pathology program were not resolved satisfactorily. Monroe also pointed out to Jenkins that there were several basic issues still unresolved concerning faculty recruitment, curriculum planning, and the lack of funds for the Health Affairs Library.[54]

On September 4, Dr. Cromartie reviewed for Vice Chancellor Holt the background of Dr. Nye's resignation, and informed him that he had arranged with the Chairman of the Department of Pathology at the UNC medical school to provide instruction to medical students during 1974-1975. He said that he did not feel it was appropriate for him also to arrange a pathology course for allied health students, and asked that Dr. Monroe be informed of this fact.

On September 9, Chancellor Jenkins forwarded a copy of Monroe's letter to President Friday, urging that they should take a joint look for answers to the problem.[55] On Thursday, September 12, Dean Christopher Fordham, at a meeting in Washington, DC, received a call from Dr. Raymond Dawson concerning the letters. Later in the day Fordham called Glenn Wilson to discuss them, and after returning to Chapel Hill met with Dr. Dawson and later with President Friday for further discussions. The next day, Fordham and Wilson met to draft a reply, which they forwarded to Dr. Dawson. Fordham thought that the letter about Nye and other issues was regrettable, and confirmed absolutely his suspicions that Monroe was behind the poisonous atmosphere and unwillingness of Greenville people to consider any program but Monroe's.[56]

On October 5, State Representative Dr. John Gamble forwarded a letter he had received on September 20 from Dr. Charles P. Nicholson of Morehead City to President Friday. Dr. Nicholson had written about Dr. Nye's resignation, which he attributed to disgust with harassment from Chapel Hill and delays in approval to hire faculty, about the exclusion of ECU medical faculty from discussions with PCMH medical staff about curriculum planning, and the adequacy, despite Dr. Fordham's doubts, of clinical resources in the east.

Dr. Cromartie wrote to Dean Fordham on October 21 about drafting an answer to Dr. Nicholson's charges. Cromartie reported that he had concluded after a meeting held on October 16 that the contracts that Dr. Nye had with ECU and with Lenoir Memorial Hospital were not a sound arrangement. He also said that the ECU medical faculty had participated fully in curriculum development, and had been completely informed about discussions with PCMH representatives.

Again on October 28, Dr. Cromartie wrote to Holt about a report he had made to Chancellor Jenkins on October 24, in which Holt had said that Dr. Nicholson's statements were somewhat inaccurate, and that Nye resigned mainly because of not having pathology faculty to help him with teaching and service responsibilities. Cromartie felt that there had been no failure on the part of the UNC administration to communicate to Dr. Nye about his requests for more resources, the appointment of new faculty, and the definition of program objectives.

Although the Nye debacle was concerned with a single department, ultimately with a single individual, it consumed a great deal of time and effort on the part of Dr. Cromartie, Vice Chancellor Holt, Dr. Monroe, Dr. Wooles, and eventually Dean Fordham, Chancellor Jenkins, President Friday, and Representative Gamble. It took meetings, correspondence, and numerous telephone calls to resolve a situation in which it had perhaps been unnecessary for Dr. Cromartie to involve himself so deeply. The questions he raised about the contracts with Nye were arguably needless, and led to nothing constructive. On the other hand, Dr. Nye's frustration and his communicating over Cromartie's head with Dean Fordham had doubtless made Cromartie's involvement unavoidable. Most importantly, the case was emblematic of the general atmosphere of discontent at the lack of decisions and of clear lines of authority that interfered with the faculty's carrying out their assigned responsibilities.[57]

Although uncertain that their work would not be wasted, the ECU medical faculty continued its separate planning for expansion of the medical program from mid-July through October. The first meeting of the search committee for the director of the ECU medical school was to be held on Saturday, August 24. Dr. Daniel Young, chairman of the committee, said that the first business would be to draw up procedures for contacting prospective candidates.[58]

The third class of ECU medical students began work on the ECU campus on Monday, August 26, 1974. Dr. William Cromartie said that the medical faculty were busy welcoming the freshmen aboard. Dr. Dean Hayek, director of admissions at the ECU medical school, said that all of the students, seventeen men and three women, were residents of North Carolina. An orientation program was held in the morning, and classwork would begin on Tuesday morning at eight o'clock.[59]

Dr. Cromartie added that he perceived no barriers to meeting the requirements of the legislature and the LCME for expanding the ECU medical school to two years. Planning and expansion were moving along in a productive manner, he said, with work to be completed by November as planned.[60] The work was indeed to be completed by November, but not in a way that he seemed to have anticipated at the end of August.

On September 4, Dean Fordham presented to the Medical Education Liaison Committee of Pitt Memorial Hospital, along with a draft of the ECU medical faculty plan, a proposal which he said could meet the requirements of Section 46—it was a variation of the "Indiana Plan" that the Board of Higher Education had investigated in 1970-71. It would require at least 12 full-time clinical faculty members for the second year program, along with help from the PCMH medical staff, to achieve accreditation. He also presented to the ECU medical faculty and administration an outline of the alternative approach to implementing Section 46. Under this proposal the two-year program would be set up with students attending classes in Greenville during their first year and returning to PCMH for their fourth year. They would spend their second and third years in Chapel Hill, beginning their residencies there before rotating to ECU.

There was a general discussion about the law's requirements regarding minority students and family medicine, and of the demands on hospital beds. Questions were raised concerning contracts between the hospital and pathologists, about grants to subsidize hospital operation, and about possible timetables. Dr. Cromartie was asked to have the ECU faculty meet to consider the curriculum proposals.[61]

Dr. Cromartie asked Drs. Thurber (Physiology), Schweisthal (Anatomy), Waugh (Medicine), Wooles (Pharmacology), and Hayek (Administration) for their opinions of the two curricula being considered. The members of the Executive Committee of the ECU medical faculty sent Cromartie a letter expressing several concerns about the curriculum and about the process being followed in carrying out the expansion of the school. The faculty committee had not been involved in any stage of the planning, whether of organizational structure or curriculum. No effort had been made to recruit additional faculty. The UNC-CH and the ECU faculties did not agree regarding the program needed to meet the mandate of the General Assembly. There were other problems concerning space, indecision regarding policy, and use of funds.

On the day after Dr. Cromartie received the memorandum from the faculty, Dr. Robert Tuttle, Associate Dean of the University of Texas Health Sciences Center, visited as a consultant, and observed that he found "an almost overwhelming sense of distrust and rejection" on the part of the ECU people toward the UNC administrators.[62]

Not everyone found Dr. Cromartie a vexation. Dr. Robert S. Fulghum, who with Dr. A. Mason Smith formulated the proposal for permanent facilities in the Department of Microbiology,[63] said, "They sent Bill Cromartie down as the director of the program from their point of view. There was some conflict about who was really the boss. But Bill Cromartie was a gentleman, and things worked out very well. I'm not sure maybe all to Wally's satisfaction, but generally speaking things ran smoothly." [64]

Dean Fordham observed to his log on September 8, that he was disappointed at the meeting with PCMH on the Wednesday before. He felt that the local group was changing its signals, and was almost certain that he could detect Dr. Monroe's "heavy hand" in the background. It was clear that the Greenville people were only interested in adding a second year of medical education as a transition to a four-year school. There was no commitment to an innovative effort, even though it was especially designed to have meaning for the eastern part of the state, minorities, family practice, and rural health. Fordham said it was his own opinion, although other people at UNC shared it, that the prospects were discouraging of finding any program acceptable to Greenville.[65] All of the ECU faculty who were consulted about the curriculum reported that they did not favor a curriculum that did not add the second year of medical education to the one-year program already under way.

Dr. Cromartie had submitted the two plans to the Medical Education Liaison Committee of PCMH, and on September 12 heard from them. The MELC favored the ECU faculty's proposed curriculum for the second year over the more radical one that the UNC planners had offered. It was unanimous in considering the traditional proposal the most reasonable and logical.[66]

The curriculum plan developed by the UNC planners was not satisfactory to either the PCMH medical staff nor the ECU faculty, all of whom preferred to have the students complete the first two years of a conventional curriculum at ECU, then transfer to UNC for their last two, more clinically oriented, two years. Faced with such opposition, the UNC planners dropped the controversial plan and returned to a more traditional one for the second year. It was still not clear that there would be adequate clinical facilities at PCMH.[67]

1 Link, p. 239. Memorandum from William C. Friday to Leo Jenkins, July 16, 1974, Leo Jenkins Papers, ECU Archives.

2 Letter from Reginald McCoy to J. P. Huskins, July 22, 1974 ECU-Med School File, Folder "J. P. Huskins - MMPC".

3 *Raleigh News & Observer,* March 9, 1974.

4 Link, p. 239; William C. Friday Papers, Subgroup 1, Series 1, "Medical Education, June-Aug. 1974.

5 William C. Friday Papers, Subgroup 1, Series 1, "Medical Education, June-Aug. 1974", Dean's Log, July 26, 1974.

6 Letter of Edwin W. Monroe to Chancellor Leo Jenkins, July 25, 1974, in ECU School of Medicine Files, Folder "EWM Correspondence;" William C. Friday Papers, Subgroup 1, Series 1, "Medical Education, Nov. 1974," paper "The Planning Effort on the Implementation of Section 46, Oct. 31, 1974.

7 On July 17, 1974, Dean Christopher Fordham instituted a record which he called "Dean's Log on the Planning Effort for the Implementation of Section 46, July 17, 1974-November 7, 1974," in which he made entries almost daily. A copy of that log is in ECU School of Medicine Files, Folder "UNC Administration and Board of Governors." It is also found in William C. Friday Papers, Subgroup 1, Series 1, "Medical Education."

8 *Winston-Salem Journal,* July 30, 1974.

9 Associated Press, July 30, 1974, reported in *Asheville Times* and other newspapers.

10 AP report in *Statesville Record & Landmark,* July 30, 1974.

11 William C. Friday Papers, Subgroup 1, Series 1, Sept.-Oct. 1974, "The Planning Effort on the Implementation of Section 46;" Dean's Log for July 1974.

12 *Greensboro Daily News,* July 31, 1974; Dean's Log, July 30, 1974. There is a conflict between newspaper reports and Dean Fordham's log, which says the he and Jenkins had lunch in Chapel Hill, with Dr. Monroe "ordered" to attend by ECU Trustees' chairman, Robert Jones; Jenkins said he was not responsible.

13 "Planning Effort," October 31, 1974, William C. Friday Papers, Subgroup 1, Series 1, "Medical Education, Nov. 1974."

14 *Greensboro Daily News,* July 31, 1974.

15 *Greensboro Daily News,* July 31, 1974.

[16] *Chapel Hill Newspaper*, July 30, 1974.

[17] Link, p. 240, citing Friday's memorandum of record, July 30, 1974, William C. Friday Papers, Subgroup 1, Series 1, "Medical Education, June-Aug. 1974."

[18] Link, p. 240-241; William C. Friday memorandum of record, July 31, 1974, Friday Papers.

[19] Link, p. 240; Friday Papers.

[20] Link, p. 240; Friday Papers.

[21] *Greenville Daily Reflector*, July 31, 1974.

[22] *Greenville Daily Reflector*, July 31, 1974.

[23] *Greensboro Daily News*, July 31, 1974.

[24] Link, pp. 239-40; Friday Papers.

[25] *Tarboro Southerner*, July 31, 1974.

[26] *Greenville Daily Reflector*, August 1, 1974.

[27] Dean's Log, August 1, 1974.

[28] *Raleigh News & Observer*, August 2, 1974.

[29] *Asheville Times*, August 1, 1974.

[30] Monroe interview, January 3, 1992.

[31] *Raleigh News & Observer*, August 2, 1974; *Greensboro Daily News*, August 2, 1974.

[32] *Asheville Times*, Thursday, August 1, 1974.

[33] *Raleigh News & Observer*, August 2, 1974.

[34] *Raleigh News & Observer*, August 2, 1974.

[35] Wooles interview, November 13, 1991; *Greensboro Daily News*, July 31, 1974

[36] *Raleigh News & Observer*, August 2, 1974.

[37] Dean's Log, August 1, 1974; Link, p. 241.

[38] *Goldsboro News-Argus*, August 1, 1974.

[39] *Fayetteville Observer*, August 1, 1974.

[40] *Durham Morning Herald*, Friday , 2 August 2, 1974.

[41] Dean's Log, August 21, 1974.

[42] Dean's Log, August 26, 1974; Link, p. 241.

[43] Letter from James Hunt to William Friday, August 2, 1974, William C. Friday Papers, Subgroup 1, Series 1, "Medical Education June-Aug. 1974."

[44] Letter from Sen. Ralph Scott and Rep. Carl Stewart to President William Friday, May 23, 1974, William C. Friday Papers, Subgroup 1, Series 1, Medical Education, Mar-May 1974.

[45] *Greenville Daily Reflector*, August 7, 1974; *Greensboro Record*, August 7, 1974.

46 Dean Fordham's report to President Friday, November 8, 1974, ECU School of Medicine Files, Folder "School of Medicine Approval, inside Folder "UNC Administration and Board of Governors-2;" *Greenville Daily Reflector*, August 18, 1974; *Chapel Hill Newspaper*, August 18, 1974.

47 Link, p. 241; Associated Press, published in many newspapers.

48 ECU School of Medicine Files, Folder "Affiliation Agreement;" interview with Wilson, April 22, 1992.

49 Associated Press, August 21, 1974, printed in *Greensboro Record*, *Raleigh News & Observer*, many other newspapers.

50 *Raleigh News & Observer*, August 24, 1974.

51 *Raleigh News & Observer*, ibid.; *Greenville Daily Reflector*, August 25, 1974.

52 *Greenville Daily Greenville Daily Reflector*, August 21, 1974.

53 From notes on a conversation with Dr. William E. Laupus, October 26, 1995.

54 Jenkins Archives, letter of August 30, 1974 from Edwin W. Monroe to Leo W. Jenkins.

55 Copies of Monroe's letter and covering letter to Friday in Jenkins Archives.

56 Dean's Log, September 12, 1974.

57 The Nye matter is outlined in detail, with supporting documents, in the William C. Friday Papers, Subgroup 1, Series 1, Sept.-Oct. 1974, in "The Planning Effort on the Implementation of Section 46," and in Christopher Fordham's "Dean's Log on the Planning Effort for the Implementation of Section 46, July 17, 1974-November 7, 1974."

58 *Raleigh News & Observer*, August 24, 1974.

59 *Greenville Daily Reflector*, August 26, 1974.

60 *Greenville Daily Reflector*, August 27, 1974; story also carried by Associated Press.

61 William C. Friday Papers, Subgroup 1, Series 1, "Medical Education, Sept.-Oct. 1974;" Dean's Log, September 3, 1974 and September 8, 1974.

62 Link, p. 242; "Dean's Log," September 10, 1974.

63 "Planning Effort on the Implementation of Section 46," p. 42.

64 Fulghum interview, November 6, 1991.

65 Dean's Log, September 8, 1974.

66 "Planning Effort," p. 38.

67 Link, p. 242.

Chapter 14
Toward a Four-Year School

On Tuesday, September 10, 1974, a kick-off dinner was held at the Greenville Golf and Country Club for a fund-raising campaign, aimed at raising $1 million over a four-year period to help support construction of the new Pitt County Memorial Hospital. Lieutenant Governor James Hunt made a speech in which he said he believed that there were certain people in North Carolina who did not want to see the medical school at ECU succeed. They were, he said, "continuing to resist its expansion and the addition of a second-year program despite the mandate of the General Assembly that this be done."

He continued, "I would simply say to these people that this school is going to succeed. It is going to expand. It is going to become a full, four-year medical school, just as the General Assembly intended. And I would hope that the people who have for so long opposed the East Carolina University School of Medicine will now, in the wake of the most recent actions of the General Assembly, abandon their opposition and join with us in building the best medical school that we possibly can and putting it to good service for our people." [1]

Hunt's optimistic pronouncement rang hollow to the ECU faculty and administrators and to the planners from Chapel Hill. Tension between the two groups became higher and higher, with increasingly rancorous arguments between Monroe, Wooles, and other ECU administrators on one side and Fordham, Sheps and Cromartie on the other. Monroe found it difficult to communicate with Wooles, Hayek, and the ECU medical school faculty because of interventions by Cromartie and Fordham, who were "pushing hard on control." Monroe and Cromartie had shouting matches in Dean Robert Holt's office, which was in Spilman Building across the hall from Chancellor Jenkins's office. Jenkins held back from taking an active role in a situation which Fordham and the other UNC planners found just as intolerable as the ECU staff did.[2]

Chancellor Jenkins lost patience on September 10, 1974, and sent a memorandum to Dean Robert Holt, Cliff Moore, and Dr. William Cromartie, asking for resumés of the points covered at all meetings, typed and signed by all the participants. In a covering note to a copy of the memorandum sent to President Friday, Jenkins wrote: "Dear Bill: Sorry I had to come to this. I am hearing too many different versions of the same conference." [3] After seeing Jenkins's memorandum and the note to President Friday, Dean Christopher Fordham wrote to Dr. Raymond Dawson that they were a "direct affront to Dr. Cromartie's integrity, and unfortunately an ironic twist to the truth." [4]

On September 16, Fordham noted in his log that the messages from Greenville "tend to indicate a concerted, if not orchestrated, effort to discredit our work in Greenville." It seemed clear that only the ECU medical faculty proposal to implement Section 46 was acceptable to ECU faculty or the staff of Pitt County Memorial Hospital. President Friday's memorandum of July 16, 1974 was not being followed. The effect was to treat the UNC group's suggestions and opinions as unworthy of serious consideration, making the group "simply agents of the ECU faculty."

He concluded that virtually no plan other than the ECU plan was acceptable to the Greenville medical community. If a plan was not acceptable to that community, it was unfeasible there. However, the ECU plan failed to address minority opportunity and family practice in any effective way. Dean Fordham was gradually approaching the conclusion that the state perhaps should consider a four-year, separately accredited program, even though it was costly, would be marginally productive, and would block more promising alternatives.[5]

The Area Health Education Center concept that had been put forward as an alternative to expanding the ECU medical school was receiving national attention. During the second week of September, Dr. Clark Kerr, chairman of the Carnegie Council on Policy Studies in Higher Education and former president of the University of California in Berkeley, told the governors attending the Southern Governors Conference in Lakeway, Texas, that the US might be developing too many medical schools. He said that the country needed a vast increase in the supply of nurses and paramedical personnel. However, because of the present rate at which new medical schools were being developed, the country could run into a surplus of doctors in the 1980's.

When Arch A. Moore, Jr., Republican governor of West Virginia, challenged his statement, Kerr admitted that there was a great problem of distribution, but said that a response to the problem was developing area health education centers rather than adding new medical schools. He praised North Carolina, which had done the most so far in developing such centers.[6]

Frustration at the apparent lack of progress was not restricted to the planning panel and the medical school. In its September meeting, the East Carolina Board of Trustees passed a resolution asking for definite answers by October 28 from the UNC Board of Governors "to questions clouding the status of the ECU medical school." They asked for a report on the status of faculty, capital improvements, including the architect, land, and interim facilities, and on the objectives that were being sought at the school. Trustee Ashley B. Futrell of Washington, N. C., in introducing the resolution, said, "We are traveling on a road on which we know no destination."

The executive committee of the board commended Chancellor Leo Jenkins for his cooperation with Dean Christopher Fordham in the initial planning of the expansion.

In response to an objection from Dr. Edwin W. Monroe that making the medical school a component of the UNC-CH School of Medicine had caused budgetary problems for the ECU nursing school, School of Allied Health and other Health Affairs Division units, the trustees voted to ask for a separate budget code to be set up for the Division of Health Affairs. A committee was set up to formulate plans, consult with President Friday, and advise the Board of Governors about ECU's views and problems in developing the medical school. If the present stalemate in setting up the school continued, some trustees said, it would have to be resolved by the General Assembly.[7]

Earlier in the summer, Fordham had refused to allow ECU officials to use any of the allocated $15 million to purchase land near the new PCMH so that designing of the new medical science building could begin. Although Fordham, Sheps, and Cromartie were nominally in complete charge, by early in September Fordham still had not released the funds. He told Chancellor Jenkins and Robert Jones that he had passed their request to purchase land on to President Friday several weeks back, and that a decision from the Board of Governors, with General Assembly authorization of funding, was needed before a purchase could be made. The ECU Trustees would have to originate the request.[8]

Dr. Andrew Best of Greenville, chairman of the ECU trustees' site selection committee, recommended on September 12 to accept an option on property of nearly 50 acres adjacent to the new PCMH for the proposed ECU medical school complex. The option to purchase the land for about $7,000 an acre, or a total of about $338,000, would run until December 1, 1974. Best said the Old Stantonsburg Road location was "a prime site, the best available in the area" for locating the basic medical sciences complex for which the 1974 General Assembly appropriated $15 million. He said other possible land in the locality was much higher priced.

Dr. Edwin Monroe observed that the property had been evaluated by the medical school faculty and administration, and found to be the most desirable site. The land had been bought some months before by a group of Greenville doctors planning to use it for medical buildings and offices near the new hospital. They agreed to extend an option for its use by the medical school.[9]

Fordham did not reply to the site selection committee, but on the following day, President Friday told the Board of Governors that the UNC medical school officials were working with ECU officials on several aspects of the program in Greenville. These included, he said, searching for a permanent dean, availability of clinical facilities for training, and plans for building a medical sciences building at the Greenville campus. A report was being prepared on the expansion plans, for presentation to the board in October.[10]

The controversy intensified when, on Friday, September 13, Dr. Cromartie presented the UNC planning panel's proposal for an eight-year program for the ECU medical school, beginning after the sophomore or junior year in college, and running through a three-year residency in family practice. Students would spend their first and fourth years at ECU, and most of the second and third years in sophomore and junior courses at the UNC School of Medicine in Chapel Hill.

Chancellor Jenkins, after cursory examination of the draft, said the legislature intended a sophomore year should be added to the ECU school, and that only adding a second year to the medical school would satisfy the General Assembly's mandate. He also noted that the plan would mean only ECU undergraduates could enroll, since it would begin in the middle of ECU's undergraduate curriculum. He objected to this restriction on admissions.

Dr. Cromartie was interviewed by the *Raleigh News & Observer* on Saturday, September 14, and said that the proposed curriculum plan was at one end of a range of several alternatives being considered. The traditional second-year program proposed by an ECU medical faculty committee was at the other end. He said UNC would not push for a program unacceptable to ECU officials and medical faculty.

Senator Ralph Scott and Representative Carl J. Stewart, co-sponsors of the legislation ordering the school's expansion, were also interviewed, and both said that the legislature intended to establish a regular sophomore year, and not to add some other year to the ECU program.

Scott said he was willing to look at the plan, or talk about it with anyone, but there had already been enough misunderstandings about a lot of things. In answer to a question, he agreed that ECU backers were suspicious of the motives of UNC officials. "I've got a lot more confidence in President Friday than that. I think President Friday is going to make a conscientious effort to carry out the law, but if Jenkins opposes (UNC's plan) as not doing what they want, then I think the legislature is going to be more inclined to go along with him."

Stewart agreed there was a fundamental mistrust among many members of the General Assembly, with causes in history and in former problems. The legislators were suspicious of the kind of response the Board of Governors might make to the legislature. Stewart thought, as others in the legislature did, that the response of the Board would be along the lines of providing a traditional second year program. The legislature would consider an alternative plan if the UNC board could show that a good faith effort was being made, but anything other than a sophomore year would have to be justified very clearly.[11]

On Friday, Dr. Cromartie had said that the proposed plan could begin more quickly than a traditional one because of limitations on clinical facilities in Greenville. On Saturday, September 14, he emphasized to his interviewer that the draft plan was for the "initial phases of the expansion of medical education at ECU."[12]

Lieutenant Governor James B. Hunt, Jr., raised two questions about the draft plan:

1. Is it "what the legislature mandated?"
2. Does it "help break the bottleneck" that has been limiting the supply of doctors being trained in the state?[13]

On Monday, September 16, the *Greenville Daily Reflector* (of which David Whichard II was editor) commented about the "so-called plan" that the Chapel Hill medical administration, through Dr. Cromartie, had advanced in an interview with a reporter. The editorial said, "Even though the UNC board of governors was meeting that very day not even the board members were informed—in the meeting at least—of this so-called plan."

The plan was presumed to represent what Chapel Hill wished to do with the ECU medical school from the beginning: hold it to the existing one year program, and develop AHECs in Greenville and elsewhere for training senior medical students.

The editorial concluded:

> We believe that if Dr. Friday and Dean Fordham insist on
> attempting to proceed with this circuitous plan the answer is
> going to be loud and clear from the people of North Carolina
> and from the elected legislators. It will be that the 'plan' does
> not conform with the action taken by the Legislature earlier
> this year. They will be told that they must proceed with in-
> creasing the class size and adding the second year of medical
> education at ECU and developing an AHEC program at Pitt
> Memorial. It will be made clear that the funds were appro-
> priated for construction of a medical sciences building at
> ECU and that must be done.
>
> All of this should have been clear long ago and it was, to
> almost everyone in the state of North Carolina. Somehow,
> though, communication from the Legislative building to
> Chapel Hill seems to be difficult. If government is going to
> continue to work, however, all government agencies, includ-
> ing Chapel Hill, will have to comply with the legislation ap-
> proved by the General Assembly. We think that ultimately
> that is going to be done, even in this matter.[14]

On Tuesday, the *Greenville Daily Reflector* published a collection
of responses, mostly negative, to the draft plan for medical school reorganization that the UNC planners had proposed. The newspaper
said that ECU officials, state legislators and other leaders were concerned that the plan might not conform with the 1974 General Assembly's intentions when they authorized expanding the one-year
program at ECU. This was in part a reaction to Dr. Cromartie's
statement that the expansion plan being studied might not techni-
cally meet the legislature's mandate, but could be put into effect
more quickly than a traditional second-year program. The proposal
would not include a traditional second-year of medical school, but
would begin after a student's sophomore year of college. For two or
three years afterward, students would take classes related to rural
family practice, such as rural sociology, along as basic science
courses. The following two years they would be mostly at UNC-CH
medical school, then would return to Greenville for their senior year
and a three-year family practice residency.

Dr. Cromartie, questioned on Monday, September 16, about the
proposed plan, had said, "I would actually prefer not to comment on

this at this particular time. I think it has been given pretty full treatment. I don't feel we've made enough progress to have anything else to release. I think we will be moving ahead, and additional information will be released" when more progress has been made. "We were hoping to have a little time to let things develop." [15]

Chancellor Jenkins, having more carefully examined the draft proposal, still contended that only a traditional second-year class added to the ECU program would meet the General Assembly's mandate for expansion. He said, "I feel I'm honor bound to do everything I think is in keeping with the wishes of the General Assembly. I'm convinced the legislature had in mind the sophomore or second year, as a next step down the road to a degree-granting, self-standing medical school, and departure from this decision will have to be made by the legislature." Dr. Jenkins also noted that under the proposed plan, only ECU graduates would be able to enroll in the program. This was not in accordance with the legislature's intentions. [16]

Senator Ralph Scott, interviewed a second time about the UNC proposal said, "I couldn't understand all this new thing they are talking about. If it's agreeable with Dr. Jenkins, then it's agreeable with me. Otherwise, I'm expecting them to go through with the first year expansion and then get the second year accredited." He said it was the legislature's intention for a regular second-year program to be added at ECU. "All this other stuff they are talking about, I'll be glad to listen, and if it's agreeable with Dr. Jenkins, I'll go along with that. Otherwise, I wouldn't."

Scott said that he did not expect the ECU medical school to be an issue in the 1975 General Assembly unless the UNC planners did something that the legislature had not intended for them to do. He was confident that President Friday would do just exactly what the legislature had directed. [17]

David Whichard reported that nothing had been mentioned at the previous week's Board of Governors' meeting about the proposed expansion plan's not complying with the General Assembly's mandate. He said, "In my opinion, the General Assembly intended to expand the first year and add the second year. Friday has made the statement that he is committed to carry out the legislative mandate. Fordham has made no such statement. It would be my hope that Friday and the Board of Governors carry out the wishes of the General Assembly."

Dr. Edwin Monroe said the proposed plan was rather confusing, splitting the first year into two years. What he understood was that the intention of the General Assembly was to add the second year.

The elective student rotation and the family practice residency program were supposed to be the responsibility of the AHEC, and the Eastern AHEC was now involved setting these up. On the other hand, planning for anything relative to medical education was separate and apart from AHEC planning.[18]

Representative J. P. Huskins said that the legislature had authorized the enlargement of the first-year class and beginning a second-year program at East Carolina. It had appropriated $15 million to carry that out. Anything short of that did not meet his understanding of what the Legislature intended and did not satisfy him as a legislator. "From what Cromartie said, they're planning sort of a glorified AHEC program at East Carolina. That was a compromise the Medical Manpower Commission and the Joint Committees on Health rejected time and again during the debate in the Legislature. We could have had that at any time we wanted to accept it."

He had talked with a few other members of the legislature and found that they were proposing to wait and see what the Board of Governors actually proposed to do. If what they suggested appeared to subvert what the legislature intended, they could remove the program from the Board's hands and put it in the hands of a legislatively appointed commission to carry out the statutory mandate.[19]

Representative Horton Rountree said that if President Friday and Dr. Fordham and Dr. Cromartie would take the time the read Huskins's committee report recommending a two-year medical school at East Carolina, they would realize their present proposal did not comply with the legislature's intentions.[20]

Dean Christopher Fordham and Dr. William Cromartie said in a telephone interview that UNC planners hadn't found much interest in their unorthodox draft plan for expanding the ECU medical school. They were exploring the question of whether clinical facilities in Greenville would suffice for a conventional second year program, but had not yet made a final determination.[21]

On Friday, September 20, Glenn Wilson, AHEC Centers Program Director, and Dr. Edwin W. Monroe, as president of Eastern AHEC, Inc., signed a contract under which funds were to be provided to support EAHEC operations for the remainder of the fiscal year.[22]

The Medical Liaison Committee of Pitt County Memorial Hospital, after careful consideration of the pre-affiliation agreement offered by the UNC planners in August, came to the conclusion that it was not acceptable to allocate seventy-five beds for teaching under the administration of the ECU medical school. The agreement had proposed that, as a sufficient basis in clinical teaching for a traditional second-year medical program seventy-five beds should be designated as teaching beds. With this, the hospital would accommodate thirty to forty medical students, sixteen full-time clinical teaching faculty and two non-physician professionals, provide an outpatient facility, and six to eight pathologists. It was suggested that hospital staff doctors should be available for teaching, with individual exceptions if necessary.

Dr. Jack Wilkerson, chairman of the Liaison Committee, said the committee had made a counter-suggestion that the EAHEC provide the outpatient clinic, and that office space for the clinical teaching faculty be provided in the $15 million basic science building to be constructed, but that these matters were outside the committee's purview.[23]

PCMH administrator Jack Richardson said to a reporter after the committee's proposal was announced that before an agreement could be reached there was still a lot of clarification needed as to how patients were to be admitted and to what service. Medical school faculty would have admitting privileges, Richardson said, but the hospital administration and trustees did not feel it would be wise to designate specific beds.

Richardson also said some other points had to be ironed out before an agreement could be completed. More information was needed about what facilities were being planned in the medical school clinical science building, for the outpatient facility, and for office space for the teaching staff. In order to plan wisely for the use of hospital facilities, they needed to know what the funding plans were for the medical school's building.[24]

Dr. Wilkerson said in a telephone interview with the *Raleigh News & Observer* that the Medical Education Liaison Committee had a meeting scheduled for the night of October 1 to review its response to the agreement submitted by UNC officials to the hospital. The pre-affiliation agreement was based on a 400-page draft plan for the second year of training drawn up by the ECU faculty. Wilkerson said he had previously endorsed the "ECU approach," but not the plan's details. He said that the hospital's position had not yet been formally stated, but he expected the committee to recommend alternatives to two of the proposals in the pre-affiliation agreement. The committee would probably make the recommendation that no beds be designated, but all be available for teaching, if patients and attending physicians were willing. The question was jurisdictional; the committee felt that it was essential that the hospital retain administrative control over all its beds.

According to Wilkerson, hospital construction was about a month behind, so would not be completed in October 1976 as planned. The first students could be admitted for clinical training in the fall of 1977, he said. He also said that some of the hospital's staff very strongly opposed the UNC policy of paying hospital staff for teaching only after the first fifty hours a year, which were donated on a volunteer basis. With the reservations he mentioned, the committee was agreeable to providing the clinical facilities the agreement called for. There was no problem with the number of students, the medical school clinical faculty, an outpatient facility, pathology service, and staff availability for teaching. The entire hospital staff had given the committee a vote of confidence to proceed with the negotiations.[25]

Dean Fordham commented, "Pretty obviously you've got to have a teaching service if you're going to get accredited." Not having a clinical teaching facility would make it difficult to hire faculty. Since the hospital committee had not yet made its final decision, and he did not know just what they would propose, he declined to be more specific.[26]

Although it was becoming obvious to all the planners that their effort to reach an accommodation was a futile exercise, no one was ready to announce publicly that the attempt should be jettisoned. Dean Fordham was doubtful that anything positive was to be accomplished, however hard they tried. The ECU faculty continued to work stubbornly on a plan for expansion into the two-year medical program, for presentation to the UNC Board of Governors in October, as President Friday had promised.

On October 3, the Medical Education Liaison Committee of PCMH sent Dr. Cromartie a letter responding to the pre-affiliation agreement presented at the September 18 meeting, with copies to President Friday and UNC Board of Governors Chairman William A. Dees, Jr. The letter reiterated the hospital's primary goal of serving Pitt County residents, and endorsed the ECU medical faculty program. It said that no beds would be allocated solely for use by the faculty of the medical school. Dr. Jack Wilkerson, chairman of the committee, Dr. John Wooten, PCMH Chief of Staff, and Jack Richardson, administrator of PCMH, who signed the letter, said the committee unanimously supported the curriculum that had been proposed by the ECU medical school faculty. The curriculum was similar to those used successfully at other schools, was economical in terms of faculty and resources, and was more compatible with the expertise of the PCMH staff and with the hospital's resources than the suggested draft proposal. That draft did not appear to comply with the legislature's clear directions to add a sophomore year to the medical school. The hospital's Liaison Committee urged that the Executive Committee of the ECU medical school faculty should be involved in further deliberations about the school's program and PCHM's participation in it.[27]

Also on October 3, the committee to locate a director for the ECU medical school met, and heard Chancellor Jenkins proclaim that he believed the ECU program should be an independent one, with a dean whose primary loyalty would be to East Carolina. He counseled the committee to challenge UNC's exercise of power, to disregard the structure laid down by President Friday and Dean Fordham, and proceed toward establishing a four-year medical school. He said that he foresaw the possibility the General Assembly might mandate a change in the rules under which the committee was presently working.[28] Dr. Daniel Young called Dean Fordham on October 4, and reported what had been "virtually a shocking experience." He said that Chancellor Jenkins doubted the validity of the committee's authority to function, and complained about Friday's arrangements, whose necessity and legitimacy he questioned. Jenkins had said he might seek redress from the General Assembly in 1975. He had also said that expending funds for Cromartie's leadership was possibly illegal, because he (Jenkins) had not authorized their use. He intended to check this out with the state auditor.[29]

In a statement to a *Greenville Daily Reflector* reporter, Dr. John Wooten, chief of staff at PCMH and a member of the hospital's Medical Education Liaison Committee, repeated the committee's position against committing seventy-five beds to teaching, as recommended by the UNC planners. He said, "Pitt County citizens are building the new hospital, and we're not about to relinquish control of a large part of the facility before it's a reality. The ECU people tell us it's not necessary for the medical school to control the beds in order to teach in a hospital, and we know there are hospitals in the country used by medical schools which do not have such an arrangement.

"This is not to say that our answer now on this matter is our final one. Perhaps eventually, when the merit is shown, some arrangement can be worked out, but not now when things are so nebulous. We don't even have UNC's commitment to a two-year program, yet they're asking us to commit seventy-five beds." He said the committee would probably meet in a few days with Dr. William Cromartie.[30]

On Monday, October 7, at a meeting of his Advisory Committee on the ECU School of Medicine called to discuss the correspondence from the PCMH Liaison Committee leading up to their letter of October 3, Dean Fordham told the UNC-CH administration that he was almost certain that ECU would not accept any supervision by UNC, any changes, or any ideas. Any LCME team that might visit the Greenville campus would observe the hostility of the East Carolina faculty and administration toward UNC, which made very doubtful any cooperative arrangement between the two campuses with Chapel Hill in command. In his frustration, Fordham was beginning to wonder whether establishing a free-standing four-year medical school at ECU could be avoided.[31]

On Wednesday of the same week, Dr. Jenkins wrote an editorial for "Other Opinion" in the *Raleigh News & Observer*, to explain ECU's view of the intent of the General Assembly in the 1974 legislation. The essentials, he said, were expanding the first-year program, adding a second year, emphasizing family practice, and encouraging recruitment of racial minority students, while working toward full accreditation for the school. No plan, such as the curriculum recently proposed by the UNC planners, would be acceptable that did not comply with all of these requirements. Jenkins also wrote that Section 46 of the 1974 General Appropriations Act appropriated $15 million for a medical science building and directed the ECU medical school and UNC medical school to cooperate in seeking full accreditation of the expanded program. Discussions with President William Friday had led him to the assurance that he shared ECU's understanding of the mandate.

He wrote further that the tentative proposal from the UNC planning group, splitting the first-year program into two years, with fourth-year elective rotations at Pitt County Memorial Hospital, would circumvent the law passed by the General Assembly. It would not implement the specific recommendations of the Medical Manpower Study Commission and the Senate-House Health committees on which the General Assembly had based its decision to expand the ECU program to a second year and enlarge entering classes from twenty to forty as rapidly as possible. Plans developed several months before by the ECU medical faculty, when it was assumed they would be responsible for initial planning, were in full compliance with the Legislature's intentions. The faculty's plans were innovative and not merely traditional, and they should be given the opportunity to describe them.

The medical staff and trustees of Pitt County Memorial Hospital, he said, had been working for several weeks with UNC officials, to

reach a specific affiliation agreement that would provide for education of second-year medical students. Further, PCMH had joined fifteen other eastern hospitals to develop an area health education
center program. The board of directors of this Eastern AHEC had endorsed plans to establish a Family Practice Residency Program and
elective clinical rotations for senior medical students.

He said that ECU was ready and committed to working with UNC
to reach the common goal until accreditation was achieved. Jenkins
invited everyone, especially the press, to join in a positive approach
to developing the medical school, "to serve the needs of the people
and to become a model for the rest of the nation." [32]

In Chapel Hill the next day, Dr. Daniel Young, professor of
medicine at UNC-CH, and chairman of the search committee for director for the East Carolina University Medical School stated that the
list of candidates should be narrowed from fifty to two or three within
a matter of weeks. He said UNC planners hoped to have the director
on the job by July 1975, but he could not predict when the committee would present its recommendations. They were looking for someone with a sense of dedication to North Carolina, but not necessarily
a person from North Carolina, and wanted a medical doctor rather
than a Ph.D., Young said, because clinical knowledge was essential.
The director should have both teaching and administrative abilities.

The committee had received recommendations from ECU and
UNC faculty, deans of medical schools throughout the country, and
from answers to advertisements in professional journals. Candidates
were still being accepted. Young said that having the structure of the
school defined would make the committee's job easier, but they were
not trying in any way to influence the school's direction.[33]

No doubt remained that the four months of striving by Dr. Cromartie and other UNC medical school planners to carry out Dean
Fordham's charge from President Friday had been a failure. Section
46 had directed the Board of Governors (1) to expand the first-year
program at ECU, (2) to add a second-year program at ECU, (3) to
concentrate on training family care physicians, and (4) to encourage
recruitment and medical education of racial minorities.[34] The ECU
administration, the faculty of the ECU medical school, and more
compelling still, the legislators who had formulated the law were
feeling that Dean Fordham's efforts were aimed at getting around
rather than implementing the legislature's mandate regarding the
School of Medicine at East Carolina. They thought President Friday
had done everything he could to counter Chancellor Jenkins's goal of
establishing a medical school in Greenville independent of the UNC

School of Medicine in Chapel Hill. By now it was clear that there was nothing to do but accept the inevitable.[35] The Chapel Hill group were thoroughly frustrated by what they saw as the General Assembly's intention to hold them as hostages until they could wear the issue out.[36]

On October 7, Dean Fordham had reported that he and his team had been unable to formulate a program which would meet the requirements of Section 46, maintain control by the UNC School of Medicine, and elicit cooperation from the ECU medical faculty and administration. He raised the question whether the inescapable outcome might not be setting up a free-standing, degree-granting four-year school in Greenville.[37]

On November 8, he submitted *A Report to President Friday on Planning for the Implementation of Section 46*, in which he described the planning effort that had been going on from July through September of 1974. The program he finally proposed was explicitly the one which the ECU medical faculty had developed, and not what he and his planners had wished to offer.

The final results of the planning process were summarized in four points. First, Fordham cited a letter of October 11 in which ECU Vice Chancellor Robert L. Holt proposed modifying the administrative organization of the medical program to meet the requirements of the law. The ultimate responsibility for the program would remain with UNC in Chapel Hill. The authority for administering the program would be given to the ECU administration, with the chief administrative officer being a Dean rather than Associate Dean and Director. Fordham noted that this organization was similar to that which the LCME had already rejected.

Second, by the time the two medical classes reached fifty students each, there should be a medical faculty of sixty-six members, following a curriculum of the traditional variety, discipline-oriented. Of the faculty, six would be pathologists and sixteen would be clinicians.

Third, space requirements as outlined by the ECU medical faculty were submitted to President Friday's office, at an estimated cost of about $25,245,000. A preliminary estimate put the cost of the operating budget for the 1976-77 year at about $3.5 million.

Fourth, without identifying facilities, the ECU medical faculty plan called for the pathologists and clinicians mentioned before, two additional laboratory scientists, designating an inpatient teaching environment, and making a commitment to residency training. Dean Fordham noted that at the time of his report, hospital facilities for the clinical faculty and teaching were not available.

Fifth, carrying out the ECU faculty's proposal would necessitate constructing additional hospital facilities. Present planning for the new hospital did not appear to Dean Fordham to meet the requirements of the LCME for a teaching program. He could see no alternative to building a university teaching hospital if the legislature's mandate was to be fulfilled. A two-hundred bed hospital would cost at least $20 million, along with a substantial yearly operating budget. Additionally, Fordham concluded, "implementation of Section 46 as described will not add to the output of doctors for the state." [38]

When the Committee on Education Planning, Policies, and Programs and the Committee on Budget and Finance of the Board of Governors met jointly on November 8, 1974, President Friday had formulated a set of recommendations based on Dean Fordham's report and on the discussions that had gone on in the Advisory Committee on the ECU School of Medicine. He briefly reviewed his efforts to develop a medical education program at ECU under the direction of the Chapel Hill medical school, emphasizing the provisions of Section 46 of the Appropriations Act.[39] He described his initial agreement with Chancellor Jenkins to assign him planning responsibility, the LCME ruling that necessitated transferring responsibility to Chapel Hill, with Dean Fordham in authority, and the subsequent efforts to develop a curriculum and plan facilities for the two-year medical school.

Friday reported that the four-month endeavor to comply with legislative requirements to expand to a two-year program, meet the criteria of the LCME, including control from Chapel Hill, satisfy the faculty and administration of the ECU school, and achieve an affiliation arrangement with Pitt County Memorial Hospital had ended in a program proposed by ECU that would not provide the state with any additional physicians (because UNC would have to limit its own enrollment to make places for the ECU transfers). It would also require substantial expenditure for a teaching hospital. At the same time that PCMH had informed Dean Fordham about problems in reconciling its community service commitment with support of the medical education program, Dr. Cromartie had recommended to Dean Fordham that the ECU administration should be given authority to administer the medical school there. He also recommended that UNC in Chapel Hill should retain, in some obscure fashion not specified, the ultimate responsibility for the medical program.

President Friday then drew an unavoidable though hardly welcome conclusion that to implement Section 46 pointed directly to a further major step in the new situation, if the mandated expansion of the ECU medical program was to have any effect upon opportunities for medical education and upon the output of physicians. He proposed that the Board of Governors authorize the development of a four-year, degree-granting School of Medicine at East Carolina University, with classes increasing from thirty to fifty over the five-year period from 1975 to 1979, and culminating in a total enrollment of 200 in the 1981-82 school year. Funds additional to those already voted by the legislature would be needed, about $5 million for capital improvements, and $5 million a year for operations.

Upon approval by the Board of Governors of his recommendations, President Friday proposed to request immediately that the LCME set up an accreditation site visit early in 1975, with the purpose of separately accrediting the East Carolina University School of Medicine. Since their criteria provided for considering the accreditation of "new basic science programs in institutions with a commitment to establish a full M.D. program with their own resources or as part of a consortium," such an action by the LCME would be appropriate, and the Liaison Committee could take action by June 1975. Once accreditation was obtained, a construction schedule for the basic medical sciences building and the teaching hospital could be set up. If the LCME should decline to take the requested action, or ECU should be unable to proceed as scheduled, then the thirty first-year students could be enrolled in the UNC School of Medicine, with spaces reserved for them.

Friday closed with these words: "If these recommendations set forth above are approved and funded, we can increase the output of physicians and expand opportunities for medical education in North Carolina. If we go no further than the implementation of Section 46 as planned, no comparable benefits can be realized from the required investments of resources." [40]

A majority of the committee members found Fordham's and Friday's conclusions convincing, although there were protests. George Watts Hill, Sr., ever the opponent of the ECU school, supported President Friday's proposed implementation of Section 46, although he found the law "crazier than hell." Victor Bryant of Durham said a four-year program at ECU would "cripple the UNC School of Medicine." If adding a second year to ECU was not feasible, he said, the school should not be expanded at all.[41] President Friday replied, "If we do not move forward on the lines we suggest or something like them, I don't really believe we would be carrying out the legislature's intent." [42]

The final vote of the planning and finance committees favored his proposal, with only Bryant voting against it. ECU Chancellor Leo Jenkins, who was at the meeting, said, "This is what we should have done 10 years ago. I think we can develop a marvelous junior-senior relationship by complementing each other. The sophisticated and bizarre programs will be in Chapel Hill and the family care program will be in Greenville." He applauded the action, and said "we are now ready to move ahead and finish the job." [43]

During the following week, reactions to reports of President Friday's presentation to the Planning Committee were uniformly favorable. Several influential legislators reached by the Raleigh *News and Observer* on Monday said that the General Assembly was likely to go along with a UNC Board of Governors' proposal to develop a four-year medical school at ECU. Senator Ralph H. Scott said, "If the Board of Governors is for it, I don't think they would have any trouble." He said that providing the money all at one time could be a problem. For the UNC board to approve a four-year school at ECU, he said, "is smart all around, politically and because of the needs of the people."

Senator Thomas E. Strickland, D-Wayne, a member of the Advisory Budget Commission said, "I don't know if we can put it all in the budget this time. I don't think we even need to do it at one time."

Representative William T. Watkins, D-Granville, House majority leader in 1974, said a four-year medical school at ECU was just kind of what everybody expected, and that the General Assembly intended for ECU to go to four years. Everyone thought a two-year medical school would never be successful.

Representative C. Kitchin Josey, D-Halifax, predicted the General Assembly would authorize and direct that the four-year proposal be carried out. "I don't think we will be able to say we have a lot of money, therefore, you build it as fast as you can," he added.

Two UNC Board supporters said opposition to the ECU medical school would no longer be practical. Representative John W. Stevens from Buncombe County said, "They (ECU supporters) didn't have much trouble when they had opposition." He was not, however, quite ready to change his mind. President Friday's recommendation surprised him, and he felt he would have to examine the facts that the board members did before committing himself to any specific action in 1975.

Representative George Miller of Durham said that opponents of ECU expansion now had to be big enough to acknowledge that the legislature had decided in favor of expansion, and that from a practical and an economic standpoint, the board had little alternative but to recommend the four-year school.[44]

On November 15, William A. Johnson, Vice Chairman of the Committee on Educational Planning, Policies, and Programs (Chairman Dr. Hugh Daniel, Jr., being absent) reviewed the President's report to the planning and finance committees, which was made part of the Board's minutes under the title *The Expansion of the East Carolina University School of Medicine.* Then he made a motion, seconded by Dr. E. B. Turner, "That the Board of Governors authorize the development of a four-year, degree-granting School of Medicine at East Carolina University . . ." approving the schedule proposed in the President's report, and that the Board should recommend to the 1975 General Assembly the additional appropriations that were specified there. President Friday was to be authorized to take the steps necessary to carry out the expansion. William Dees, board chairman, said, "A lot of us have felt from the beginning there was no practical way to have a two-year medical program that would benefit the state. . . . There is something to the idea that a medical school program oriented to family practice is a different emphasis than the kind of medical training we are giving at Chapel Hill." The discussion on the proposal from the joint planning and finance committees of the board lasted more than an hour.

Chairman Dees commented that it seemed to him that a two-year program would not enhance the overall medical education program. Through adoption of the Committee's recommendation, the Board was saying to the General Assembly, "This is the only way to approach it."

Some Board members held that the cost would probably be a great deal more than the $50 million estimate presented by President Friday to the joint planning and finance committees. William Johnson estimated the school would cost more than $100 million in the end, if it was to be first class. Several members, including Charlotte banker Luther Hodges, Jr., had doubts that the state could afford to spend that much without diluting support to other schools.

Victor Bryant presented a lengthy statement in opposition, suggesting that the Board do no more than report the facts to the legislature, without any recommendation, since the legislature had initiated the expansion, and it should remain a legislative decision. Thomas J. White submitted a statement in favor of the President's proposal, as the first one that had been put forward that was fiscally sound.

When, after some further discussion, the motion was brought to a vote shortly after 11 a.m., it passed by a large majority, opposed only by Mrs. Albert A. Lathrop, Mrs. Hugh Morton, Mrs. George D.

Wilson, Victor S. Bryant, and Phillip G. Carson.[45]

Arnold King wrote, "President Friday was overheard to remark, after the approval of his recommendations, that the university could not tolerate a second-class medical school. If East Carolina was to have a four-year, free-standing medical school, he stated that he intended to do all that he could to make it an excellent school."[46]

As late as 1992, President Friday was still dissatisfied with the decision that was forced on him. In particular, he believed that it was a mistake to enter into an agreement to use facilities at Pitt County Memorial Hospital for teaching, rather than having the medical school establish its own teaching hospital. He said, "I didn't have any doubt about the need for the hospital—that had to be there. I think we made a bad decision in how we set it up administratively—it ought to be a part of the University and ought to have been from the beginning."

He said of the long struggle between Chapel Hill and Greenville over the ECU School of Medicine, ". . . the thing that I regret most about it was the politicalization of it. It was not settled as an academic question, never was from the beginning. And I tried desperately to keep the University of North Carolina out of politics. It's in the political process because it's a public institution, but it never should take sides, choose up or draw . . . You pay a terrible price in the public mind, though, when you go at an issue politically, I don't care which side you're on. You also draw strength away from the main campus. For example, here at Chapel Hill, when the decision was made to go to four years, I don't think they built a building on the main campus for seven years, because all the money had to go into the medical school."

Before making his decision to give up the joint planning effort, Friday talked with Senator Ralph Scott, telling him that the months of fruitless striving showed there could be no satisfactory solution on educational grounds. He told Scott, "It is clearly going to be resolved politically, so tell me what you want to do. Because . . . there's no point carrying this on any further. We've carried it on for months. There's a weariness out in the state that's bad for East Carolina, it's bad for the University. People are fed up with hearing all of this bickering, and we've got to bring it to an end." There was a clear possibility that all their exertions had been wasted. He added, "I just saw it all unraveling."

He thought that Chancellor Jenkins also realized this in the end, because things had gone too far, there had been too much tension on both sides, and too much acrimony. He said, "And then when I knew that it was going to happen, I went to see Senator Harrington. He and I had been friends. And I said, 'Now, Monk, you and I have been on opposite sides of this question. But I want you to understand something. If you legislate this, and you make it a part of the University, and we have anything to do with it, I want you to know we're not going to be second class. I want you to know that, if it's my job to oversee this in a general way, that we're going to do what is required down there, not only for accreditation, but for the people of the state who will be served by that place. We can't have second-rate operations when it comes to medical care. We don't do it anywhere else, we're not going to start down there. And I said now, if you want to have that understanding okay, but don't, when the yelling starts, and I come in here asking for moneys . . . I want you to remember this conversation.' Because I knew what was going to happen. And that's why I did it. He did, he accepted it, and we went from there." [47]

---

[1] *Greenville Daily Reflector*, September 10, 1974.

[2] Interview of Dr. Edwin W. Monroe, January 3, 1992.

[3] Jenkins Archives.

[4] Dean's Log, September 12, 1974.

[5] Dean's Log, September 16, 1974.

[6] *Raleigh News & Observer*, September 11, 1974.

[7] *Raleigh News & Observer*, September 12, 1974.

[8] Dean's Log, September 19, 1974.

[9] *Greenville Daily Reflector*, September 12, 1974.

[10] Durham *Sun*, September 13, 1974.

[11] *Raleigh News & Observer*, September 15, 1974.

[12] *Raleigh News & Observer*, September 15, 1974.

[13] *Raleigh News & Observer*, September 15, 1974.

[14] *Greenville Daily Reflector*, September 16, 1974.

[15] *Greenville Daily Reflector*, September 17, 1974.

[16] *Greenville Daily Reflector*, September 17, 1974.

[17] *Greenville Daily Reflector*, September 17, 1974.

[18] *Greenville Daily Reflector*, September 17, 1974.

[19] *Greenville Daily Reflector*, September 17, 1974.

[20] *Greenville Daily Reflector*, September 17, 1974.

[21] *Greenville Daily Reflector*, September 20, 1974.

[22] *Greenville Daily Reflector*, September 20, 1974.

23 *Greenville Daily Reflector*, October 1, 1974.

24 *Greenville Daily Reflector*, October 1, 1974.

25 *Raleigh News & Observer*, October 1, 1974.

26 *Raleigh News & Observer* and *Greenville Daily Reflector*, October 1, 1974.

27 Letter from Jack W. Richardson, John L. Wooten, M. D., and Jack W. Wilkerson, M. D., to Dr. William Cromartie, October 8, 1974, ECU School of Medicine Files, Folder "Affiliation Agreement with PCMH;" William C. Friday Papers, Subgroup 1, Series 1, "Medical Education, Sept.-Oct. 1974," *The Planning Effort . . .*', p. 38.

28 Link, p. 242; letter from Dr. Daniel T. Young to Dean Christopher Fordham, William C. Friday Papers, Subgroup 1, Series 1, "Medical Education, Sept-Oct. 1974."

29 Dean's Log, October 4, 1974.

30 *Greenville Daily Reflector*, October 7, 1974.

31 Link, pp. 242-3; Dean's Log, October 7, 1974.

32 *Raleigh News & Observer*, October 9, 1974, Editorial: "Mandate on ECU Medical School Must Be Carried Out," By Leo W. Jenkins; King, p. 188.

33 *Raleigh News & Observer*, October 10, 1974.

34 Senate Bill 977 [embodied in the Appropriations Act, Chapter 1190 of 1973-74 Session Laws].

35 Link, p. 243.

36 Glenn Wilson, cited by Link, p. 243.

37 Link, p. 243;

38 "A Report to President Friday on Planning for the Implementation of Section 46, Submitted by Dr. Christopher C. Fordman, III, Dean, School of Medicine, University of North Carolina at Chapel Hill," November 8, 1974, in ECU School of Medicine Files, Folder "UNC Administration and Board of Governors—2," inside folder "School of Medicine Approval."

39 General Assembly North Carolina, 1973 Session (2nd Session, 1974), Chapter 1190, Senate Bill 977.

40 "The Expansion of the East Carolina University School of Medicine: Recommendations of the President to the Committee on Educational Planning, Policies, and Programs and the Committee on Budget and Finance, Board of Governors," November 8, 1974. In ECU School of Medicine Files, Folder "UNC Administration and Board of Governors," inside folder "School of Medicine Approval;" see also William C. Friday

Records, Subgroup 1, Series 1, "Medical Education, Nov. 1974."
[41] Link, p. 243.
[42] *Raleigh News & Observer*, November 9, 1974.
[43] *Raleigh News & Observer*, November 9, 1974.
[44] *Raleigh News & Observer*, November 12, 1974.
[45] Minutes of the Board of Governors for November 15, 1974, William H. Friday Records, Subgroup 2, Series 2, Subseries 3.
[46] King, p. 191.
[47] Interview with William C. Friday, July 7, 1992.

Chapter 15
Through the Open Door

In late September or early October, 1974, the ECU medical school faculty and administration had heard rumors that President William Friday might stop fighting and accept what they believed to be inevitable. However, when he proposed to the Board of Governors in November that East Carolina University School of Medicine should become a four-year medical school, it was a surprise. They were taken aback in particular by the scope of his proposal. They had hoped to achieve the proximate goal of a two-year program, with further expansion to four years somewhere in the future. Now, unexpectedly, the President and the Board of Governors had recommended that the General Assembly fund the full expansion right away, had presented the best arguments for it, and requested the necessary funds.

President Friday's reversal was a mystery to Dr. Edwin Monroe, who speculated that it had taken place in response to pressure from legislative leaders.[1] Senator Harold Hardison was fairly sure that this was true, but remembered only one occasion when Friday had been pressed about the medical school. Senator Hardison, Senator Kenneth Royall, Senator John Burney and possibly Representative Horton Rountree had suggested to Friday that unless he released funds so Leo Jenkins could buy land and get on with the school, the appropriations to the entire sixteen-campus system might have to be "rearranged." That suggestion occurred in a conversation when they were sitting in front of the Brownstone Inn in Raleigh, probably too early to have entered specifically into Friday's November decision.[2]

Dr. Wallace Wooles thought that Friday had "fought this as long as he could. As soon as he counted the votes, and he knew he was beaten, he said, 'There's no way I can let this run over me.' So in fact he made the recommendation to make this a four-year school."[3] Dr. Raymond Dawson, when asked years later about the recommendation for a four-year school in Greenville, glided over the question of Friday's dramatic 180 degree shift with, "The decision had been made."[4]

It does not appear that President Friday was under any new and sudden pressures from legislators, nor that he was reacting to a tally of the members of the General Assembly. He was fully aware of the unremitting resistance from ECU medical faculty and ECU administrators, and of the support they had in the legislature. Dean Fordham's report of early November—the contents of which were no sudden revelation to Friday—made explicit that the strategy he had been following would not satisfy the requirements of Section 46 or those of the Liaison Committee on Health Education.

These requirements were in fact mutually contradictory. The initial plan of having Chancellor Jenkins direct the ECU medical program would have met the legislature's requirements. This was made impossible by the LCME's demand that control remain in Chapel Hill, which would unavoidably have eroded the effectiveness of the medical school there, taking up student slots without increasing the number of physicians graduated. The proposal approved by the Board of Governors and submitted to the legislature was probably the best available solution for East Carolina University, a victorious outcome to the long struggle to establish a medical school in Greenville. President Friday reluctantly accepted the political judgment of ECU's organized political supporters, in and outside the General Assembly, against what he believed to be the best educational judgment in the situation. He did not, however, compromise in the slightest his determination to preserve the University's excellence.

President Friday's capitulation could be, and was, interpreted as a defeat. If so, it was the loss of only a single battle. He and UNC did not lose the campaign; the medical school was consolidated into the University system, and its establishment ended both East Carolina's pressure to expand, and intervention by the legislature in University governance, at least for the time.

With the Board of Governors' decision, the field of action shifted. Chancellor Leo Jenkins lost no time in consulting the officials of the Liaison Committee on Medical Education. Toward the end of November, Jenkins announced in a news conference that he had talked with national accreditation officials, and foresaw no problems with accreditation for the four-year medical school in Greenville. He said he had "no idea" when the accreditation team would visit the school.

He acknowledged that accreditation had been a problem, but said that the Board of Governors' endorsement of a four-year school provided the support necessary for accreditation. In any case, the state had the authority and the ability to build the school, he said.

He informed reporters that a committee had been formed to search for a dean for the medical school, and that it would probably take "a couple of months" for the selection process. Jenkins said that UNC officials had dissolved the original committee because of the change in the conditions for the position. A different charge would be given to the new committee, which would seek not just a director for a limited program, but a dean for a full-fledged school of medicine. Jenkins said the dean would be someone dedicated to training doctors for family practice, and not "specialty conscious," and that ECU wanted to hire "the best qualified man in modern medical education today."[5]

Some of the members of the reconstituted committee were from the old group who had searched for a director of the UNC satellite medical education program, and some of the original panel's findings would be used, he said. UNC medical school professor, Dr. Daniel T. Young, who had been chairman of the earlier search committee, was to be an advisor to the new twelve-person group. Its members were Dr. Wallace R. Wooles, Associate Vice Chancellor for Health Affairs, and other ECU faculty members—Dr. Hubert Burden, Dr. James McDaniel, Dr. Evelyn McNeill, and Dr. William Waugh—ECU Trustees Dr. Andrew Best, Dr. Donald Copeland, and Troy Pate. Pitt County Memorial Hospital was represented by Woodrow Wooten and Drs. Frank Longino, Earl Trevathan, and Jack Wilkerson. Dean John M. Howell, Vice Chancellor Edwin W. Monroe, Vice Chancellor Robert L. Holt, and other members of the ECU administrative staff were to serve as nonvoting members. Dr. Wooles would have a vote on the committee only in case of a tie.[6] The search committee began meeting on December 2, met once more that month, and continued to meet each week through the first half of 1975, with few interruptions of their schedule. The committee considered more than seventy candidates, during a period when twenty-one medical schools were seeking deans, before settling on the two whom they referred to President Friday for decision.

One might anticipate that with the action of the Board of Governors in approving President Friday's recommendation, the campaign against the ECU medical school would have ended. This was by no means the case. There was still the possibility, remote though it might have been, that the legislature would reverse itself, or at least find that in view of the need for stringent budgeting, the Governors' recommendations could not be carried out. The carping and criticism from newspapers in the Piedmont, in particular the *Raleigh News & Observer*, continued with little, if any, abatement, with the ECU News Bureau and the *Greenville Daily Reflector* continuing their support of East Carolina.

The first salvo in the new stage of the struggle was reported in the *Daily Reflector*, which noted that there were some who felt the price tag of $50.2 million estimated by President William Friday was too low. With construction costs rising, it was said, many believed the $26 million recommended for building the basic science building and the $20 million for a 200-bed teaching hospital were unrealistic. It was recalled that Friday himself had said that the figures were conservative. Chancellor Jenkins responded that estimates the school might cost as much as $100 million were "scare figures," and that he had confidence in the $50.2 million estimate that President Friday gave. [7]

On the Wednesday before Thanksgiving, the Advisory Budget Commission confirmed that it had recommended that the ECU medical school be fully funded. In three days of closed meetings, the Commission had drafted a budget for the four-year school. It had also recommended a $3.8 million appropriation in the 1975-77 budget period for medical school operation.[8]

President Friday said that the school could graduate its first class of medical doctors as early as 1979, if it was accredited by June 1975. This would call for a tight construction schedule without delays. He also said he hoped the new dean would be on campus by July 1, 1975. He had, as he had stipulated, committed spaces at UNC so that ECU students would be able to continue their training even if the four-year school should be delayed.[9]

Just after Thanksgiving, a statement by First District Congressman Walter Jones appeared in the *Greenville Daily Reflector*. He said, ". . . a new and developing medical school is eligible to apply for federal funds to assist in its establishment, its facilities, and its operations." The school "must have reasonable assurance of accreditation, which I personally view as not difficult if a state authorizes the development of the medical school and provides for adequate basic funding for facilities and for faculty and staff. The developing medical school is eligible automatically for a direct capitation grant based on the number of students enrolled."

He said that he understood that the East Carolina School of Medicine had received a proportionate share the year before, through the University of North Carolina-Chapel Hill Medical School, based on twenty medical students enrolled at East Carolina. Because of the change implemented in the administration of the program, no capitation funds had been transferred to East Carolina for use during the current year.

The capitation grant program, he said, had been funded through the Health Manpower Training Act of 1971, which he was certain would be renewed during the upcoming congressional session. He also explained that there was another federal program, Special Projects Grants, which would provide funds to a medical school to innovate, to establish family practice programs, to increase enrollment from rural areas and from minority or low-income groups, and to train physician assistants.

Jones continued, "In spite of comments I have heard or read these past two years to the contrary, there are still federal funds appropriated and available to assist in the construction of facilities for a new medical school," he said. They "are not automatically doled out. Applications for them must be made and reviewed in competition with applications from other medical schools. My point is simply that a new and developing medical school is eligible to apply for federal funds to supplement the basic state funds appropriated to it. Let me emphasize, however, that the developing school of medicine must reach independent status to receive the maximum funds possible. This is one more reason for action leading to an independent medical school at ECU." [10]

The day after Thanksgiving, Steve Adams, a staff writer, wrote in the *Raleigh News & Observer*, "The expansion of the East Carolina University medical school is expected to be delayed by at least a year, even though the N. C. Advisory Budget Commission has recommended fully funding of the school, the *News & Observer* has learned.

"Unless ECU is able to develop plans for a four-year program more quickly than is expected, accreditation of the school probably will be delayed until 1976, according to reliable sources. If the expected delay occurs, ECU's present one-year medical program would be discontinued and students admitted to ECU for the fall of 1975 would be transferred to the University of North Carolina medical school at Chapel Hill."

Adams quoted one unidentified source as saying that to meet the proposed schedule of opening as early as June, 1975, ECU would have to move "in record time." Another source said that when he met with accreditation officials in Washington, ECU Chancellor Jenkins agreed to delay accreditation until 1976, contradicting his statement that there had been no firm decision on when to invite the accreditation team's visit. The newspaper could not reach the accreditation authorities by telephone, but in a telephone interview from Atlantic Beach, Jenkins had said the decision as to timing would be up to the school's new dean.

Adams continued by noting that before accreditation could be sought, ECU must hire several clinical department heads and make detailed curriculum plans. He also mentioned the possibility that there might be difficulties in getting approval from the North Carolina Office of Comprehensive Health Planning for the 200-bed hospital which accreditation authorities have said is necessary. He had talked with Lawrence Burwell, director of the state health planning office, who told him that he was concerned that building a new hospital in Greenville could draw patients away from other hospitals in the area and increase hospital care costs. Many eastern North Carolina hospitals were already operating below their capacity, and losing more patients could make it necessary for them to increase their fees, he said.

Without approval by Burwell's office, the hospital would not be eligible for federal reimbursement through such programs as Medicare and Medicaid. Approval was based on need, impact on other hospitals in a region, impact on health care cost, and the efficiency of the proposed hospital.

The article reported that President Friday had said on Thursday, November 28, that he stood by his statement to the Board of Governors that ECU could graduate its first doctors in 1979, assuming early accreditation and a tight construction schedule. It was in that same statement to the Board that Friday had said that UNC-CH might enroll the thirty first-year students if the ECU program was not accredited. He had also said on Thursday that construction on the planned teaching hospital and basic sciences building could not begin until the school had received at least provisional accreditation. Other "unidentified sources" told Adams, "It is unlikely that ECU will be awarded provisional accreditation in time to admit students in 1975 and the accreditation of ECU's one-year program is not expected to be renewed." [11]

The *News & Observer* article was widely quoted in newspapers all across the state. In response to the renewed furor about the medical school, Chancellor Jenkins, issued a statement about the medical school's progress toward accreditation. He wrote:

> The question of when accreditation will be granted for a four-year degree-granting School of Medicine at East Carolina University depends upon a number of factors. We are progressing as rapidly as possible toward fulfilling all conditions and requirements which we are confident will result in our achieving provisional and then full accreditation within the next year or two. The first step is to select a dean and I

have this week appointed a Search Committee which is already conscientiously pursuing this matter. In informal discussions with officials of the accrediting body in Washington, D.C., last Monday and in other conversations and correspondence we have been assured that we are approaching the matter of applying for and achieving accreditation in a manner which is both procedurally correct and expeditious. We have been assured of full cooperation and guidance by the accrediting officials and we are working as rapidly as possible to fulfill, step by step, each and all of the necessary requirements.

I see no cause at all for alarm about undue delay and I wish to remind the public of the many instances over the years in which our critics have attempted, unsuccessfully, to mislead, to undermine and try to block every effort we have made to provide this much-needed, urgently-needed addition to our state's medical education program. The people of North Carolina, through their collective voice and through their elected representatives, have made clear that they want a fully-acceptable, four-year degree-granting School of Medicine at East Carolina University, and we are pledged to that end. I can assure you that in spite of our detractors, we are going to move ahead. [12]

The *News & Observer* apparently felt a need for more support in its campaign against the ECU medical school than North Carolina could produce. At the beginning of December, staff writer Steve Adams was sent to Charlottesville, Virginia, to attend a conference of medical school officials on the national doctor shortage, sponsored by the Southern Newspaper Publishers Association. On December 2, an article appeared on some of the presentations at that conference. There was a consensus among attendees at the meeting, the article reported, that there was a shortage of physicians in rural areas everywhere. They could not come up with a solution for the problem, but did not think that simply educating more doctors was the solution. Lack of facilities and social pressures kept doctors from practicing in rural areas, they observed. There seemed to be agreement that new medical schools in this country might at least reduce the influx of poorly-trained foreign doctors.

Virginia state Senator Edward E. Willey, a conservative and chairman of the state senate's finance committee, said he thought that producing more doctors would drive doctors into rural areas because of competition in the cities.

Thomas H. Hunter, University of Virginia professor and former vice president for health affairs, declared wisely that doctors were not willing to practice where the facilities are inadequate. They either leave rural areas or take the attitude "I'll do the best I can, let them rot," he said. He said that rotating residents through rural areas provided only a temporary solution to the health care problems there. Also, when medical students were given loans repayable by practicing in rural areas, they chose instead to repay them in cash.

Two University of Virginia health officials who served on the Bennett Committee were in attendance at the meeting, and were interviewed. It appeared that they still stood by the panel's recommendations. Dr. Jules I. Levine, assistant dean for allied health programs, said the solution to inadequate health care in rural areas was not necessarily to provide doctors for every community. He said that even if producing more doctors meant that more would practice in rural areas, there was no evidence this would substantially improve the health of people there. He said that health indicators such as infant mortality were more closely related to family income and other socioeconomic factors than was the availability of doctors. Neither he nor the interviewer explicitly drew the conclusion his analysis implied, that it would be more beneficial to community health to raise family incomes than to provide them with more doctors.

The other Bennett Committee member, Dr. Kenneth Crispell, UVA vice president for health science, agreed with Levine. He said that when Argentina drastically increased its capacity to educate doctors, graduates who could not practice in urban areas emigrated to practice in urban areas in other countries, often in the US. That created a problem in this country, where doctors from other countries, often inadequately trained, already comprised about half of those beginning practice.

Dr. James F. Kelly, executive vice chancellor of the State University of New York, and former assistant secretary of Health, Education and Welfare, said that rotating young doctors for two-year stints on Indian reservations had lowered infant mortality there from a much higher level down to the national average. He had other things to say more useful to the *News & Observer*'s purposes, according to a second article on the Charlottesville meeting. He said that the projected operating budget of $10 million a year for the ECU medical school was about half the national average for facilities of similar size. The national average for constructing hospitals was about $150,000 per bed, where the UNC estimate for the 200-bed hospital in Greenville was $20 million, or about $100,000 per bed. This confirmed UNC President William C. Friday's recent acknowledgment that the $50.2 million estimate for expanding the school was probably too low.[13]

The work in Greenville on the new medical school went ahead steadily. On November 21, Dr. Wallace Wooles had received a call from Dean Harold Wiggers of the Albany University College of Medicine. Dr. Wiggers had been dean of the Albany, New York, school for twenty-four years, the longest continuous service of any medical school dean in the country. Having recently retired, he planned to move to Greenville where his daughter and her family lived. He had heard about the school's expansion, and offered to help in the endeavor. He had no interest in any kind of full-time position, but was willing to serve as a resident consultant or other such capacity. Wooles immediately told Dr. Edwin Monroe about the availability of Wiggers. Monroe arranged to talk with Wiggers when he came to Greenville in December to spend Christmas with his daughter's family.[14]

During the weekend of December 7, there was a meeting in Chapel Hill of North Carolina editorial writers. On Sunday morning, December 8, during a breakfast meeting with those attending the conference, President Friday gave a talk saying that he hoped that the UNC Board of Governors would be allowed to complete its plan for higher education without having its power curtailed. Just before the breakfast, he had heard from Representative Herbert L. Hyde of Buncombe County that a study commission of the General Assembly had been considering taking away the budgeting power of the governing board, negating its power to set educational priorities. The proposal being considered, the *News & Observer* learned from a source on the study commission, grew out of the East Carolina Medical School controversy.

Though he did not specifically discuss the information which Representative Hyde had given him, Friday told the editors:

> When the restructuring act setting up the UNC system was passed, it was stated that three to five years would be required to implement successfully the statutory requirements enacted by the General Assembly. The Board of Governors is in the third year of the implementation effort, and it has invested enormous time and energy in what has been, in my

judgment, a successful and accountable effort so far. I earnestly hope the board will be permitted to complete these significant and important legislative assignments and establish for the state a plan for higher education that is both sound and effective.[15]

On December 11, ECU announced that Dr. Harold C. Wiggers was being appointed as a senior consultant to assist in developing the four-year medical school. Among his responsibilities would be to assist in selecting a dean and architects for the new hospital and medical sciences building, in hiring key staff, and in planning the curriculum.

Dr. Wiggers was a native of Ann Arbor, Michigan. He had graduated from Wesleyan University and received his Ph.D. degree from Case-Western Reserve University in 1936. He attended the Harvard Medical School as a W. T. Porter Fellow of the American Physiological Society. Before becoming Professor and Chairman of the Department of Physiology and Pharmacology at Albany Medical College in 1947, he taught at the College of Physicians and Surgeons, Columbia University, at the Case-Western Reserve School of Medicine, and the College of Medicine, University of Illinois. In 1953, he became dean at Albany.

Dr. Wiggers was founder of the Albany, NY, Heart Association, chairman of the advisory group for the Albany Regional Medical Program, science advisor to the New York State legislative committee, and had been active on committees and councils of the National Heart Institute. His experience as a consultant to the National Institutes of Health for proposed medical school construction was a special advantage that ECU gained from having him join in the medical school effort.[16]

When he was interviewed in Albany by telephone after the announcement of his appointment, Dr. Wiggers told a reporter from the *Raleigh News & Observer* it would take a remarkable effort for ECU to win accreditation as an emerging four-year school in time to admit students by the next fall. But he added, "I wouldn't say it's impossible . . . I've seen some apparently impossible things happen."

Wiggers said he was such a neophyte to the accreditation process that he could not predict whether the program would be accredited by June. He agreed with Jenkins's earlier statements that little could be done before the new dean was named, and said that the dean could begin planning before he arrived in Greenville. Also, key faculty members could be named once the dean was appointed.

It was Wiggers's opinion that the ECU medical school was "no panacea" for North Carolina's rural health care problems. "I think the ultimate solution is going to be for doctors to learn to use physician extenders." He explained that this did not mean that producing more doctors would not be necessary, since paramedical personnel could work only under a doctor's supervision.[17]

The Advisory Budget Commission met in secret session on Monday, December 16, to consider the budget allocations for the ECU medical school. There had been speculation that the commission would reconsider a recommendation to allocate all capital improvement money to the school in the 1975-77 budget period. Senator Ralph H. Scott said Governor James E. Holshouser called the special session of the twelve-member commission, and was expected to make some recommendations to them.

The commission was expected to consider proposals to increase aid to private colleges from $200 to $400 a year per student. Scott said there might be other requests for the state university system. "If additional funding is recommended, it's hard to say where it'll come from. It's going to be hard because you've got to take it from someone."[18]

Chancellor Jenkins said ECU would not delay planning and the search for a dean of the medical school. "The planning must be done first. We do the planning, we continue the plan because we have the authorization and money is in the reserve to cover it."[19]

The *Charlotte Observer* reported that a source close to the budget commission had said the closed-door session was called because "what the budget commission has recommended allocates all capital improvement funding to the ECU medical school, leaving the other fifteen campuses without a penny. This includes the Charlotte campus, which is the fastest growing in the state. And the hike in state aid to private colleges should boil down to whether or not the hike should be scaled down and how to handle the allocation of capital improvement funds."

The Advisory Budget Commission, in a meeting of about an hour, rejected an effort by some of its members to trim $35 million from ECU medical school's $50 million recommended funding, leaving only the $15 million reserve. It shelved about $100 million in capital improvement requests from the other state colleges and universities, including a request for a $9.2 million building at UNC-C.[20]

UNC President Friday said on Monday that funding for top priority capital improvement items and salary increases for faculty and staff would be sought in the General Assembly. It was necessary to go back to the legislature because during the previous session the budget commission and legislature had bypassed the usual lump sum budgeting procedure for the university system. Instead of allowing the board of governors to set the priorities, the General Assembly had provided for the ECU and veterinary school requests by specific directives.

The UNC Board of Governors had recommended at least a twelve percent raise for faculty and staff, but the budget commission recommended only five percent for the two years beginning the next July. Funding was withheld for a major classroom building at NC State, a women's gymnasium at UNC-CH, and a new law school building at NC Central. It approved a $2 million increase in state aid to private colleges, and planning funds for a veterinary school.

A UNC-Charlotte spokesman said the office-classroom building the university had hoped to have funded the next spring was "so critical that we cannot make any appreciable increase in students until we have it." Friday said, "I view it as one of the major items of the University budget. That facility is badly needed." [21]

On December 19, Chancellor Jenkins announced he was setting up a fifty-five-member group he called the Chancellor's Advisory Committee on Medical Education, to counsel him on the planning of the medical school. The persons he invited to serve on this committee—there were actually sixty-two—were community and state leaders who had demonstrated time and again that they were supportive of the ECU project. Members included US Senator Jesse Helms and Senator-elect Robert Morgan, Lieutenant Governor James B. Hunt, Jr., NC House Speaker-elect James C. Green, former Governor Robert W. Scott, and state Representative Walter Jones. Jenkins named a number of other legislators, physicians, businessmen, and educators to the committee.

The editors of seven publications were included: Hoover Adams, editor of the *Dunn Daily Record*; J. Marse Grant, editor of *The Biblical Recorder* in Raleigh; Henry A. Dennis, editor of the *Henderson Daily Dispatch*; Joe M. Parker, editor of the *Ahoskie Herald*; Eugene Price, editor of the *Goldsboro News-Argus*; David J. Whichard, editor of the *Greenville Daily Reflector*; and H. Clifton Blue, editor of the *Sandhills Citizen* in Aberdeen.[22]

On Wednesday, December 18, the state Department of Revenue reported that revenues for November resumed their steady growth, reversing the downturn of the previous month that had given some legislators grounds to question whether funds would be available for the medical school. On the same day, the Board of Governors released $2.5 of the $15 million medical education reserve fund to ECU, for use primarily for planning. The board authorized $698,000 for planning a 200-bed teaching hospital, $853,000 to plan the $26 million basic science building, $55,000 for planning an outpatient facility, $50,000 to plan interim clinical and library facilities, $350,000 to purchase land adjacent to the new PCMH for the hospital and basic science building, and $550,000 to renovate Ragsdale Hall, a dormitory, to house the medical program temporarily.

UNC President Friday said the $2.5 million funding was needed if ECU was to have any chance of meeting the schedule he had recommended to the board of governors in November. Under his plan, the first students would graduate from the four-year school in spring 1979.

Dr. Ed Monroe commented on the board's action, "It is very gratifying that the Board of Governors and President Friday's office are just as interested as we are in trying to implement the November 15 action of the Board of Governors (which authorized the medical school), and we are proceeding with the necessary planning just as quickly as possible." He noted, "We have initiated a discussion process with the (Pitt Memorial) hospital authorities and county officials to help us determine what additional hospital resources are going to be needed." He noted that the university had an option on a fifty-acre tract of land west of the new hospital's site, but said two to three months of study might be needed to decide whether the land would meet the medical school's needs.[23]

The search committee for the medical school dean in its early meetings formulated a set of qualifications for candidates. They started from Chancellor Jenkins's charge in the letter he sent to each committee member, acknowledging his or her willingness to serve. Jenkins had said, "Your objective in this search is to identify the candidate with experience in medical education and medical school administration qualified to develop and to administer a degree-granting school of medicine. This candidate should be firmly committed to the concepts of the education and training of family care physicians and the recruitment and the education of minority students in medicine."

The committee decided that clinical training and a major interest in family medicine were needed, and sent letters to all the medical school deans in the United States, as well as to clinical academic departments, inviting nominations. They posted advertisements in the major medical journals, in the *Affirmative Action Register*, and in *The Chronicle of Higher Education*. They wrote letters canvassing the medical staff of PCMH for nominations and recommendations.

Early in 1975, they set up a schedule for initial two-day visits by candidates who, on the basis of their curricula and recommendations, were considered to be serious possibilities. During this visit, they were to meet the search committee members, university administrators, and the department chairmen already at work in the medical school, with as many other faculty members as was feasible. Candidates who were judged after their first visit to be good prospects were invited to visit Greenville again. On their second visit, candidates were scheduled to meet with local physicians and with local members of the legislature. President Friday was consulted, and indicated his interest in interviewing any serious candidate, and having UNC Vice Presidents Raymond Dawson, Felix Joyner, and John Sanders do so also. The committee interpreted this as meaning those who returned for a second visit.

Chancellor Jenkins informed Dr. Wooles on March 3 that he and the chairman of the ECU Board of Trustees, Robert L. Jones, did not want all the candidates returning for a second visit to be scheduled for interviews by President Friday and his staff. Only the committee's first choice from among the candidates was to be interviewed by the officers of the General Administration, unless Jenkins decided that the second and third choices should be taken to Chapel Hill.[24]

On March 20, Dr. Edwin Monroe granted an interview to the ECU student newspaper, *The Fountainhead*, which provided a capsule summary of the progress that had been made toward recruiting a dean for the medical school. In the interview, Dr. Monroe said that before the end of April at least two candidates for the post of Dean of the ECU School of Medicine would be recommended. The selection committee for the dean's post had been working since the first of December, and was narrowing the field of candidates to a few. He said they had reviewed the credentials of seventy to eighty candidates from around the country, had interviewed several prospects once, and some twice. However, the field had not yet been narrowed down to the final few.

Dr. Monroe noted that if the recommendations were made by the end of April, the new dean could be doing some work with the medical school by late spring. If the committee were to complete its work on schedule, it would be something close to a record for choosing a medical school dean. It usually took from eight to twelve months. The committee had been meeting at least once a week since it began its search in December, but had been hampered by the fact that twenty other medical schools in the country were searching for deans at the same time. He described the qualities the committee had sought in candidates: strong backgrounds in clinical medicine, medical education, administration, and attunement to the primary mission of the ECU school, whose emphasis was to be on family practice.[25]

Earlier in the year, Dr. William E. Laupus, chairman of the Department of Pediatrics at the Medical College of Virginia, had come to Greenville as one of three consultants brought in to assist in planning for teaching facilities.[26] The consultants agreed that ECU should not build a separate hospital, but work out an affiliation agreement with PCMH, and reported this to Chancellor Jenkins, Dr. Monroe and Dr. Wooles.

While Dr. Laupus was at ECU, Dr. Wooles, who had worked with him in Richmond, suggested that he should apply for the deanship of the medical school. He said that he felt Laupus would give credibility to the effort. Laupus had just completed working on a major project at the Medical College of Virginia—a planned addition to the MCV Hospital and thought that his contribution to MCV had probably peaked, and he needed to go elsewhere if he hoped to do much more. So, he submitted his name for consideration by the search committee. As he said, he felt he had one good general contract left in him before he retired. Dr. Wooles distributed copies of Dr. Laupus's résumé at the Search Committee's April 7 meeting, and the committee decided unanimously to invite him and his wife for a visit.[27]

On April 25, the Search Committee met to evaluate and rank the five candidates who had been called back for second visits, and to select two candidates to recommend to Chancellor Jenkins. Three alternates were included in the report to the Chancellor, but not recommended for consideration unless the first two did not work out. From the two proposed, Dr. Jenkins chose Dr. William Edward Laupus, and arranged to have him meet with President Friday and other members of the General Administration early in May.[28]

On June 4, Jenkins held a news conference and announced that the recommendation of the search committee for a dean of the ECU school of medicine would be considered by the UNC Board of Governors' personnel committee on June 18. Chancellor Jenkins, President Friday, and members of the search committee would attend the meeting. In a telephone interview from Chapel Hill, President Friday said that, depending on the committee's action, the recommendation could go to the full board the next day. He said he was in favor of the search committee's recommendation.

Both Friday and Jenkins declined to reveal the name of the leading candidate, or salary, working conditions and other details of the position, which would be negotiated later. The committee had recommended a leading candidate and several alternates, Jenkins said, and added, "If this doesn't work out, we will get another man." [29]

Chancellor Jenkins said on June 6 that he hoped the announcement of a dean for the ECU medical school could be made "right soon." He had met with UNC President William Friday the day before, to introduce a candidate for the position. Jenkins said, "President Friday and the candidate and I are studying the details of the appointment." He also said, "He is the only person we discussed. And I don't want to reveal his name at the moment." [30]

On June 13, 1975, Chancellor Jenkins announced that the UNC Board of Governors had appointed Dr. William E. Laupus dean of the ECU School of Medicine. His appointment was to be effective July 1, 1975, and he would assume full-time duties on August 1.

Bringing in Dr. Laupus, who had no enemies in either Greenville or Chapel Hill, made it possible to put an end to many political and personal conflicts that had plagued the campaign for the medical school. It had been unavoidable that the many skirmishes about large and small issues would generate a great deal of rancor. Laupus's recruitment provided an opportunity to go beyond the bad feelings and enmities generated out of a multitude of heated battles.

President Friday commented later, "I think the key to the whole business, and the one decision that really did enter into settling this whole issue, was bringing Bill Laupus there. His temperament, his background, his method of working—he and I hit it off with the first conversation we ever had. And I knew then that he trusted what I would say, and I trusted him. And we had to build on that. We had to create a new environment, looking toward the building of the school, because the other environment had so jaundiced so many people that no one was willing to trust anybody." [31] Laupus's first duties would be to select faculty members for the medical school and see that it met requirements for accreditation.

Jenkins said, "Dr. Laupus is not only a distinguished member of his profession but also is recognized as an outstanding medical educator and administrator. We sincerely believe that the selection committee and all those who have been involved in the careful and thorough search are to be congratulated and commended." [32]

Jenkins congratulated the search committee and everyone who had assisted them for doing a thorough screening and a careful selection procedure. He mentioned that the Personnel Committee of the UNC Board of Governors had acted on the appointment of Dr. Laupus before it went to the full Board. He said, "This has been a very tedious and complex procedure in addition to the many months of work necessary to find the right man for this very important task."

Dr. Laupus had been professor and chairman of the Department of Pediatrics at the Medical College of Virginia in Richmond since 1963. He was born in Seymour, Indiana on May 25, 1921. He earned his bachelor's degree at Yale University, graduated from the Yale University School of Medicine in 1945, and completed internship and residency at New York Hospital, Cornell Medical Center. He practiced privately for seven years in Detroit and Dearborn, Michigan, and was assistant pediatrician at Wayne University School of Medicine.

From Detroit he went in 1959 to the pediatrics department at the Medical College of Georgia, as an assistant professor, a position he held for about six months, then became associate professor for another six months before being promoted to full professor. From the start, he was also director of pediatric cardiology.

His department head in Georgia, Laupus said, "pushed me out of the nest" to become chairman of the Department of Pediatrics at the Medical College of Virginia in 1963. He also became chief of children's services at the Medical College of Virginia hospital, and in 1974, chairman of the Virginia Pediatrics Society.

Chancellor Leo Jenkins mentioned at his news conference in Greenville that Laupus had close ties to eastern North Carolina through his wife, the former Evelyn Fike of Ahoskie, and they had four children. The Laupuses had for some years owned a house in Kitty Hawk.

Early in his career, Jenkins said, "Dr. Laupus was cited for exceptional experience in opthalmoscopy of small infants and young children while [he was] engaged in research in Retrolental Fibroplasia at New York Hospital, Cornell Medical Center." He was president-elect of the American Board of Pediatrics and has been an official examiner of the board since 1966. He had authored or co-authored more than twenty papers and book chapters.[33]

When, on July 1, Dr. Laupus was appointed Dean of the ECU school of medicine, some of the people who most strongly opposed the expansion of the school said of him, "They got a pretty good man." Laupus replaced the strident boosterism surrounding the medical school during the ten-year battle for its establishment with cautious optimism.

A few weeks after his arrival, Laupus was interviewed for a profile in the *Raleigh News & Observer*. He talked about the advantages of living in a small southern town, and of attracting faculty from big cities that are no longer good places to raise a family. He thought that it was regrettable that there was a heritage of political controversy, because he would like to see everybody supporting the school now it was a reality. He needed time to work out the best ways to set goals and wished to avoid the stupidity of making extravagant claims that would be blown to pieces by an accreditation visit.

"We're trying to avoid having things set in concrete at this point, to avoid making hasty decisions," he said. "This takes some time and education on my part. In many ways, I was pleased to find that the program here is as advanced it is—after reading reports in the newspapers."

He thought that adhering to the September, 1976, schedule was reasonable, though he realized that many pieces had to fall into place in order to meet that goal.

About his decision to come to ECU, Laupus said, "I could give you all kinds of platitudinous statements about this. But really the things that appealed to me most were, first, the newness of the project; secondly the renewed emphasis on primary care; thirdly, the ability to function constructively in solving the health care problems over a large area; and, fourthly, I like this area of North Carolina generically." He was attracted by the golfing in the area, by fishing in streams, surf casting for blues, croakers, spots, roundheads, jack, and "an occasional pompano," His wife came from Ahoskie, only sixty miles from Greenville, and they owned a cottage at Kitty Hawk. He said he figured that the school would attract other medical educators for some of the same reasons he found Greenville attractive.

"I sincerely think there are a great many people in academic medicine who would like to move to this area," he said. "We emphasize first the uniqueness of the local situation in terms of an opportunity to participate in the planning and development of the new medical school and the advantages of living in a community the size of Greenville, with its educational and recreational opportunities. And we stress also the basic kinds of values that exist in a small southern city."

The medical school, he said, had been born out of the unavailability of health care in eastern North Carolina. Since 1900, there had been a search for a way to stop the flight of doctors away from rural areas. It had been generally agreed that doctors and their families avoid rural areas because of the lack of medical facilities, social and cultural activities, and other services.

The UNC Board of Governors held the same opinion when they voted in 1973 to oppose expanding the ECU medical school. They argued that educating doctors in Greenville would not increase the number of rural medical practitioners in eastern NC. They made the counter-proposal of establishing AHEC's to provide education for interns, residents, physicians already in practice, and other health care workers. In the EAHEC, based in Greenville, the alternative program turned into a cooperative arrangement with the ECU medical school.

"You know, there are a lot of communities that want to have health care that can't really support it," Laupus said. "I don't mean to be unfair, but they simply don't have enough people in some communities needing care to support a hospital setting. Most physicians prefer to practice near a hospital.

"From a regional standpoint, North Carolina is a very long state—do you say long or wide? Anyway, transportation and other things are really not as simple as people thought they were. When you get beyond fifty miles, regional health care systems begin to break down very quickly.

"Many organizations are part of the regionalization of health care. One alternative is to develop a medical school and regional health care system simultaneously. This is what I believe has been chosen as an appropriate goal by the people of eastern North Carolina. Pretty soon, we'll know how much the AHEC can do—we're partners."[34]

---

[1] Monroe interview, January 3, 1992.

[2] Hardison interview, March 26, 1992.

[3] Wooles interview, November 13, 1991.

[4] Dawson interview, June 10, 1992.

[5] *Red Springs Citizen*, November 27, 1974.

[6] Georgette Hedrick *Chronology* p. 71; *Greenville Daily Reflector*, November 27, 1974.

[7] *Greenville Daily Reflector*, November 28, 1974.

[8] *Raleigh News & Observer*, November 28, 1974.

[9] *Raleigh News & Observer*, November 28, 1974.

[10] *Greenville Daily Reflector*, November 28, 1974.

[11] *Raleigh News & Observer*, November 29, 1974.

[12] *Raleigh News & Observer*, November 30, 1974.

13 *Raleigh News & Observer*, December 2, 1974 and December 4, 1974.

14 Monroe interview, January 3, 1992.

15 *Raleigh News & Observer*, December 9, 1974.

16 *Greenville Daily Reflector*, December 11, 1974.

17 *Raleigh News & Observer*, December 12, 1974.

18 *Jacksonville Daily News*, December 16, 1974.

19 *Jacksonville Daily News*, December 16, 1974.

20 *Charlotte Observer*, December 17, 1974.

21 *Charlotte Observer*, December 17, 1974.

22 *Chapel Hill Newspaper*, Thursday, 19, 1974; ECU School of Medicine Files, Folder "Chancellor's Advisory Committee, 1974-75."

23 *Greenville Daily Reflector*, December 19, 1974.

24 ECU School of Medicine Files, Folder "Search Committee for Dean of ECU School of Medicine."

25 *ECU Fountainhead*, Thursday, 20, 1975.

26 Dr. William E. Laupus said on November 13, 1995 that the other two consultants were Dr. Lee Clough from the University of Florida medical school, who became associate director and later director of the Robert Wood Johnson Foundation, and Dr. Charles Eckert, a surgeon from Albany, NY.

27 From notes on a conversation with Dr. William E. Laupus, October 26, 1995; Minutes of the Search Committee for the Dean of the ECU School of Medicine, April 7, 1975.

28 ECU School of Medicine Files, Folder "Search Committee for Dean of ECU Med School."

29 *Raleigh News & Observer*, June 5, 1975.

30 *Greenville Daily Reflector*, June 6, 1975.

31 William C. Friday interview, July 2, 1992.

32 *Greenville Daily Reflector*, June 13, 1975.

33 *Rocky Mount Telegram*, June 14, 1975; Curriculum Vitae of Dr. William E. Laupus in ECU School of Medicine Files.

34 *Raleigh News & Observer*, August 10, 1975.

Chapter 16
Back into the Arena

By the time the General Assembly met in January, 1975, little doubt remained that it would approve the UNC Board of Governors' proposition in favor of a four-year, degree-granting medical school at ECU. There were legislators who raised the question whether, because of the economic recession and attendant low revenues, funds would be available to complete the project. With some members concerned about the shortfall in taxes, and some inveterately opposed to expanding the medical school, the legislature returned to a continuing controversy about the ECU School of Medicine.

There were those in the legislature who advocated reorganizing the UNC Board and removing its budgetary powers. On the other side, supporters of the Board, including Governor James Holshouser, were arguing that the legislature had already violated the Board's authority in the 1974 legislative session when it overrode its recommendation not to expand ECU's medical school. Holshouser did not conceal his opposition to the school, even after the Board gave up its resistance and agreed to President William Friday's proposal of expanding it to a four-year program. Perhaps the Governor did not believe that, by prolonging its resistance to the legislature's clear intentions, the Board might permanently undermine its viability.[1]

James B. Hunt, Jr., who as Lieutenant Governor appointed Senate committees and controlled their assignments, predicted that the legislators would reassess the role of the Board of Governors, because of concerns about the coordination of higher education. He said, "I've talked to enough (legislators) to know nobody wants to go back to the old days with everybody in here lobbying for everything." Control of the community college system by the Board of Education and not the Board of Governors, he said, had led to absence of a coherent policy regarding allocating resources to higher education. Hunt favored a study to determine what the needs and resources were, and this might, he said, lead to a change in the administration of higher education—he would not speculate about what sort of change.[2]

After a meeting of the Commission to Study the Elimination of Waste in State Government on Friday, January 3, 1975, some of its members said that the commission would not recommend to the General Assembly that it should refrain from reinstating its authority to add or strike some priority items from the UNC board's budget request. The proposal to impose these limitations on the board was a result of the legislative battle over the ECU medical school, a source close to the commission had said.[3] In spite of the conflicts of the previous year, the legislature was, as Hunt had said, not prepared to return to the bad old days of rivalry between the various colleges and universities in different areas of the state, with the political maneuvering that had resulted.

In an interview published in the *Chapel Hill Newspaper*, Dr. Edwin W. Monroe said it was not surprising to him that some people were still opposed to ECU's medical school. "Just about every new med school faces vigorous opposition from the already established med schools." He also said it was unfair to compare startup costs at ECU with costs in other parts of the country. "You have to remember we are an established institution," he said. "If we were to go out in the middle of nowhere and try to start a Duke University, then the $100 million cost for starting a med school under those conditions *might* be correct. But that's not what we're talking about at ECU."

Dr. Monroe said he believed the $50 million figure mentioned by UNC President William Friday was valid. He also observed that when critics actually learned what was being accomplished at ECU, their complaints subsided. He mentioned Dr. John Gamble, legislator from Lincoln County, who had strongly opposed the medical school, but who, after visiting the campus and seeing firsthand what was being done, had became a staunch supporter of the program.[4]

On the night of Monday, January 20, the Advisory Budget Commission presented to the General Assembly its recommendations to provide funds for expanding the ECU School of Medicine. About $17.5 million of new funds were proposed for the 1975-76 budget to use in building ECU's basic science building, and $21.5 million were to be used in 1976-77 for construction of a teaching hospital. The $15 million reserve already appropriated would make available a total of $54 million for capital expenditures at the expanded medical school. In addition, the Budget Commission allocated $4 million for operating expenses.

No money was specifically recommended for new building at any other university campus, though $23.8 million for the current year and $30.7 million for the following year were included for unspecified capital expansion, with the Board of Governors to decide on its allocation.[5] The Commission also recommended only $14.6 million for renovations and repairs on the other fifteen campuses.

There were immediate complaints. Dr. Charles Lyons, Chancellor of Fayetteville State University said that his institution and others in the UNC system would suffer substantial setbacks in development if the legislature approved the Advisory Budget Commission's proposals regarding funding the ECU medical school expansion. He said, "East Carolina's Medical School will unquestionably require a substantial amount of funding. However, if that funding is done by channeling funds from other institutions, those campuses will find their development grinding to a halt." [6] While avoiding direct criticism of the Advisory Budget Commission, chancellors at the schools whose requests had been cut out of the budget request began quietly lobbying the legislators from their districts. They expressed their concern that their schools might be forced to limit enrollment if the new buildings were not funded.[7]

On the following Friday, H. Horton Rountree, Representative from Pitt County, noted that the entire $54 million set aside for the medical school by the Advisory Budget Committee might not be needed because of arrangements still being discussed with Pitt County Memorial Hospital for locating clinical training facilities in the new hospital. If this could be done, it would be unnecessary to use all of the $20 million budget for a teaching hospital. Representative Rountree said, "There is no doubt but what money is tight in the General Assembly this year, but the base budget people are cutting some funds. I think in the final analysis, there will be sufficient funds to get started with the four-year med school at ECU."[8] The next day, he commented further, "Let's face it, we're not increasing the number of first year medical students. There's got to be a four-year med school in Greenville. I think the Legislature believes this to be the case. The question will be, in my opinion, how much of the $35 million [that will be needed beyond the $15 million already in reserve] we'll get. There could be some savings if we could dovetail the med school program with existing facilities, rather than having to build a new teaching hospital." [9]

Chancellor Jenkins said it would be premature to say that the $20 million would not be needed, but it might be a possibility, and East Carolina would welcome any means of saving money.[10] A few days later, he announced that he and other officials involved in planning the expansion of the medical school would be meeting in Raleigh on Wednesday night, January 29, to discuss whether any money could be cut from the budgeted $54 million. About $20 million of the proposed appropriation had been earmarked for a 200-bed teaching hospital, but Jenkins said that the planners would be looking into the possibility of replacing the teaching facility with an added wing at the PCMH. The medical school planners were divided over the question of building an independent teaching hospital or utilizing the facilities in the county hospital.[11]

Jenkins said that a firm decision would be up to the dean of the medical school, still not selected at the time, to the accreditation officials, and the hospital staff. "If there can be any economies, ways to cut the cost, the decision will be made." [12]

At the meeting on Wednesday of the Chancellor's Advisory Committee on Medical Education and the medical school planners, Dr. Edwin W. Monroe said accreditation officials had convinced him and other ECU administrators that the full $20 million allocated for a teaching hospital would be needed, even if some arrangement could be worked out with PCMH about clinical teaching there. At the same meeting, Chancellor Jenkins said the $35.2 million 1975-77 appropriation for ECU's four-year school was "absolutely essential." He told the Advisory Committee, "We must have assurances of adequate appropriations before such a school can be accredited. We will, of course, explore all possible avenues and approaches to use the appropriated funds wisely.... The time has arrived to provide the bricks and mortar in terms of the full amount of the recommended appropriations." [13]

On Sunday, March 2, 1975, Senator Tom Strickland, an ECU supporter and member of the Advisory Budget Commission, told a reporter from the *Raleigh News & Observer*, "There are other worthy projects, for sure, but somewhere we have to set priorities—and the ECU medical school is the top priority." He and other legislators said that money for the North Carolina Central University law school was a major concern, and the chairmen of three committees of the legislature came out in favor of appropriating money for a new building for the law school.

It appeared very unlikely that money could be found for the thirteen other buildings given high priority by the UNC Board of Governors. Among these were a $10.4 million general academic building at NC State University, a $5.3 million womens' physical education facility in Chapel Hill, and a $45.2 million business and economics building at UNC-Greensboro.

Representative Lane Brown III of Stanly County said, "In the normal course of events, other projects would have been funded routinely. But ECU is a single-shot deal and because of that—and a tight budget—other things just had to be affected adversely. . . . The philosophical debate over ECU is over. But maybe the economic debate—especially this year—should now begin."

The Budget Commission's decision to recommend no new capital funding other than that for the Greenville campus continued to stir up a flurry of activity in and outside the legislature. Representative Mickey Michaux of Durham prepared a bill to require financing of the North Carolina Central University law building. In doing so he broke away from the normal procedure for handling requests from the Board of Governors for specific projects. He took as his precedent the procedure for handling the ECU medical school's funding. Faculty and students at UNC-Charlotte started a letter-writing campaign to the Mecklenburg legislative delegation asking them to push for funding of the classroom-office building that campus had requested from the Board of Governors.

Some legislators wanted to go so far as to challenge the ECU appropriations, an effort that supporters of the medical school believed was bound to fail. Senator Strickland said, "We've been at it for ten years. I realize that this is a tight budget year, but there's really no argument left—we've been waiting so long, this year it's our turn to have the top priority."[14]

UNC Chancellor N. Ferebee Taylor told the board of trustees that Chapel Hill would bear more than a fourth of the $73 million decrease recommended in the university's budget by the state Senate's appropriations subcommittee. That subcommittee had voted the week before to raise in-state tuition by $200 and out-of-state tuition by $300, and to eliminate funds for increased enrollment. Their proposal would also require the university system to give up to the state $5 million, including surplus grant money and Chapel Hill utility revenues amounting to $3.4 million. Another subcommittee recommendation would end the practice of charging in-state tuition rates to students recruited for special talents and given special scholarships, including athletic scholarships.

Taylor protested that freezing enrollment would block expansion of the medical school by thirty medical students next year and another thirty-eight the following year. "It is inconceivable to me that a General Assembly so conscious of the state's need for physicians would knowingly deprive the state of, in essence, eighty-eight more medical students," he said.

The UNC-CH trustees named a six-member committee chaired by state Senator Hargrove "Skipper" Bowles of Greensboro to lobby against the proposals. Bowles said "the further along something like this gets, the harder it is to stop. What we ought to do is point out some specifics and the way to do that is on an individual basis. What they're doing is painting with a very broad brush and we need to point out some of the specific problems."[15] Specifically, what needed to be pointed out was the impact of the cuts on individual legislators' districts.

The many discussions about the budget kindled interest in the expenditures for salaries at the ECU medical school, and how they compared with other state salaries. State Budget Officer S. Kenneth Howard said that maximum salary levels for clinical department chairmen were set in the budget at the same level as those at UNC-Chapel Hill medical school, $52,000 a year. This compared favorably with the highest state employee salary, that of Dr. N. P. Zarzar, director of the Division of Mental Health Sciences, who was being paid $49,536 a year, according to a report prepared by state budget officials for the General Assembly. Dr. Zarzar's salary was paid entirely from state funds, however, and an ECU faculty member receiving $52,000 would earn part of his salary from fees for treating patients.

According to the budget office, the second highest state salary was that of Dean Christopher Fordham, who received $49,000 a year; third highest was Dr. Jacob Koomen, state director of health services, at $48,601 a year; fourth was President William Friday, with a salary of $48,500; and Governor Holshouser was fifth, at $38,500. Both Friday and the Governor were provided with housing and other expenses, while the doctors were not.[16]

A confidential source revealed to the *Raleigh News & Observer* that UNC President Friday had told the Board of Governors personnel committee in a closed meeting on January 10 that until 1979, when the medical school's hospital would begin to generate revenue, ECU doctors' salaries would have to be paid from state funds. He had set the salary for the dean of the ECU medical school at $38,000-45,000, though Chancellor Jenkins, he said, had requested a range of $48,000-$58,000. Friday said his recommendation was based on the salary range of deans of other southern medical schools, and that he would reconsider this range in the spring when new data became available. He also said that while the maximum was set at $45,000 a higher figure could be negotiated to recruit a particular individual.

Chancellor Jenkins said in a telephone interview that the salary for the new dean would be negotiated and, "If the salary does not fit the man, he probably wouldn't take the job." He said he had interviewed four candidates and would interview several more. He expected to announce an appointment about March 15. He said he was very impressed with all the candidates.

Friday had told the Board that the maximum salaries for clinical professors at ECU would range from $27,000 for instructors to $51,000 for full professors and $52,000 for department chairmen.

The average salary would be much less than that. Jenkins request had ranged from $27,000 for instructors to $58,000 for department chairmen.

The maximums set by President Friday were the same as those at the UNC medical school, except for the dean's salary. The average clinical instructors' salary in southern medical schools was $15,000 a year, and the average clinical department chairman's was $46,000. Medical school deans ranged from $32,000 to $57,000. The maximum salaries for basic sciences faculty at East Carolina ranged from $16,500 for an instructor to $44,000 for a department chairman.[17]

Revenue forecasts for the state at the end of March were increasingly pessimistic, and the General Assembly was steeling itself for tough choices to make in order to balance the budget. Lieutenant Governor James B. Hunt, Jr., said that everything was in question, and that almost any item in the $6.89 billion budget for 1975-77 might be cut. The $20 million hospital planned for ECU medical school, a five percent raise for state employees, and many other large and small items had to be scrutinized.

Governor James Holshouser withdrew his recommendation to repeal the sales tax on food in response to the impact of the recession on the state's revenue. He said his figures showed there might be $100 million less than expected over the two years beginning July 1, 1975.

An analyst in the legislature's Fiscal Research Division, Lloyd O'Carroll, projected that the revenue shortfall might range from $225 million to $382 million over the next two years. Another economist, Al Smith of North Carolina National Bank in Charlotte, predicted the deficit in the state's total revenue during the current budget year and the 1975-77 period might be more than $300 million. Both House and Senate committees were looking for places to cut, but there was not enough "fat" in state programs to provide places to cut as much as $300 million. There was speculation that the $20 million teaching hospital at ECU might be in for some cuts.

Lieutenant Governor Hunt said he would prefer for the medical school to use the existing facilities at PCMH rather than build a new teaching hospital. The $15 million budgeted for the rest of the ECU school was less in doubt, Hunt said, and would probably survive any budget cuts. The legislature could reject such continuation increases as the nearly $26 million budgeted to handle increased enrollment in the UNC system.[18]

"At the moment there are no federal funds available that we are aware of for a teaching hospital," UNC Vice President for Finance,

Felix Joyner, told the *Chapel Hill Newspaper*. "The federal government has been extremely bearish on building new teaching hospitals lately." He said UNC administrators could only assume ECU had been unsuccessful in obtaining federal assistance because government projections showed insufficient need for the hospital. [19]

Another source within the university system who asked not to be identified said chances of East Carolina's gaining federal assistance were remote. The competition was terrible between hospitals seeking federal funds, he said. ECU would have a problem proving another hospital was needed because the four closest urban areas, Wilson, Rocky Mount, Goldsboro, and Kinston, had new, underutilized hospitals. The Division of Facility Services of the NC Department of Human Resources had reported that all four cities were served by hospitals less than ten years old, and three of the hospitals averaged thirty-five to forty percent empty beds. The source said that those empty beds were a barrier for federal funding of a teaching hospital in Greenville.

Claiborne Jones, UNC vice chancellor for business and finance, also interviewed by the *Chapel Hill Newspaper* said, "I doubt if any medical school-teaching hospital has been constructed without the aid of federal money and private donations. It's almost taken for granted you need outside help." If the state spends the money budgeted for the four-year medical school and 200-bed teaching hospital, it would amount to $50.2 million in one capital outlay. And according to figures obtained from the University accounting Office, he said, it would have spent more money at one time than was spent in twenty-three years on developing the medical school and teaching hospital in Chapel Hill.

Jones said that at the Chapel Hill campus, facilities larger than those at ECU but otherwise comparable had cost $95 million, of which only forty to forty-five percent came from state funds. The amount appropriated between 1952 and 1975 was between $38 and $42.75 million, he said, less than the ECU capital budget for the biennium. The $95 million had been spent on the hospital and medical school only, and did not include the Schools of Public Health and Nursing, or any other related programs. Some funds were yet to be spent on buildings under construction. Cost overruns at the UNC-CH campus, Jones said, were made up from private and federal sources. The UNC medical school had recently received a federal grant for one-third of the cost of a new addition to the hospital, allowing its completion.

Because of inflation between 1952 and 1975, the costs at

Greenville and Chapel Hill were not comparable, according to President Friday. He said earlier that the state appropriation for the ECU hospital would probably prove to be conservative when the actual construction bids came in. The plans for the hospital had not yet been drawn.

Representative Patricia Hunt of Orange County suggested that there might be another debate about funding the ECU medical school expansion, if no federal funds were likely to be available. "When we get down to the financing of it, we may very well see more discussion on ECU," she said, "in the context that we perhaps should go with what we have and not begin anything as expensive as a medical school." [20]

The Senate held a series of hearings on the budget bill it had received from the Advisory Budget Commission. On Tuesday, April 29, Raymond Dawson, UNC vice president for academic affairs, informed legislators that if the ECU medical school reached an agreement to use PCMH facilities rather than building a teaching hospital, $6-8 million could be cut from the $20 proposed for a new 200-bed facility. The state would add 100-150 teaching beds to the new Pitt hospital, which was about a third complete.

On April 30, UNC President Friday appeared before the Senate appropriations subcommittee on education to recommend ways to cut the UNC budget. The subcommittee accepted his recommendations and voted to cut $7 million from the request for $35.2 million in new funds for constructing facilities at ECU medical school. Friday said the money would not be needed because of plans to use the new PCMH as a teaching facility by adding a 100-bed tower to the new hospital instead of building an independent teaching hospital. He said that the ECU faculty and administrators had almost reached agreement with Pitt County officials and the PCMH medical staff over terms of an agreement. Under the subcommittee's recommendation to the General Assembly, East Carolina would receive $28.245 million for new medical school construction. [21]

Freshman Senator Jack Childers of Lexington suggested delaying the construction of the medical school, saying, "I think we ought to take a look at whether a state that is fortieth in per capital income should get into what seems to me ought to be a luxury." He said that the first ECU graduates would not begin practicing until the 1980s, that some eastern NC hospital were already underused, and that the federal government was discouraging new medical schools because the doctor shortage was expected to be over by 1990.

Senator Thomas E. Strickland answered him, "That sounds like a playback of what we heard last year. I think the decision has been made, and we should move ahead."

Childers received support from Senator McNeill Smith of Guilford County, who said, "We have a whole new economy, and we ought to look at this question again." The subcommittee quickly dismissed the suggestion, with only Smith and Childers dissenting.[22]

During May, the opponents of ECU, most of them the same persons who had taken sides against the medical school in 1974, took advantage of the new opportunity given them by the state's economic setbacks. Chancellor John T. Caldwell of North Carolina State University, speaking to a group of alumni on Friday, May 2, said that the proposed veterinary school and the planned expansion of ECU medical school should be delayed or financed through bond issues. He attacked the legislature's proposal to double state aid to private colleges and universities while increasing tuition at UNC campuses. He claimed that the quality of NCSU was being reduced and hardship imposed on students to pay for expansion elsewhere. Caldwell, who was retiring on June 30, said he was talking as NCSU chancellor and a person knowledgeable in higher education in North Carolina, and not speaking for the university system. UNC President Friday was present when Caldwell gave his speech, but declined to comment on it, except to remark, "He wanted his say, and this was it." [23]

On the following Monday, ECU Chancellor Jenkins said, "I have utmost respect for Chancellor Caldwell as a university administrator and wish him well in his retirement. However, I do not quite understand his suggestion to delay both the School of Veterinary Medicine and the ECU School of Medicine, as if they are in the same stages of development. . . . Surely, he of all people must realize the difference. The School of Veterinary Medicine is an idea heading for federal court adjudication and is hardly more than in the planning stages, an idea on paper. By contrast, the School of Medicine at East Carolina has been more than ten years in planning and has actually been in operation for the past three years with faculty on hand. Also, as he well knows, the Pitt Memorial Hospital is now under construction and this is the appropriate time to add the medical school wing at the least possible expense to the state.

"To delay the medical school would obviously cost far more in the long run than to complete it now. The good Lord has told us he who puts his hand to the plow should not look back. Our only course now, it seems to me, is to move ahead and be done with it." [24]

At a meeting of the Senate Appropriations Committee on Tuesday, Senator Jim McDuffie of Mecklenburg County took a new tack in opposition to funding the medical school. He suggested the possibility of a referendum which would give the people a chance to vote on the concept of a medical school at East Carolina. Senator D. Livingston Stallings, chairman of the subcommittee, replied that the legislature had already gone too far on ECU to turn around. Before McDuffie made his suggestion, Senator Lawrence Davis of Forsyth County had questioned the expenditure of $28 million for the ECU medical school, with only $14.6 million for university-wide improvements and renovations. Because state collections had continued to fall below the level predicted, legislators were still seeking to cut $232 million off the proposed 1975-77 budget.[25]

That night, in a speech to a Pi Sigma Alpha honorary fraternity banquet, Mayor Howard Lee of Chapel Hill said that he thought that funding the full amount requested for the medical program this year would be a mistake, and would not help the medical school in the long run. The ECU medical school expansion could be carried out only by postponing other capital projects requested by the UNC system. Lee, who was a longtime supporter of the four-year medical school concept, whether it was built at ECU or elsewhere, was apparently spreading his bets. He was expected to decide in the fall whether or not to run for Lieutenant Governor in the next election.[26]

The state House of Representatives began steps to impound all funds appropriated for capital improvement projects. This would shut off all construction plans for the ECU medical school and all other building programs for at least one year. House Speaker James C. Green had mentioned the proposal several weeks before, and it was decided in a strategy session late Thursday afternoon, May 8, between Green and a few House members, to make it into a resolution. The delay was in part occasioned by some of Green's associates' trying to convince him that if he played an active role in the matter, he would damage any future political plans he might have.

Green said, "I don't know what the political implications of the action will be, but I do know this is the responsible thing to do at this time. We are doing the same thing for all the programs and are not singling out any particular one. This is certainly something which we have been most deliberate with, and it is merely a stopgap measure. We're not saying don't build the facilities, but are saying it is responsible to hold up until we know what accurate revenue figures will show.

"It makes no sense to me to build a medical school at East Carolina or anywhere else while at the same time we're voting to raise tuition fees for university kids. It makes no sense to spend money on brick and mortar while at the same time cutting back on money for classroom teachers.

"If the revenue figures show we can go ahead, then fine. But I want to see the figures. We don't have to go through with the resolution if the funds are available. I don't think this is a slap at any pet project."

The resolution would prohibit spending funds appropriated but not spent, or for which no contract has been let. Its two chief sponsors were Representative Herbert Hyde of Asheville and Representative John Ed Davenport of Nash County.

Some senators had said they thought reopening the past construction authorizations would lead to maneuvering by supporters of various pet projects. They cited a lack of coordination between House and Senate, which were, for the first time, considering the budget separately, at the insistence of House Speaker Green. One of the senators suggested that Green was motivated by his plans to run for governor or lieutenant governor in 1976 against Jim Hunt. But Green denied vehemently that there were any political considerations, saying that if he was accused of playing politics with the budget, he would just have to live with it. He said also that he did not want to be a party to a reversal of policy on ECU.[27]

On Saturday, May 10, Senator Jack Childers said that building a medical school at ECU would be expensive and was not necessary, considering that the state already had three good medical schools. He said that powerful legislators from down east wanted a medical school in Greenville no matter how much it cost. The price tag for the school, he said, was one of the best kept secrets in North Carolina, and he thought it would be better to spend the taxpayers' money elsewhere.[28] He said he would like to submit the issue to a bond referendum, which he was confident the people would defeat.[29]

On Tuesday, in spite of opposition from members who were in favor of the ECU medical school, a House committee approved legislation to freeze all state construction money, and sent it to the floor of the House. The resolution, sponsored by Representative John Ed Davenport of Nashville, would hold up all capital expenditures until the General Assembly studied revenue projections and sorted out priorities for projects funded previously.

Representative Samuel D. Bundy of Farmville argued against the proposal as a dangerous precedent, under which every General Assembly would be going back and undoing what the last General Assembly did. Representative Davenport agreed it might set a precedent, but thought it would be a good precedent for each legislature to re-examine the capital improvements for which appropriations were made during previous sessions.[30]

Chancellor Jenkins told a Wednesday, May 14, meeting of the Williamston Chamber of Commerce that a few diehard enemies were making a last ditch effort against expansion of the ECU medical school. "We are seeing new attacks by those few who have always opposed the medical school and who fought it every step of the way. Now, using the same scare tactics and biased, unfounded argument, the big lie techniques and distortions, they are mounting a campaign of confusion in a last-ditch effort to delay or even kill the medical school at East Carolina University.

"We have every confidence that our General Assembly will keep faith with the people of North Carolina and will respond to the wishes and the needs of our state in a positive, constructive way. I am sure our legislators will not be fooled or misled by these few die-hard enemies but will continue to listen to the people." [31]

On Tuesday, Representative Liston B. Ramsey of Madison County introduced a bill for a referendum of $41.8 million to finance capital construction in the UNC system. It would not include funds for the NCSU school of veterinary medicine or for expansion of ECU medical school. He expected the bill to be referred to the House Finance Committee of which he was chairman, where a bill introduced the week before by Representative Carolyn Mathis of Mecklenburg County, with forty-seven co-signers, was being considered. Ramsey said he would guess the committee might consolidate the two bills before sending them to the floor.

Representative Horton Rountree of Pitt County called Mathis's bill "a political stunt which will get her a lot of votes in Charlotte," and Representative W. T. "Billy" Mills of Granville, said the bill was fiscally unsound. Chancellor Leo Jenkins, reached for a telephone interview at his house at Atlantic Beach, said that he would prefer that the medical school funding remain in the legislature the way it already was. He said, "I talked to her (Representative Mathis) about it and said, in effect, it has gone through the legislature and the legislature has processed it and talked about it for a long time and I don't see a bond issue at this time in its progress." He declined to speculate about the outcome of a bond referendum, and when he was asked whether he felt certain the legislature would fund the medical school if the bond referendum did not pass, said, "I hope so—we've worked hard on it."

UNC President Friday endorsed Ramsey's bill. He said "I'm out to get the money, if the General Assembly decides that's the way they want to finance it." [32]

Representative Horton Rountree said on May 21 that both bond proposals before the state House or Representatives were, in his opinion, financially unsound. He mentioned the present state debt service of $27 million which, with $300 million in school bonds and $150 million in clean water bonds, would go up to $41 million in the next three or four years. Rountree thought the ECU expansion funding would be approved, but that it was a question of how much support it would be given by the legislature.[33]

Chancellor Jenkins made headlines when he announced on Tuesday, June 2, that he planned to ask that the UNC policy limiting political activity by administrators—said to have been devised in re-action to his politicking on the medical school issue—be changed. He said he did not think it was good for the state. The newspaper added the comment, "He has often been mentioned as a potential Democrat candidate for governor." [34]

Toward the end of the first week in June, a Senate finance sub-committee chaired by Senator Ralph Scott, which had been reviewing the state budget all week, approved the full operating budget request for ECU school of medicine. State budget officer Kenneth Howard suggested trimming $750,000 to $1 million from the budget for the current operation for the 1975-77 biennium, but the subcommittee ignored his suggestion.

"We've done settled this issue. Let's move on," Senator Scott said. After the meeting, he commented, "We've been on this medical school so long. We've got to give them the money to keep it going." He noted that the UNC Board of Governors voted the fall before to ex-pand the school from two to four years, and said, "We are doing ex-actly what they recommended."

The Greenville school was to open its first class in the fall of 1975, but because planning for the four-year program had not pro-gressed rapidly enough for it to be accredited by the fall of 1975, the opening was delayed until the fall of 1976. The one-year program, which had started in 1972, was closed in June 1975, because it would no longer have the accreditation it had been given as a part of the UNC-CH medical school. During the following year, there would be no medical students on the Greenville campus. The time to pre-pare for the opening of the four-year school was more than welcome to the faculty and administrators.

During the Senate subcommittee session on Thursday, June 5, Senator Cy Behakel of Mecklenburg asked whether the operating budget could be reduced because of the delayed opening of the school. He inquired, "What are the actual dollar needs?" Senator Vernon White answered that he had spoken with ECU officials in the past few days, and "They say it's impossible to get the faculty aboard (without the money). They will be working. The money won't be wasted."

Before the vote the next day, State Budget Officer Kenneth Howard, who earlier in the week had made his suggestion about trimming the budget, tried to get Senator Scott's attention, but was not recognized until after the vote. He then threw up his hands in disgust and said, "What you have approved is sixty-seven positions with not a single student enrolled."

UNC President Friday was quoted during the debate as saying the ECU budget should not be cut, but when he was reached by a reporter on Thursday afternoon, said some cuts might be made. He had recently, at House Speaker James C. Green's request, called accreditation officials in Washington to ask what effect, if any, cutting the budget would have on accreditation. He said that the officials declined to take a position.

The subcommittee did not alter the $43 million capital construction recommendation, including the $15 million set aside in 1973 and 1974 in the medical education reserve fund. It had already been cut from $50 million at President Friday's request, when building a bed wing on PCMH was substituted for a proposed 200-bed teaching hospital.[35]

The effort to resolve the urgent financial questions facing the General Assembly was complicated by a budget planning procedure introduced by House Speaker James Green that was quite different from past years. In other years, a joint House and Senate "super-subcommittee" had worked out a version of the budget that both houses could accept. In the 1975 session, Speaker James Green insisted that the House write its own budget, with differences between it and the Senate's version to be ironed out after the bills cleared each chamber.

The House Base Budget Committee took up the continuation budget line by line, with the House Appropriations Committee dealing only with expansive items. During the weekend of June 7 and 8, Base Budget chairman Representative Billy Watkins of Granville County, and House Appropriations chairman, Representative Jimmy Love of Lee County, met to bring the entire budget together. The continuation budget had already been cut by $95 million, and $193 million more had to come out of the expansion proposals.

Senate Appropriations Chairman Senator Ralph Scott, of Alamance County, Senator John Henley, of Cumberland, Senator Kenneth Royall, of Durham, and Senator Billy Mills, of Onslow, in a Senate "super-subcommittee" tried to cut out $11 million in the first year of the 1975-77 biennium in order to balance the budget. They had $11 million uncommitted for the second year, but could not bring that forward to the first year.

Scott was aggravated about the arrangement Green had initiated, saying it complicated and delayed the budgeting process. "There are too many people running for governor around here," he said on Friday. He was a supporter of Lieutenant Governor James Hunt, who expected a challenge from Green.

Scott had asked Green to combine for a conference committee on the budget " so they could go to the floor united," but Green had refused. "He says there's more participation the other way," Scott commented.

Frank Justice, adviser to House and Senate budget committees, said the two houses seemed to be racing each other to see who could get to the floor with a budget first. Linda Powell of the legislature's Fiscal Research Division, who was working with Love and Watkins on the House version, said the two budget bills would look alike when they reached the floor. When budget cuts were discussed, the committees were not sympathetic to Republican-controlled state agencies.[36]

On Wednesday, June 11, the House Finance Committee voted twenty-four to twenty-three in favor of Representative Carolyn Mathis's bill to hold a referendum on issuing $32 million in bonds for expanding the ECU medical school, and $43.2 million more for capital improvements at other institutions in the UNC system. The bill was sent to the house floor, where a sharp fight was expected and the bill's future was in serious doubt. It was strongly opposed by eastern legislators. Representative Larry Eagles of Edgecombe County, said "It's just another way the Mecklenburg delegation has of keeping us from getting a medical school at East Carolina University."

Representative Mathis denied that the bill's purpose was to kill the medical school. She said that if the people should vote down the bond issue it would be up to the General Assembly to fund the medical school expansion out of regular tax funds. She estimated that if the bill was passed it would free $28 million to restore appropriation cuts.[37]

On Thursday morning, Representative Horton Rountree said, "We're not worried about that angle of it (about the bond proposal). I don't know if it will be on the calendar or not, it got out with such a slim vote." He said the legislature was "in the throes of trying to close things out. Both the Senate and House (appropriations) bills have the med school moneys in there." He said he expected "there will be a move on the floor of the House . . . and Senate, I assume . . . by people from the Charlotte area to pull it (medical school funds) out of the appropriations bill. We're in real good shape in the Senate." However, he said, there were forty-three new people in the House who were not familiar with the fight that had been going on for ten years. "The issues have never really been debated. Maybe they will be debated today." [38]

That night, the House of Representatives tentatively approved a $6.6 billion 1975-77 budget. The budget the House proposed had been cut by nearly $290 million from the original $6.9 billion budget the Advisory Budget Commission recommended. There was virtually no money in it for new programs, 700 state-funded jobs were eliminated, and capital improvement funds were much less than in the past.

Medical school supporters decided they would attempt to re-refer Representative Mathis's bill to the House Finance Committee. They hoped that sending the bill back to committee would kill it, since fourteen members of the committee were absent when it had been favorably reported out by a one-vote margin. The move to re-refer the bond issue bill came after Representative Carl J. Stewart, Jr. of Gaston County, had lined up medical school supporters for the effort. Those who supported the bond issue, many of them medical school opponents, urged that there should be an opportunity for the House to debate the issue. The only argument offered by those seeking re-referral was the closeness of the vote in the Finance Committee.

Representative Mathis contended that the tight biennial budget justified a bond issue, arguing, "The Appropriations and Base Budget committees have worked very hard to get a balanced budget, cutting out may things for which we are all accountable." She repeated her claim that the referendum, to be held early in the next spring, would not delay the medical school if it failed, since the legislature would make an appropriation when it came into session just afterward. She said she would like to have the legislature consider an alternative to a direct appropriation.

Speaking in favor of re-referral, Representative Horton Rountree of Pitt County said that failure to pass the appropriation as a part of the proposed budget could jeopardize provisional accreditation of the medical school. Representative George Miller of Durham, argued against sending the bond bill back to committee. He said it was a legitimate issue that required floor debate. He said the motion to re-refer was intended to send it back so it would not be heard from again. Representative Robert A. Jones, D-Rutherford, asked that the bill not be sent back to the "funeral committee."

The motion to re-refer had valid grounds, according to Representative John R. Gamble, Jr., from Lincolnton. The bill against which it was directed had come out of committee by a margin of only one vote, with thirteen or fourteen absent. He said the bond bill's backers had one intention, to torpedo the ECU med school. He said that they were prejudiced, determined that if they couldn't have the medical school [in Charlotte], then no one should have it.

Mecklenburg Representative Ben Tison, an official of NC National Bank in Charlotte, said, "I've been here three years and have not yet had an opportunity to vote on this matter, or an opportunity . . . to debate it."

The vote was initially fifty-eight to fifty-three against sending the bill back to committee, but Representative Hugh C. Sandlin of Onslow County, changed his vote, so that in the end the vote to kill the motion to re-refer was fifty-seven to fifty-three.[39]

On Friday, four pro-ECU legislators were planning to be away, Representatives A. Harwell Campbell of Wilson County, William T. Watkins, of Granville, John Ed Davenport of Nash, and T. W. Ellis, Jr., of Vance County. They were among a group of seven legislators planning to spend the weekend in Nassau with their wives and some legislative secretaries.[40]

Anticipating the absence of the four ECU supporters the anti-medical school forces, mostly from urban and Western districts, on Thursday night held off their move against the $28 million capital improvements appropriation. Representative Tison told reporters, "We've got everything going for us tomorrow." He predicted a net gain of two votes for the med school opponents, but would not estimate their overall strength.

In Friday's session, Representative Tison made a motion to strike the $28 million medical school appropriation from the $87 million capital appropriation bill. Tison suggested that the funds ought to be removed to give the people a chance to decide for themselves.

House majority leader, Kitchin Josey of Halifax County, spoke against the amendment, saying it would "deal an absolute death blow to the East Carolina University medical school." He made a motion to table the amendment, and the house approved his motion seventy to forty-two, effectively killing the amendment. This left the way open for the ECU cause to prevail in the House.

Finally, on that Friday, June 13, 1975, the House approved without change the $6.6 billion state budget presented by the Appropriations Committee. The budget included $28 million in capital funds to expand the ECU medical school. Representative Herbert Hyde of Buncombe County, made a last-ditch effort to change the budget, by an amendment to eliminate state aid to private colleges except when a student has been denied admission to a state school because of lack of facilities. He maintained that the proposed state aid of $400 per student was unconstitutional. His amendment was tabled without debate on a motion by Appropriations Committee Chairman, Representative Jimmy Love.

The Senate's budget bill also passed, in spite of an attempt by Senator Ollie Harris of Cleveland to amend it. He proposed to take $100,000 from ECU medical school operating funds and use it for salary adjustments for other state employees. His motion was rejected thirty-six to nine.

Senator Ralph Scott, chairman of the Senate Appropriations Committee, commenting that it was Friday, the 13th, said, "Considering the tight money situation, it's easy to see why some folks have regarded this budget as an ill-fated budget from the word go. They profess to see black cats and spooks and all kinds of dark things in it. But I don't think we ought to look upon this day as Black Friday. I think we ought to look upon it as a case where we found a silver lining in some dark clouds." He said the budget was balanced, continuing, "It is as forward looking as we could make it under the circumstances. And I am proud of it."

There were major differences between the House and Senate budgets, but the upper chamber was expected to substitute the House version for its own. House Speaker James Green insisted that any changes in the House's budget would have to be approved by the full House Appropriations Committee. He told the House members, "You can say this is one session when one or two people did not run into a corner and write a budget."

Under pressure of revenue shortfalls caused by poor economic conditions, both versions of the budget cut spending proposals made by Governor Jim Holshouser and by the Advisory Budget Committee. Retaining ECU's capital improvement appropriation of $28 million would make a total of $43 million available for expanding the medical school, including the $15 million appropriated by earlier legislatures.[41] Between the legislature's action and the reconciliation of the two budgets by a House-Senate conference committee there was a flood of partisan editorials and of news stories, few of which were unbiased.

The chairman of the UNC Board of Trustees, Henry Foscue of High Point, said that the General Assembly had been misled to think it was possible to graduate doctors "like you grow peanuts." He asserted that the ECU medical school would cost $150 million, and not $43 million as the legislature estimated. "It will be like a rathole, taking more and more money," he said. "North Carolina is the only poor state in the southeast with three medical schools. It does not need and cannot afford a fourth one." He mentioned that New Mexico had spent $60 million in starting its new medical school, and Connecticut $24.5 million on a 200-bed hospital that had not yet admitted a single patient. Some trustees said they felt that Foscue's point of view was a mistaken one.

Chancellor N. Ferebee Taylor's criticized the legislature's taking $960,000 received at the Chapel Hill campus from overhead on federal research and training grants, one of his major concerns. He said, "It is an absolute shame to deprive the crown jewel of money it has earned and husbanded, to build a medical school which at best can be mediocre." He believed that the Chapel Hill trustees had been gentlemanly and silent too long. He asked the board members to convey the facts and their feeling to legislators from their areas.[42]

On Monday, June 16, the House approved a referendum on a $43 million bond issue for capital construction on UNC campuses. It had, of course, to be passed by the Senate before it could be placed before the people. This was done, and on June 25, it was ratified by the General Assembly as the "State Institutions of Higher Education Capital Improvement Voted Bond Act of 1975." Representative Mathis got her bill, but without delaying progress on the School of Medicine at ECU.

The representatives, in a technical parliamentary move, voted on June 16 to amend the Senate budget bill by substituting the House version, but the Senate declined to go along with it. Accordingly, the General Assembly's leadership prepared to establish a House-Senate conference committee to work out differences (mainly in the appropriations for prisons, universities, public schools, and general capital improvements) between the two versions of the proposed $6.6 billion budget for 1975-77. The conference committee was expected to concentrate mostly on reconciling differences, but Senator Ralph Scott, chairman of the Senate appropriations committee, said "I think it (the committee) can do anything they want to."

Representative Love, chairman of the House appropriations committee agreed with Senator Scott, saying, "I assume the whole bill is up for perusal, but I feel the differences will be focused on. If we have money left over, we'll put it where it can be used the best." [43]

On June 26, the General Assembly enacted a compromise version of the $6.6 billion budget worked out during the previous week by the joint conference committee, to become effective on July 1, 1975. It included $32.76 million for capital construction for the ECU medical school and funds to operate the school during 1975-76 and 1976-77. No expansion funds were allocated to any of the sixteen campuses. It appropriated almost $12 million for AHECs. [44]

The next day a news conference was held on the Greenville campus. Chancellor Jenkins said, "This is an historic moment for the citizens of North Carolina and for generations to come. The funds for the four-year medical school . . . which will emphasize family practice and primary health care, have been approved by the State Legislature. We can now proceed with building the school, gaining its accreditation, and beginning its important work."

Dr. Edwin Monroe said, "We are grateful to the General Assembly and the Board of Governors for bringing to fruition what we've all worked so hard for. We don't see any insurmountable problems with gaining accreditation." He expected it to be forthcoming in the spring, with the first four-year medical students starting in the fall of 1976. The $32 million appropriated, along with funds appropriated earlier, was ample money to provide the clinical facilities and basic medical science building for the school, as well as operating costs. He indicated that there was no urgency about beginning the bed tower, on which work should start sometime during the year ahead. Money for the medical science building would become available July 1, 1976. In the meantime, renovating Ragsdale Hall, a $500,000 project to provide labs for basic science teaching as well as faculty office space, was scheduled to begin in August.

Dr. Monroe explained that all the construction and recruitment of faculty and staff had to be tied together under the leadership of the new dean, Dr. William Edward Laupus, who would be in Greenville by July 1. [45]

[1] "A Victory for North Carolina and for Chancellor Jenkins," *North Carolina*, Vol. XXXIII, No. 9 (September 1975) p. 48.

[2] *Raleigh News & Observer* , January 2, 1975.

[3] *Raleigh News & Observer* , January 4, 1975.

[4] *Chapel Hill Newspaper*, January 16, 1975.

[5] *Greensboro Daily News*, January 21, 1975.

[6] *Monroe Enquirer-Journal*, January 23, 1975.

[7] *Raleigh News & Observer* , March 2, 1975.

[8] *Charlotte Observer*, January 25, 1975.

[9] *Statesville Record & Landmark*, February 26, 1975.

[10] *Charlotte Observer*, January 25, 1975.

[11] Monroe interview, January 3, 1992.

[12] *Chapel* Hill *Newspaper*, January 28, 1974.

[13] *High Point Enterprise*, January 30, 1975; Same article in *Chapel Hill Newspaper, Durham Sun, Greensboro Daily News*, etc.

[14] *Raleigh News & Observer* , March 2, 1975; *Charlotte Observer*, same date.

[15] *Charlotte Observer*, March 2, 1975.

[16] *Raleigh News & Observer* , March 2, 1975.

[17] *Ibid.*

[18] *Raleigh News & Observer* , March 30, 1975.

[19] *Chapel Hill Newspaper*, March 31, 1975

[20] Ibid.

[21] *Raleigh News & Observer* , April 30, 1975.

[22] *Raleigh News & Observer* , May 1, 1975.

[23] *Raleigh News & Observer* , May 3, 1975.

[24] *Greenville Daily Reflector*, May 5, 1975.

[25] *Durham Morning Herald*, May 7, 1975.

[26] *Greenville Daily Reflector*, May 7, 1975.

[27] *Greensboro Daily News*, May 9, 1975; *Raleigh News & Observer* , May 10, 1975.

[28] Georgette Hedrick's *Chronology*, p. 76.

[29] *Lexington Dispatch*, May 12, 1975.

[30] *Asheville Citizen*, May 14, 1975.

[31] *Raleigh News & Observer* , May 15, 1975.

[32] *Raleigh News & Observer* , May 21, 1975.

[33] *Greenville Daily Reflector*, May 21, 1975.

[34] *Raleigh News & Observer* , June 5, 1975.

[35] *Durham Morning Herald*, June 6, 1975.

[36] *Greenville Daily Reflector*, June 9, 1975.

[37] *Durham Sun*, June 11, 1975.

[38] *Greenville Daily Reflector*, June 12, 1975.

[39] Vote on the move to re-refer was as follows: <u>For</u>: Baker, Barbee, Barker, Barnes, Beard, Bell, Breece, Bright, Brown, Bumgardner, Bundy, Campbell, Chapin, Chase, Collins, Cullipher, Davenport, Debruhl, Eagles, Ellis, Enloe, Gamble, Gardner, Gentry, Gregory, Hightower, Holt, Hunter, Hurst, Huskins, Hutchins, James, Jernigan, Lachot, Lilley, Love, Mason, Messer, Oxendine, Quinn, Ray, Rountree, Sandlin, Sawyer, Schwartz, Smith of Rowan, Soles, Stewart, Ward, Watkins, White, Woodard, and Wright. <u>Against</u>: Adams, Ballenger, Bissell, Blackwell, Cobb, Cook, Creech, Deramus, Diamont, Dorsey, Erwin, Farmer, Foster, Frye, Gilmore, Griffin, Hairston, Harris, Heer, Helms, Holmes of Chatham, Holmes of Yadkin, Hung of Orange, Hyde, Johnson of Robeson, Johnson of Wake, Jones, Jordan, Lawing, Leonard, Long, McMillan, Mathis, Michaux, Miller, Morris, Nash, Nesbitt, Parnell, Phillips, Plyler, Prestwood, Pugh, Ramsey, Rhodes, Setzer, Short, Smith of Forsyth, Smith of Wake, Spoon, Stevens, Tally, Tennille, Thomas, Tison, Varner, and Webb. <u>Not voting</u>: Auman, Davis, Edwards, Falls, Hunt of Cleveland, Josey, Revelle, Rogers, and Wiseman]. *Raleigh News & Observer,,* June 13, 1975.

[40] *Greenville Daily Reflector*, June 13, 1975.

[41] *Greenville Daily Reflector*, June 13, 1975.

[42] *Durham Sun*, June 13, 1975.

[43] *Raleigh News & Observer* , June 17, 1975.

[44] *Raleigh News & Observer* , June 26, 1975.

[45] *Greenville Daily Reflector*, June 26, 1975.

Chapter 17
The Area Health Education Program

As the renewed struggle to establish funding for the four-year medical school in Greenville went on, the faculty and administration were busy at beginning to carry out the plans they had been preparing for years. The dean's search committee worked diligently, screening the numerous candidates, and interviewing those they found likely. Discussions continued about joint arrangements with Pitt County Memorial Hospital, discussions that had begun even before medical school plans crystallized, in connection with nursing and allied health programs at East Carolina University. By 1972, general talks had turned to specific negotiations aimed at an affiliation agreement between the ECU medical school and the hospital, which was preparing to move to a new facility. In 1975, a decision would have to be made between building a new hospital and affiliating with PCMH, and funding decisions by the legislature hinged on that decision.

The original alternative to a second medical school, proposed by the Bennett Committee to the Board of Governors and gratefully accepted, had still to be worked through. The concept of Area Health Education Centers was not incompatible with that of a medical school, but rather a logical extension, especially when primary medical care was a central goal of that school. There was a natural partnership between AHECs and the new school in the endeavor to provide more family practitioners and improve medical service in small communities and rural areas.

The panel led by Bennett had strongly supported the concept of AHECs, its first recommendation being that the Board of Governors should develop a system of medical and health education utilizing hospitals all over the state. Duke and Bowman Gray Schools of Medicine, the consultants advised, should be included with UNC-Chapel Hill in the development of the system. Resources should be provided to utilize "the expertise, experience, and educational resources of all three institutions in an organized fashion, integrated into a Statewide effort."

The UNC administration, in particular the School of Medicine, welcomed this first recommendation of the Bennett Committee. It was entirely in accord with undertakings the medical school already had in hand, such as the NC Regional Medical Program and the affiliation agreements that had been set up with hospitals in Charlotte,

Greensboro, Raleigh, Rocky Mount, and Tarboro before 1970. President Friday was doubtless influenced in his energetic support of area health education centers by recommendations of the Carnegie Commission on Higher Education, on which he served from 1967 to 1971. In the chapter dealing with health manpower education in their 1970 report, the Commission had recommended the development of 126 new area health education centers nationwide.[1]

The Commission's description of an AHEC's functions were closely paralleled by those of the centers established in North Carolina. An area health education center was associated with a community hospital or group of hospitals. It conducted educational programs under the supervision of a university health science center with which it was affiliated. The programs included residencies, clinical instruction for medical and dental students, clinical experience for paramedical personnel, and continuing education programs for physicians and other health workers.[2]

In the spring of 1970, Glenn Wilson had been brought to Chapel Hill for the purpose of helping the University with what was to be the Orange-Chatham Comprehensive Public Health Center. He was also appointed Associate Dean to serve as director of an office of community health services. The Division of Community Health Services which he established in the Dean's office later formed the nucleus of the AHEC program.

The program began in 1972, with AHECs in Charlotte, Wilmington, Raleigh, and Asheville, set up with a five-year federal grant of $8.5 million awarded in June of that year to the UNC-CH School of Medicine under the Comprehensive Health Manpower Training Act passed by Congress in 1971.

In the spring of 1972, as was mentioned earlier, Glenn Wilson, statewide AHEC director, had talked with Pitt County hospital's medical staff about setting up a family practice residency under an Area Health Education Center. He proposed that the same arrangement would be used in Greenville as in the other centers that had already been set up across the state. The standard residency arrangement was to make every patient in the hospital available for teaching. Local physicians were not to be paid for the time spent directing residents, on the assumption that the residents would take over some of their routine duties of the medical staff. Some staff doctors, however, objected to "having students messing around with their patients."[3]

Wilson submitted a specific proposal on April 5, 1972. The hospital staff, with Dr. Jack Wilkerson taking the most negative position, voted against an immediate affiliation. They complained that not enough time had been given for them to study the details of the AHEC proposal, and they could not make an immediate decision. A nine-person Medical Education Committee comprised of hospital staff, administration, and trustees, with ECU and UNC representatives, was set up to develop a plan.[4]

Since there were time constraints on the federal grant under which the AHEC program was being established, Wilson could not wait while the committee studied the proposal. He gave up on Greenville for the time being and proceeded to set up an AHEC with its headquarters in Tarboro, also serving community hospitals in Rocky Mount, Wilson, and Roanoke Rapids.[5]

In 1973, Wilson and his staff again asked the committee to join a program for Greenville and at least five surrounding counties. If the hospital joined immediately, the committee was told, it would receive up to $5 million for new facilities. The $5 million carrot did not bring about an agreement. The PCMH medical education committee asked for time to consult with surrounding counties to plan for the hospital's possible role in the AHEC program.

For a second time, no agreement came out of the negotiations. The Medical Education Committee reported that the hospital was already working with ECU in many clinical training programs, and had agreed to expand services if the medical school expanded. The hospital, they said, had been functioning as a health education center except that there were no advanced medical students, residents, or full-time faculty there. (In 1969, the hospital's trustees had made the decision to become active in education, and from that time on had cooperated with East Carolina University on programs that were considered to be mutually beneficial).

In January 1974, Dr. Jack W. Wilkerson of Greenville, a member of the board of trustees of Pitt County Memorial Hospital, made a statement about the hospital's participation in the AHEC program. He said that a remark to newspaper reporters by William A. Dees, chairman of the Board of Governors about rebuffs by the hospital of AHEC proposals was simply false. In a letter to Dees, Wilkerson also disputed statements by AHEC director Glenn Wilson, that the hospital and its medical staff had rejected a proposal to set up an AHEC in 1972. He said that the medical education liaison committee, made up of hospital personnel and others from the community, had been given only eight days to respond to a proposal that would have cost $75,000 or more a year. The committee had voted to continue planning and to investigate ways to fund the program other than having patients or taxpayers pay.

Furthermore, he reiterated the report that PCMH and ECU had been cooperating in clinical programs, and the hospital was willing to expand services. He also restated that PCMH had been functioning as a health education center although without advanced medical students, residents, or full-time faculty. Wilkerson said ECU should play a major part in the AHEC program because of existing services and potential ECU development.[6]

The 1974 General Assembly that funded the expansion of the ECU medical school also authorized and funded a statewide network of nine AHEC's, to be administered by the Office of Community Health Services of the UNC-CH.[7] During the spring and summer of that year, negotiations between PCMH and Glenn Wilson's office continued.

On Friday, August 10, 1974, at a meeting in Belhaven, Dr. Edwin Monroe was elected president of Eastern AHEC, Inc., heading a board made up of representatives of ECU and of hospitals serving twenty-two eastern counties. Local AHEC committees were to be set up by each hospital to determine area health needs and plan programs to develop health manpower for consideration by the EAHEC board of directors. Other officers included Joseph J. James, Jr., administrator of Wayne County Memorial Hospital, as vice president; John P. Davis, administrator of Beaufort County Hospital, as secretary; and L. Daniel Duval, director of the Lenoir Memorial Hospital, as treasurer. Member hospitals were Albemarle Hospital, Beaufort County Hospital, Bertie County Hospital, Chowan Hospital, Carteret General Hospital, Columbia Memorial Hospital, Craven County Hospital, Lenoir Memorial Hospital, Martin General Hospital, Onslow Memorial Hospital, Pitt County Memorial Hospital, Pungo District Hospital, Roanoke-Chowan Hospital, Washington County Memorial Hospital, and Wayne County Memorial Hospital. [8]

The executive committee of EAHEC, Inc., held its first meeting in Greenville on August 20. One item on the agenda was selecting a full-time administrative director, and a search was initiated. After the meeting, Dr. Monroe said that EAHEC represented "a unique partnership between hospitals of widely varying size in a large geographic area; university, community college, and technical institute health professional education programs; and community-based human resources agencies and health professionals in private practice."

In September, 1974, Glenn Wilson again attempted to negotiate to establish an AHEC in Greenville. His transactions now were with EAHEC, Inc., which was independent of both the Pitt County hospital and the East Carolina medical school, and had been incorporated especially as a vehicle for an AHEC. Its purpose was to implement the elective student rotations and the family practice residency programs to be carried out by the area health education center. AHEC planning was to be held separate and apart from anything relative to the education programs at the medical school.

On September 23, Dr. Monroe signed a contract with Glenn Wilson under which funds were to be provided to support EAHEC operations for the remainder of the fiscal year.[9] The EAHEC would be the ninth center, and would serve the largest area of any center in the state, comprising twenty-three counties and seventeen community hospitals. Like the other AHECs, it had been authorized and funded by the 1974 General Assembly, and would be centrally administered by the Office of Community Health Services of the UNC-CH School of Medicine.

The contract worked out was, in the end, quite a favorable one for Eastern AHEC. Wilson grumbled about it, saying that Greenville declined the arrangement that Charlotte Memorial, New Hanover, Wake Memorial, and all the rest of the hospitals had accepted. He said, "There is, to my detriment, an AHEC contract signed with Pitt County that would not have been signed any place else in the state. There is an agreement for the University to pay and pay and pay for that hospital."[10]

During the fall, disagreements between medical school planners and the PCMH staff about sharing facilities caused some difficulties in setting up the AHEC program. A permanent family practice center was still needed, as well as adequate facilities for the AHEC administration. The failure of efforts by UNC planners and the ECU medical school faculty and administration to reach agreement on expanding the school had its effect on AHEC planning.

There were advantages in having EAHEC under an independent corporation. Still, Dr. Monroe spent considerable time negotiating for the university, as one of the main proponents of sharing facilities with the existing hospital. He managed also to make some progress toward inaugurating the area health education center programs. On October 9, Chancellor Jenkins, in an invited article in the *Raleigh News & Observer*, said that Eastern AHEC was supporting plans for a residency in Family Practice and for rotations for senior medical students, which were to be extended to other eastern area hospitals.[11]

Dr. Monroe announced on Friday morning, January 3, 1975, that Dr. F. M. Simmons Patterson of New Bern, director of the Cancer Control Program of the Duke University Comprehensive Cancer

Center, had been appointed executive director for the Eastern Area Health Education Center. Dr. Patterson's appointment was advantageous to the EAHEC program, from his wide experience as well as his extensive network of collegial contacts in the state's medical establishment.[12]

One of Patterson's first tasks would be to plan for rotations of students and residents from the medical schools of the state into hospitals and clinics in the AHEC's twenty-three-county area. The EAHEC would provide for undergraduate, graduate, and post-graduate education not only for physicians, but also for dentists, nurses, pharmacists, and allied health and public health workers. The program would be administered through the contractual arrangements that had been set up with UNC School of Medicine.

Patterson had been a member of the faculty of both the Department of Surgery and the Department of Community Health Sciences at Duke University School of Medicine. As part of his agreement to become the AHEC Executive Director, he was appointed to the faculty of the ECU School of Medicine. Patterson's office was to be located on the campus of East Carolina University. He said he would begin his work at EAHEC February 1. His first priority would be to visit the seventeen participating hospitals. He wished to learn first hand from the physicians. and the administrators of the hospitals what their priorities were. He said EAHEC was a partnership between the medical schools and the community hospitals in the area, to improve the quality and increase the number of health care personnel. Patterson anticipated that some medical students might begin rotations in area hospitals during the coming year.

Patterson announced that he had asked Joel E. Vickers from the faculty of the ECU School of Allied Health and Social Professions to be Deputy Director. He said he would soon appoint three other staff members, a Director of Family Practice Residency Programs, an Associate Director for Nursing Education, and an Associate Director for Allied Health Education.

Dr. Patterson, a New Bern native, was the grandson of Furnifold M. Simmons, who had been US Senator for the first thirty years of the twentieth century and leader of the Democratic political machine that had replaced Reconstruction Republicans. Patterson had received his undergraduate degree from the University of North Carolina in Chapel Hill, and graduated from the University of Pennsylvania Medical School in Philadelphia. He was Chief of Surgery and Chief of Staff at Scotland County Memorial Hospital in Laurinburg between 1946 and 1952. He had been President of the Craven

County and Second District Medical Societies, and chief of Staff and Chief of Surgery at the Craven County Hospital. He had also served as President of the NC Surgical Association.

Patterson was a Diplomate of the American Board of Surgery, a Fellow of the American College of Surgeons, and President of the North Carolina Surgical Association. He was a member of the Board of Directors and Executive Committee of the North Carolina Division of the American Cancer Society, and had been a member of the Board of Trustees of UNC in Chapel Hill. Before becoming Director of Duke's Cancer Control Program, he had been Executive Director of the NC Regional Medical Program. He came from a family of physicians, both his father and his brother being doctors.[13]

Interviewed at the Duke Cancer Control Center for a "Tar Heel of the Week" feature in the *Raleigh News & Observer*, Dr Patterson agreed that EAHEC had not been able to escape political controversy, because of its close affiliation with the ECU School of Medicine, but said he hoped to avoid getting involved in politics when he took the job. He had been negotiating with Eastern AHEC for a while, but not until the medical school was approved by the UNC Board of Governors and the contracts for an AHEC in Greenville were signed had he accepted the position.

The interviewer noted that Dr. Patterson was sixty-one years of age, but looked closer to fifty. "His body is compact and his thick black hair is streaked with gray only at the temples," he said. Patterson described his career mostly in terms of moving from challenge to challenge. "It was a very difficult decision to make," he said. "My life up here [in Durham] and my associations up here have been very happy ones. But I think a man ought to move occasionally and accept new challenges. The challenge that was offered to me there was something I wanted to meet."

Like most doctors, who tend to practice in the areas where they do their residency and prefer urban areas with medical schools and big hospitals, Patterson first joined the surgical staff of a hospital in Abington, PA, after doing six years of internship and residency there. In 1968, he came to Duke, with access to two medical schools.

"In 1952," he said, "I moved back to my home down in New Bern and entered practice in surgery with my brother, Dr. Joseph Patterson. We were the first two people in that area who limited ourselves 100% to surgery. It seems like I've come and done things, accepted a challenge and then moved on. In 1968, I felt like I wanted to make a change. In the life of a surgeon, other things get pushed back—like your family, your children, and so forth. I wanted to see them and spend some time with them."

"One reason I came back to North Carolina is that North Carolina means so much to me—particularly eastern North Carolina," he said. He said there was a tendency for doctors to go to medical centers and large cities instead of rural areas. The doctors in rural areas were intellectually isolated to a large degree, and cut off from engaging social activities. In many small towns, there were valid reasons for physicians to worry about getting a good education for their children.

"We've got to do everything in our power to improve the medical climate in eastern North Carolina to get people there," he said. "The medical school is going to help—and the AHEC is going to be a tremendous attraction. It's not only that they will help to stimulate them intellectually. A man does have to be stimulated intellectually. If he does not have a challenge, he's not effective. But also, if a physician is out in a rural area by himself, he doesn't have another physician to consult with."

In eastern North Carolina, students would be exposed to the realities of practice. But the AHEC system would also enable the doctors with whom the students were associated, and who taught them, to stay abreast of the latest developments in their fields. Also, the system would provide continuing education for community hospital staffs, and would recruit technicians and other paramedicals from community colleges and technical institutes. Patterson stressed that the AHEC program would involve people in all areas of health care, and not only physicians.

One argument that ECU supporters had made during their campaign to bring the medical school to Greenville was that medical students who came from rural areas were likely to return to them when they began their practices. The school would try to enroll students from small towns, and concentrate on family practice and other primary care fields. While these arguments, he said, had been lost on medical educators, the public and the members of the General Assembly had listened to them.[14]

[1] Carnegie Commission on Higher Education, *Higher Education and the Nation's Health*, (New York: October, 1970), p. 59.

[2] *Ibid.*, p. 57.

[3] Wilson interview, April 22, 1992.

[4] ECU School of Medicine File, Folder "Affiliation with PCMH;" Wilson interview, April 22, 1992.

[5] Folder, "Affiliation with PCMH;" Wilson interview, April 22, 1992.

[6] *Raleigh News & Observer*, January 20, 1974.

[7] *Greenville Daily Reflector*, August 16, 1974.

[8] *Greenville Daily Reflector*, August 16, 1974.

[9] *Greenville Daily Reflector*, September 24, 1974.

[10] Wilson interview, April 22, 1992.

[11] *Raleigh News & Observer*, October 9, 1974.

[12] *Greenville Daily Reflector*, January 3, 1975.

[13] *Ibid.*

[14] *Raleigh News & Observer*, March 9, 1975.

Chapter 18
Hospital Facilities

When President William Friday called on the Board of Governors on November 9, 1974, to recommend a four-year medical school at East Carolina University, he projected that it would have its own 200-bed teaching hospital in Greenville. That arrangement would have had advantages for the medical school, but if it had been adhered to, it is probable that the tax shortfall in 1975 would have forced postponement of funding the ECU expansion. Another delay could have given the school's opponents in the Piedmont and Charlotte new opportunities to hinder its development. The East Carolina planners had been envisioning an affiliation with Pitt County Memorial Hospital from the beginning, and were willing to sacrifice the benefits of having their own hospital to making it easier for ECU's friends in the legislature to champion immediate funding of the school, even though it was a tight year. Furthermore, a mutually productive association with the county hospital advanced relations between the medical school, the local medical establishment, and the community at large.

Dr. Edwin Monroe, in his negotiations with the PCMH trustees and medical staff, was able to make a good case for the advantages of combining forces. Shared teaching facilities promised long-term gains to the hospital and its staff, through the prestige and financial benefits that accrue to an academic medical center. Without the school, the hospital was just another county hospital, although one with a solid record of service since it had been founded as a 120-bed institution in 1951. Establishment of a separate teaching hospital would have brought competition for patients between the two hospitals, with the advantage on the side of the university hospital.

When he started work part-time in 1968 as Director of Life Sciences and Community Health at ECU (later to become Dean of the School of Allied Health and Social Professions and Director of Medical Education), Dr. Monroe became immediately involved in the planning for a new hospital in Pitt County. He also began to discuss with the hospital administration and staff the feasibility and mutual benefits of using the hospital as a clinical training site for the various kinds of allied health professionals studying at the university.

In June of that year, Dean Monroe wrote at length to the Pitt County Board of Commissioners and the PCMH Board of Trustees, urging them to consider in their planning for a new hospital building the need for clinical training facilities which were adequate to be approved by national accreditation officials. He also emphasized the importance of the growing trend toward providing out-patient clinics in community hospitals, to meet Medicare and Medicaid requirements, and furnish facilities in which medical and nursing students, residents, and paramedical personnel could be provided experience in patient care.

He continued to press his suggestions through 1968, cooperating also with consultants brought in to assist in developing plans for a new hospital, whose funding was to be brought to a referendum on a special bond issue in 1970. In an August letter to Dr. Eric L. Fearrington, with whom he had been associated in his practice, and who was a member of the hospital staff, Monroe recapitulated his recommendations as he had set them forth to the hospital architect. In particular, he emphasized the importance of allowing for future expansion and planning for a comprehensive health complex centered on the hospital.[1]

On the evening of January 13, 1969, the hospital's consultant on planning the new facility, Charles P. Cardwell, Jr., of the Medical College of Virginia, met with the Joint Conference Committee of the Pitt County Board of Commissioners, the hospital administration, and the hospital medical staff. He had asked for the meeting in order to discuss the issue of becoming involved in educational programs. After lengthy discussion, the group agreed that, while the primary responsibility of the hospital was to provide good medical care to the area, they were "willing and even eager to negotiate with any established educational institution in working out an affiliation to use the hospital for clinical experience of their students." Such an affiliation, which they insisted must not pose any financial burden on patients or taxpayers, would extend all the way from the programs already being conducted within the hospital to a possible affiliation with the medical school if it should become a reality.

The consultants and the architects for the hospital were instructed to include educational facilities in their plans, including conference rooms, lecture rooms, and at least one large auditorium. The physicians agreed to accept the provision of outpatient services as an irreversible and inevitable trend, even though they did not completely agree that a hospital should provide such services. They suggested that communication be kept open between the hospital and East Carolina University to discuss any mutually beneficial programs that might be proposed.[2]

In 1969, there was an abortive movement led by some members

of the Board of County Commissioners to sell the hospital to a private corporation. Such an arrangement would have removed the burden of having to muster support for a bond issue, one which might easily be defeated, wasting all the time and money that had been put into planning. In a stormy meeting early in December, 1969, the hospital's consultant, Cardwell, pointed out the numerous disadvantages of turning the hospital over to a company that had to make it profitable, whatever the effect on service to the community. He emphasized the fact that private operation of Pitt Memorial would almost surely eliminate any affiliation with a medical school.[3]

Plans for the new hospital building were carried forward, and in November, 1970, the voters of Pitt County approved a special bond issue of $9 million to finance its construction. The groundbreaking for the hospital was held on February 14, 1974. The county's expenditure reached $16.7 million by the opening of the hospital in 1977, the state had provided $2.2 million for adding a regional physical rehabilitation center, and the ECU School of Medicine had supplied $5.1 million for facilities to support clinical teaching.[4]

During the climactic period of ECU's campaign for its medical school, construction on the hospital proceeded, and discussions of possible affiliation between the school and PCMH continued. Dean Christopher Fordham III and the planning group from Chapel Hill met several times with the hospital staff committee that considered affiliation with the medical school, with ECU officials and medical faculty to discuss details of the new hospital expansion.

Dr. Monroe said on Monday, August 19 , 1974, "From everything I hear, when he meets with those kinds of people, he gives the same old answers—it's the same old merry-go-round. If the legislature wants a medical school different from the one in Chapel Hill, that has a different mission, then the way to get it is to authorize a four-year medical school." Asked whether Fordham was planning towards eventually creating a four-year school emphasizing family practice, Monroe said, "If they are, I'm not aware of it. It's hard to get those kinds of answers from him." Monroe said of the cooperation President Friday had instructed Fordham to seek from him, "As it has worked so far, that means simply stay out of it."[5]

On August 28, Dean Fordham, Dr. William J. Cromartie, his deputy director, Dr. William Bakewell, and Glenn Wilson met with the PCMH medical staff. Their purpose was to discuss a proposal from the hospital that staff physicians should be paid $50 an hour for their participation in the educational program. Fordham told the group that such an arrangement would contravene UNC policy, which provided only for (unpaid) volunteer, part-time, and full-time faculty.

Fordham, with Cromartie, Wilson, and Bakewell, held three other meetings with the PCMH medical staff, trustees, and administration. The hospital was a crucial component of any medical school for Greenville, since ECU possessed no medical care facility. The questions raised were, To what extent could PCMH accommodate medical education? And how would it affect the hospital's charge? The UNC planners concluded that the number of full-time faculty and the facility requirements attendant on their presence in the hospital were seen as a threat by the PCMH staff.

On September 4, Dr. Cromartie presented to the Medical Education Liaison Committee of the hospital the two educational programs that had been proposed for the ECU school, and which he had outlined in a memorandum on September 2. One was a preliminary report by the ECU faculty, the other the UNC planners' draft plan for reorganizing the medical education program, with the first and fourth years on the ECU campus. The fifth year of the curriculum was to be pursued at ECU and at PCMH, and subsequently the graduates of the program, it was planned, would do residencies in family medicine at the hospital and other regional centers. A pre-affiliation agreement was also submitted for consideration by the hospital staff and administration. It asked that the hospital designate seventy-five beds as teaching beds, that the hospital accommodate thirty to forty medical students, fifteen full-time clinical teaching faculty and two non-physician professionals, provide an outpatient facility, and six to eight pathologists. It stipulated that all hospital staff doctors should be available for teaching, with individual exceptions if necessary.

Dr. Jack Wilkerson, chairman of the hospital's medical education liaison committee, transmitted the committee's suggestion that the EAHEC provide the outpatient clinic, and that office space for the clinical teaching faculty should be furnished in the $15 million basic science building that was to be constructed. He emphasized that these matters were out of the committee's jurisdiction. Wilkerson said that the committee had previously endorsed the concept of affiliation with ECU. Their approval, however, had been based on the understanding that a traditional second-year class was to be added to the ECU program.

The negative response of PCMH's officials, seconding that of the ECU faculty and administration, put a temporary hold on medical school expansion plans. After meeting on September 18 with the PCMH staff, to which Drs. Dean Hayek and William Waugh of the

ECU medical school faculty were invited (and Dr. Wallace Wooles was deliberately not invited), Fordham noted that the PCMH doctors were against having the ECU proposal imposed on them, but blamed the UNC planners for it. He recognized that the hospital's medical staff had a real problem. They had a responsibility to provide the community and surrounding area with health care, and a major clinical education program would present new difficulties, would distort the medical care pattern, and would affect their professional lives. On the other hand, they felt under pressure to respond to East Carolina's drive for a medical school. The result was a conflict between their community care responsibilities and the responsibilities they felt toward educating more doctors.

Fordham noted that UNC must emphasize earnestly that it did not originate their dilemma, and was sympathetic. However, carrying out the demands of Section 46 of the law passed by the General Assembly demanded provision of adequate resources for clinical teaching.[6]

On September 19, Dean Fordham met with Chancellor Leo Jenkins and the chairman of the ECU Board of Trustees, Roddy Jones, to talk about hiring an architect, acquiring land for the medical school, and general planning issues. He told them that there could be no contract with an architect until the Board of Governors approved it and the General Assembly released funds. In the meantime, anything done would have to be on a consultancy basis. He said he had turned over to President Friday some weeks back the request for permission to purchase land, and it was also awaiting approvals from the Governors and the legislature. These could not be issued without a formal request from the ECU trustees.

He also said to them that since the UNC planners' innovative proposal that articulated resources in Greenville with those of the University in Chapel Hill in other parts of the state had been rejected by the people in the Greenville medical community, they were putting all their efforts into implementing the ECU medical faculty proposal. Recruiting sixteen full-time clinical sciences faculty and providing facilities for their work raised problems.

There could be, he told them, a stand-alone accreditation of the ECU school only with a commitment by the Board of Governors and the General Assembly to build a four-year medical school. In his log of the meeting, Fordham noted, "However, I made it clear that I was not indicating to them I supported such a project for a variety of reasons." [7]

When the UNC Board of Governors in November, 1974, dropped

their opposition to the expansion, the plan they submitted to the General Assembly included a $20 million teaching hospital for ECU. For the time being, any affiliation between the medical school and Pitt County Memorial Hospital appeared to be in abeyance.

On Tuesday, January 7, 1975, Chancellor Jenkins announced in an address in Washington, NC, to the North Carolina Educators Association from District 15, that ECU's medical school would be located on a 50-acre site near the new PCMH. The land would be purchased during the following week, he said. The basic medical sciences complex and a teaching hospital would cost $40 to $50 million, Jenkins said, "as opposed to scare figures [of $100 million] that ought to be ignored." The planned facilities included a helicopter pad for emergency and other medical service in a seventy-five to a hundred mile radius, a necessity in an area where the roads were not adequate for transporting patients quickly to treatment facilities.

Jenkins said that the medical school would work closely with the Eastern Area Health Education Center in Greenville to rotate medical students from ECU teaching facilities to hospitals in the 24-county area the education center served. He predicted that the first family practice residency program would be operating in Pitt County within a year.[8]

That same week, a possible competitor to PCMH in the provision of teaching facilities to East Carolina floated a trial balloon. The Wilson County Medical Society had discussed offering a portion of the Eastern North Carolina Hospital there for use as a teaching hospital by the medical school. Dr. Robert Youngblood, secretary of the medical society, said on January 9 that the proposition had been discussed informally, without any action taken. The medical society had not yet talked with ECU officials about using part of the hospital.

The suggestion was not entirely new. In February, 1970, the Legislative Research Commission Subcommittee on Health, acting under a resolution of the House of Representatives, had considered a proposal to utilize any medical facilities at the Eastern North Carolina Sanatorium to supply the region's unmet educational needs.[9]

The hospital was one of three hospitals supported by the state, and specialized in chest diseases. It had 224 beds with another six to be opened in February for acute respiratory care. In 1975, UNC medical school already had a satellite program operating at the hospital providing medical services, diagnostic laboratory testing, educational programs, and some research in pulmonary medicine. Also there was a program in paramedical training operated jointly with ECU. Joseph S. Lennon, general administrator in Raleigh of the state's specialty hospitals, said that one wing of the Wilson facility was in good condition, but the other, built in 1942, "would take a lot of money to put it into first-class hospital shape."

Dr. Monroe thought that the discussion raised an interesting possibility. However, he said, the hospital, originally a tuberculosis sanitarium, had not been built to be used as a general hospital, or as a teaching hospital. He believed the school's primary teaching hospital had to be in Greenville, he said, especially for first- and second-year students who would otherwise miss the interaction between classrooms and the clinical setting.[10]

Faced with the shortage in revenue that the recession had brought about, the General Assembly was wrestling with the problem of identifying funds to carry out the ECU project to which a majority of legislators had committed themselves during the previous session. On Friday, January 24, Representative Horton Rountree mentioned publicly for the first time that changing plans for the ECU medical school might mean that it would not need all of the $54 million set aside for it by the Advisory Budget Committee. Possible arrangements, he said, were still being discussed with Pitt County Memorial Hospital for providing clinical training facilities of the new hospital being built at a cost of $16 million. This arrangement might make it unnecessary to use all of the $20 million budgeted for a teaching hospital.

Chancellor Jenkins, as was mentioned before, responded that it would be premature to say that the $20 million would not be needed. It might become a possibility, and ECU would welcome any means of saving money, as long as the medical school program did not suffer.[11] He said the $35.2 million 1975-77 appropriation for ECU's four-year school was absolutely essential.[12]

At a meeting in Raleigh of the ECU Chancellor's Advisory Committee on Medical Education, on Wednesday, January 28, Dr. Monroe said experts and accreditation officials had convinced ECU that the full $20 million allocated to construct a teaching hospital would be needed even if some arrangement could be worked out with PCMH about clinical teaching in that hospital.

At a meeting on the previous night, PCMH's medical staff had reaffirmed its wish to affiliate with the ECU medical school. The next morning, Jack M. Richardson, administrator of the hospital, said the PCMH medical staff had invited the School of Medicine to participate in a joint endeavor to practice medicine and educate medical students, as guests of Pitt Memorial Hospital, with both hospital staff and medical school faculty serving at the pleasure of the Board of

Trustees and the Board of County Commissioners. They hoped for a real cooperative relationship.

The medical staff emphasized, he said, that the hospital should retain its identity as Pitt Memorial Hospital and its ownership by the county, with the state bearing the cost of medical education. The medical staff were unanimous that there should be no duplication of facilities in Pitt County. The local physicians recognized the need for medical education, Richardson said, and supported that recognition by offering a set of principles as a basis for affiliation, with the understanding that the teaching program should supplement the hospital's purpose of providing medical services to the people. He also said that the medical staff recommended considering the addition of another bed tower to the new hospital, so that enough beds would be available to take care of teaching needs.

Bruce Strickland, Chairman of the Board of County Commissioners said that the commissioners would work with the medical school in any mutually advantageous way possible. He also mentioned that the county and ECU had joined in other projects beneficial to the county and the school. "We have offered them the old hospital building," he said, "but we don't want to get into competition with the medical school." Establishment of a separate teaching hospital could result in competition between the two hospitals for patients, he theorized. A committee of the board had been set up to work with the university to cooperate in working out a solution.

Strickland thought that while constructing another hospital might lead to competition, having the medical school base its clinical program at PCMH could add prestige to the county operation. The best thing for the county might be to find a workable plan for combining efforts.[13]

That the PCMH medical staff in reasserting its wish on Tuesday night, January 28, to affiliate with the ECU medical school had "substantially qualified" its proposal was not lost on interested observers.[14] The staff physicians were uneasy about competition for patients by a medical school faculty with a 200-bed teaching hospital, if one should be built, but not uneasy enough to accept any affiliation agreement that put a large portion of PCMH under administrative control of the medical school.

The *Raleigh News & Observer* commented editorially that this kind of issue often arises wherever new medical schools are proposed. What made Greenville different was the fact that the school's funding had already been approved. But planning was incomplete, and tensions between private and publicly funded medical practice might still make it difficult to recruit a medical school dean and faculty.[15]

Chancellor Jenkins, in an address to the Greenville Rotary Club on Monday, February 10, said that reports of conflict between Pitt County Memorial hospital and the East Carolina University Medical School had been contrived to create confusion. The Chancellor described as false the editorials and news stories making claims that local hospital officials in Greenville were reluctant to provide clinical teaching facilities to the medical school. He said that the reports were published by a few newspapers opposed to the school's expansion.

Jenkins denied there was any misunderstanding or disagreement between local medical practitioners, the hospital, and ECU planners. He outlined the planning that was going on. He said there would soon be residency programs in family practice, emphasizing primary care medicine. Also, residencies would be established in medicine, pediatrics, gynecology, and obstetrics, in cooperation with local physicians and the EAHEC.

UNC President Friday was quoted in news articles about the lack of an affiliation agreement as saying, ". . . a significant incompatibility exists in relating the clinical resources required for the proposed medical education program and obligations of the staff and trustees of a community-owned hospital." [16]

On March 13, 1975, the PCMH medical staff approved an agreement which would make PCMH the ECU School of Medicine's primary clinical training facility. The document, entitled "Principles of a Proposed Affiliation Agreement by the Pitt County Memorial Hospital and East Carolina University School of Medicine," would go before the hospital Board of Trustees on the following Tuesday, February 18.

Dr. Eric L. Fearrington, hospital chief of staff, said that the proposed agreement was not a legal document, but a set of principles on which to base an agreement. He explained that any affiliation agreement involved three parties: the hospital, including its staff and board of trustees, the University and its medical staff and board of trustees, and the national accrediting agency. He said the agreement being offered had been developed by the medical education liaison committee of PCMH, working with the medical school's administration, Kenneth Dews from the hospital board of trustees, and Charles Gaskins from the Board of County Commissioners.

The provisions of the affiliation agreement included these items: the PCMH board of trustees would continue to administer the hospital, with a third of its members representing the university; with the complete knowledge and consent of the patient and the attending physician, all patients would be available for the teaching program; patients from Pitt County would have priority for admission, in accordance with need; an open staff would be maintained, i.e., rights and privileges of physicians at PCMH who practiced privately in Pitt County and who were members of the hospital's medical staff could decline to participate in the program and still remain on the staff; additional beds and supporting teaching facilities would be added to the new PCMH at the expense of the State of North Carolina. The chairmen of the clinical departments at the medical school would administer hospital services, with an advisory committee including non-university physicians to provide checks, balances, and review for the system.

Fearrington reported that the medical staff had approved the principles by a decided margin, and had recommended to the hospital's board of directors that it also should approve. He said, "This approach to use Pitt County Memorial Hospital as the primary teaching center for the university will sort of obviate the need of having two separate hospitals in this community." He noted that a great deal of concern had been expressed by PCMH medical staff members and university officials that there might be two hospitals standing side-by-side each of them with about fifty percent occupancy. This would be a very expensive situation, he said. It was his opinion and that of the staff that the proposed affiliation would save money for the county's citizens. He commented that the financial side of the joint venture would be up to the Board of County Commissioners and the hospital board of trustees, and was outside the authority of the medical staff.

Jack Richardson, administrator of PCMH, agreed, and said it would be up to the trustees and commissioners to set up a formal contract agreement between PCMH and ECU. He thought the proposed agreement showed there was firm support at the hospital for the ECU medical school, with eighty-five percent of the medical staff voting to recommend to the trustees the acceptance of the principles.

Dr. Monroe, in an interview by a *Greenville Daily Reflector* reporter, said, "The university is very gratified at the tremendously positive attitude the Pitt County Memorial Hospital medical staff demonstrated. This is a major step toward the goal of developing a medical school which is closely allied with the community of Pitt County and of Eastern North Carolina. And as the necessary additional steps are taken to officially complete the affiliations and arrangements implied in this action . . ., it will be of great benefit to the university, to the hospital, and to the people."[17]

On March 19, 1975, as expected, the Board of Trustees of Pitt County Memorial Hospital approved the affiliation of the hospital with the ECU School of Medicine.[18] On Saturday, April 25, the ECU Board of Trustees, unanimously and without discussion, approved the tentative affiliation plan.[19] Approval would have to come from the UNC Board of Governors before an agreement could be entered upon.

In the General Assembly, the battle to assure funding for the medical school went on. The agreement to use PCMH facilities rather than building a teaching hospital would cut $6-8 million from the $20 million proposed for a new 200-bed facility, UNC vice president for academic affairs Raymond Dawson told the legislators. The state would add 100-150 teaching beds to the new Pitt Hospital, now about a third complete. The education subcommittee accepted Friday's recommendation, and on May 1, the Senate Appropriations Subcommittee accepted it also, voting to cut $7 million from the request for $35.245 million in new funds for constructing facilities at ECU medical school, leaving $28.245 million.[20]

When, in June, the General Assembly finally approved the budget for expanding the medical school, it was predicated on completion of the agreement to add educational facilities to PCMH. The funds for a separate teaching hospital had been deleted, and a lesser amount approved for the required changes in the hospital.

ECU Chancellor Jenkins, Vice Chancellor Monroe, and Dr. Harold Wiggers, acting dean of the medical school, went to Chapel Hill on Thursday to announce to the UNC Board of Governors Planning Committee that ECU had reached an agreement with Pitt County Memorial Hospital and the Pitt County Board of Commissioners to use the hospital for teaching. The agreement was contingent on approval by the UNC board and by accreditation officials. The hospital board would maintain control over all the beds, but ECU representatives would make up at least a third of the board. The university and the hospital would each bear the costs of their own programs.

Work was scheduled to begin the following May on a 100-bed tower for the medical school, giving the hospital a total 450-bed capacity. The addition was estimated to cost $12.3 million instead of the $20 million for a separate teaching hospital. In order for the new hospital to be eligible for Medicaid and Medicare reimbursements it would have to be approved by the Comprehensive Health Planning Section of the NC Department of Human Resources. Lawrence B.

Burwell, chief of the section, had written to say that the approval process would take at least forty-five days.

The tentative affiliation agreement included the clause "this agreement can be either terminated or amended by mutual consent of both parties." Felix Joyner, UNC vice president for finance, wondered how the university could dispose of a bed tower inseparably attached to PCMH, if the agreement should ever be terminated. He said that if the agreement should collapse after several years, the state "would probably have built the county a nice big hospital." [21]

A further impediment to the affiliation process, and to accreditation of the medical school, was still to come. On June 3, 1975, Dr. Harold Wiggers wrote to Dr. John D. Porterfield, Chairman of the Joint Commission on Accreditation of Hospitals, whom he had met many years ago, to discuss the denial of reaccreditation to the Pitt County Memorial Hospital. A single site visitor from the commission had examined the hospital in March, and had left without indicating that he had found any inadequacies, or indicating in any way that the accreditation of the hospital was in immediate jeopardy. The notice that reaccreditation was being refused because of more than seventy violations of commission guidelines had come as a great shock.

Wiggers had been led to believe that the field representative had failed to fulfill his mission properly, and must have developed a retaliatory attitude because of what may have seemed to be harassment and a refusal to cooperate on the part of a few vocal physicians in the locality. While he did not excuse their behavior, he did not think that an entire hospital should be made to suffer for the attitudes of a few of its medical staff.

He outlined for Dr. Porterfield the progress that had been made toward developing a four-year medical school in Greenville, including the decision not to build an independent 200-bed teaching hospital. Agreement had been reached to use the redesigned and enlarged PCMH facility then being built as a teaching facility. That agreement, satisfactory to the LCME, to local officials, and to the hospital, was to be submitted to the UNC Board of Governors the next week for approval. The medical school was then in the process of recruiting chairmen and faculty for clinical departments. Withdrawal of accreditation of the hospital would create a catastrophic situation, threatening not only recruitment, but also funding and LCME accreditation. If the hospital was not re-accredited well before March 1976, the date of the medical school's accreditation visit, then the entire project would be washed down the drain.

Wiggers entreated Dr. Porterfield to make sure that the appeal from the hospital was given attention quickly and fairly. In Greenville, everything possible would be done to meet the commission's standards.[22]

The trustees of Pitt County Memorial Hospital were, according to newspaper reports, not informed until June 17 that the hospital was not to be reaccredited. The trustees were shocked and indignant when they were told about it at their regular meeting. Dr. Eric Fearrington, Chief of Staff, immediately set to work with trustee chairman W. R. Duke to prepare a presentation the following week to the commission in Chicago. Fearrington said, "These people don't care a thing about how we treat our patients. We could kill every one that comes in just as long as we document it correctly. But we have to go through this to get the federal nickel." That is, Medicare and Medicaid reimbursement depended on meeting the standards of the commission.

Some of the recommendations of the commission concerned environmental services and the physical condition of the existing hospital. Some dealt with meeting new fire safety codes, which would be met when the new hospital was put into use. Eight had to do with governing body bylaws and twenty-eight with revisions of medical staff bylaws. These revisions had been delayed until some of the interrelationships between the PCMH staff and ECU's faculty could be clarified. Twenty-one violations dealt with documentation of hospital activities for which there was no record. Hospital administrator Jack Richardson said that the negative report meant the hospital was doing things for which they did not get credit.[23]

The commission's action, which would not be made final unless the appeal failed, did not affect the plans to locate ECU medical school teaching facilities in the new hospital. Dr. Monroe said that the hospital was outdated and overcrowded. No one had any illusions about this. He believed that once the situation was understood clearly by the accrediting authorities, and they were informed about the new hospital being built, the preliminary decision would be changed. It was based on only partial understanding by a site visitor. Jack Richardson said that when the site visit took place in March he tried to point out that the physical deficiencies at the present hospital were the prime reason for the new multimillion dollar plant.[24]

On June 25, the General Assembly approved the appropriation for the medical school. Dr. Monroe said to a *Greenville Daily Reflector* reporter the next morning that the funds appropriated would permit expanding the area in PCMH to accommodate the medical school's needs for a teaching hospital, would support an intensive care nursery, the Health Affairs Library, and provide a building to house all of the medical school departments and administrative units. Monroe indicated that there was no urgency about constructing the bed tower, on which work was scheduled to begin.

The UNC Board of Governors met on July 21, 1975, and accepted a committee recommendation on where to cut spending in response to budget reductions made by the General Assembly. They decided to cut out all of the system's priority items except funds scheduled for eliminating racial discrimination. The Board appointed sixty-eight members to the boards of trustees of the constituent institutions of the university system. They voted not to reappoint Roddy L. Jones of Raleigh to the ECU Board of Trustees, despite objections of David J. Whichard of Greenville. A board member who did not want to be identified said Jones has been "very abrasive" in his dealings with the board over the ECU medical school situation. This had made some of them unhappy.

William J. Stanley of Rocky Mount was proposed by the nominating committee to fill the unexpired term of a retiring member of the ECU board of trustees. Whichard nominated Jones for that post, but he was defeated in a secret ballot. The board appointed one new member to the ECU board, and reappointed three incumbents for four-year terms. Dr. Wiley T. Armstrong of Rocky Mount, chairman of the board, was also not reappointed.

Jacob H. Froelich, Jr., of High Point, who was chairman of the nominating committee, said after the meeting that the decision not to nominate Jones for another term had "nothing in the world to do" with the ECU board's efforts to expand the school of medicine to a four-year school. William A. Dees, Jr., of Goldsboro said the vote indicated only that the board thought William Stanley was "the better man."[25]

The Board of Governors also decided that the $13 million appropriated to modify PCMH to provide teaching facilities would be allocated only when (1) an acceptable agreement was reached between the school and the hospital, (2) the state hospital planning authorities had approved the planned changes in the hospital to accommodate the school, and (3) the hospital's accreditation was renewed. The plans were to modify the central portion of the hospital to provide space for x-ray, laboratory, and other facilities for the medical school, and to add a 100-bed tower.

The Board agreed to hold a special meeting in August if the requirements had been met by then. Otherwise, they would not meet again until September.[26]

Dean William E. Laupus said he considered the action taken by the board "exactly what we expected, quite routine. It's just a matter of following procedure and not releasing the funds until everything is in order. We're proceeding on all three requirements and will be ready whenever they choose to meet. This will be up to Dr. Friday, I believe."[27]

Administrator Jack Richardson announced on July 24 that Pitt County Memorial Hospital had received provisional one-year accreditation from the Joint Committee on Accreditation of Hospitals. The usual accreditation was for two years, but the full term had been withheld because the hospital's medical staff by-laws were under revision to provide for affiliation with the new four-year medical school. There were also deficiencies in the physical plant, he said, but these would no longer exist when the new building was completed in 1976.[28]

On September 15, 1975, the Governor's Advisory Council on Health Planning, after a public hearing, gave preliminary approval to a $7.6 million construction and renovation project at PCMH to provide clinical facilities and space for ECU medical school. A final decision was still to be made by the Comprehensive Health Planning Agency (CHPA) of the Human Resources Department, whose approval was necessary for the hospital to receive Medicaid and Medicare reimbursements. The planned construction would give the hospital 88,000 square feet of additional space, and include clinical laboratories, X-ray facilities, and emergency operating rooms.

No opposition was presented at the hearing, which, according to Lawrence Burwell, chief of the CHPA, was unusual for a project of its size. He saw no problem with the request, and said that if no objections were received in the next five to seven days, his agency could approve it before the deadline for the decision, at the end of September.

Dean William Laupus told reporters that no consideration was being given at the time to the construction of a bed tower. He did not know when the beds would be needed.[29]

On September 19, the *Greenville Daily Reflector* reported that the PCMH Board of Trustees had informally rejected a request by ECU medical school Dean William Laupus that the school be given fifty percent representation on the Trustees' Executive Board. The LCME had demanded such representation, Laupus said, and asked Board members to reserve judgment until the matter could be discussed at length. He had promised to send Dr. Eric Fearrington, chief of staff at the hospital, a copy of the confidential LCME report calling for the fifty percent representation.[30]

Members of the hospital board commented on its action. Dr. Fearrington said, "Apprehension is running high in the county that this hospital will be taken over by the Medical School." Mrs. Bancroft Moseley, a member of the hospital board said, "The people of Pitt County do not want this, and we are their representatives." Dr. John Wooten said he considered the LCME demand rather arbitrary. "I don't see how they can say that the Medical School will succeed if they have fifty percent representation on the hospital executive committee and will not if they have less. And I wonder if it would stand up in court if it were to be contested."

Dr. Fearrington said he believed the University group should sell their people on the affiliation agreement that had taken so much hard work and such a long time to produce.[31] He did not bring up the fact that the university had now relinquished the original objective of building an independent teaching hospital, and the legislature had decreased the medical school's funding proportionately. There was no longer any imminent threat of having a rival hospital built in PCMH's neighborhood.

On Tuesday, September 23, 1975, the Comprehensive Health Planning Section of the Department of Human Resources notified the PCMH that expansion of clinical facilities at the hospital to accommodate the medical school at ECU could proceed. The approval did not include expansion of the hospital's bed capacity, the agency said. If this was needed later on, it would have to be the subject of a separate request.[32]

Dr. E. W. Furgurson of Plymouth was recognized in the September issue of *N. C. People Magazine* for his involvement in the early campaign to bring a medical school to East Carolina University. In the article, Dr. Leo Jenkins outlined the eleven-year political fight which had come to an end with the General Assembly's approving the funding of the expansion of the school to a full degree-granting program.

He gave Dr. Furgurson credit for planting the seed for the school when he visited Dr. Jenkins one Sunday afternoon in 1964. Jenkins wrote:

> Dr. Furgurson told us he had just returned from a symposium at Duke University. The symposium dealt with the decline of medical practice in rural areas. As a family doctor in Rural Eastern North Carolina, Dr. Furgurson was particularly concerned about the growing shortage of doctors to meet the medical needs of the region.

I became concerned myself when he acquainted me with the alarming situation. It came as a shock to me to learn that in terms of the availability of medical and health care delivery, the eastern section of our state was one of the worst in the nation. The question was, what could our institution do about it? [33]

UNC President Friday said on Tuesday, October 14, that the Educational Planning, Policies and Programs Committee of the Board of Governers voted on Monday to recommend to the full board approval of an affiliation agreement between the ECU School of Medicine and PCMH. Approval of the agreement will make the hospital the primary clinical teaching facility for the medical school. Friday said the proposed agreement would be considered by the board when it met on November 14, at North Carolina A&T State University in Greensboro.

The agreement had been worked out in meetings between the Pitt County Board of Commissioners, the hospital's medical staff and board of trustees, medical school officials, members of General Administration staff and the medical school planning committee. The county officials had approved the idea of affiliation several months before, but had balked at allowing state control of the hospital, Jack Richardson said. Instead of the fifty percent representation on the executive committee of the hospital's board of trustees that ECU had sought, the agreement provided that three of the seven-member executive committee would be from the medical school, but not specifically designated as officers. This was an improvement on the earlier offer by the local officials of two positions to the medical school.

The full hospital board would be sixty percent local representatives, forty percent appointed by Pitt County commissioners from a group named by the Board of Governors. When the Board of Governors approved the agreement, about $7.6 million in state funds would become available for alterations to the new hospital building. Dr. Jenkins commented on the planning committee's action, "This brings us one step closer to our medical school, and I'm grateful for the dedication on the part of all the people concerned." [34]

The UNC Board of Governors on Friday, October 14, 1975, approved by a twenty-three to six margin the twenty-year affiliation agreement between the ECU School of Medicine and Pitt County Memorial Hospital. George Watts Hill, Sr., of Durham, strenuously objected to the action. He was doubtful that having a hospital with two medical staffs could possibly work out. He objected to the weak University representation on the hospital board of trustees and its executive committee, insisting that there should be equal representation between the county and ECU. The fact that the PCMH medical staff had not yet approved the affiliation agreement made it unacceptable for the UNC Board to approve it, Hill said.[35]

The board also approved the release of $4.8 million to expand facilities of the 315-bed hospital. It set aside a $3.8 million reserve to add a 100-bed tower to the hospital later. The agreement now had to go back for final approval by the hospital trustees and the Pitt County Board of Commissioners, who, according to Pitt County Manager H. R. Gray, had already tentatively endorsed it.

Dean Laupus, replying in a telephone interview to Watts Hill's statement, said that the agreement contained adequate checks and balances, and that he was confident it would protect the state's investment in the hospital. He said that it relied on the good faith of both university and county officials. "I don't think America got where it is by people not being willing to risk some things on faith," he said. He also said that Hill's objection to the medical school's having only forty percent representation on the board of directors of the hospital was compensated for by the school's being able to designate the chairmen of its clinical departments as chiefs of the staff in their specialty areas of the hospital.

Hill had objected that medical school faculty might be paid considerably less than their colleagues appointed by the hospital board of trustees, because of regulations about state salaries. He had complained about the agreement that ECU would pay all of the educational costs, when it is impossible to separate these from treatment costs. Laupus agreed that there were some gray areas, but said problems could be resolved by negotiation.

Laupus disputed Hill's claim that affiliation was likely to raise costs for patients, which was at the time only $48 a day at PCMH, whereas at Duke Hospital and NC Memorial Hospital it was about $200 a day, and at Watts Hospital in Durham $110 a day. He said that he did not believe costs would increase anywhere near as much as Hill estimated. The hospital was going to be in a completely different milieu from the ones with which he compared it.

[1] Letter from Edwin W. Monroe to Eric L. Fearrington, August 28, 1968, in ECU School of Medicine Files, Folder "Affiliation Agreement with PCMH."

[2] Memorandum Covering Discussion and Conclusions Reached at a Meeting of the Joint Conference Committee Held at Pitt County Memorial Hospital, 8 p. m., Monday, January 13, 1969, ECU School of Medicine Files, Folder "Affiliation Agreement with PCMH."

[3] Letter from Charles P. Cardwell, Jr., to Dean Edwin Monroe, December 9, 1969, ECU School of Medicine Files, Folder "Affiliation Agreement with PCMH."

[4] Georgette Hedrick in *Chronicles of Pitt County North Carolina*, ed. Elizabeth H. Copeland, Pitt County Historical Society (Greenville, 1982) ; p. 25.

[5] Telephone interview with *Raleigh News & Observer*, August 19, 1974.

[6] William C. Friday Records, Subgroup 1, Series 1, "Medical Education, Sept.-Oct.. 1974;" "Dean's Log," September 19, 1974.

[7] *Ibid.*

[8] *Raleigh News & Observer*, January 8, 1975.

[9] Legislative Research Commission, Subcommittee on Health, Minutes of February 27, 1970 meeting, in ECU School of Medicine Files, Folder "Legislative Research Commission (Health Subcommittee), 1969-70."

[10] *Raleigh News & Observer*, January 10, 1975.

[11] *Charlotte Observer*, January 25, 1975.

[12] *High Point Enterprise*, January 30, 1975.

[13] *Greenville Daily News*, January 29, 1975; Associated Press & United Press; *High Point Enterprise*, January 30, 1975; same article in *Chapel Hill Newspaper, Durham Sun, Greensboro Daily News*, etc.

[14] Editorial in *Raleigh News & Observer*, February 1, 1975.

[15] Editorial in *Raleigh News & Observer*, February 1, 1975.

[16] *Raleigh News & Observer*, February 11, 1975.

[17] *Greenville Daily News*, March 13, 1975.

[18] *Greenville Daily News*, March 19, 1975.

[19] *Raleigh News & Observer*, April 26, 1975.

[20] *Raleigh News & Observer*, June 2, 1975.

[21] *Raleigh News & Observer*, June 13, 1975.

[22] Letter from Dr. Harold Wiggers to Dr. John D. Porterfield, June 3, 1975, in ECU School of Medicine Files, Vice Chancellor and Dean's Office, LCME Site Visit Notebook

[23] *Greenville Daily News*, June 18, 1975.

[24] *Greensboro Daily News*, June 20, 1975.

[25] *Raleigh News & Observer*, July 22, 1975.

[26] *Ibid.*

[27] *Raleigh News & Observer*, July 23, 1975.

[28] *Raleigh News & Observer*, July 25, 1975.

[29] *Washington Daily News*, September 16, 1975; also *Greensboro Daily News, Henderson Dispatch, High Point Enterprise, Monroe Enquirer-Journal, Winston-Salem Journal, Raleigh News & Observer*, etc., for same date.

[30] *Greenville Daily News*, September 17, 1975.

[31] *Greenville Daily News*, September 17, 1975..

[32] *Winston-Salem Journal*, September 24, 1975.

[33] *Plymouth Roanoke Beacon*, September 24, 1975.

[34] *Greensboro Daily News*, November 5, 1975.

[35] William C. Friday Documents, Subgroup 2, Series 3, Minutes of the Board of Governors, October 14, 1975. The full six-page text of Hill's remarks is included in the minutes.

Chapter 19
Troubles with Accreditation

The Liaison Committee on Medical Education surveys existing and proposed medical schools in the United States and Canada for the purpose of maintaining the quality of medical education. The committee is recognized as the accrediting agency for medical schools, and a graduate of an unaccredited school would find it difficult or impossible to enter residency training, obtain hospital staff privileges, or even receive a license to practice.[1] For this reason, it was essential for the new four-year program at East Carolina University to win independent accreditation.

Under the plan that the Board of Governors authorized on November 15, 1974, the responsibility of the UNC School of Medicine for the medical school at East Carolina University would end with the conclusion of the 1974-75 academic year. On November 19, President Friday wrote to Dr. James Schofield, secretary of the Liaison Committee on Medical Education, asking him to take steps to provide for separate accreditation of the ECU medical school.

He enclosed a copy of the resolution passed by the Governors, which he understood would qualify the ECU program for separate accreditation under LCME criteria. On the same day, he informed Chancellors Leo Jenkins and Ferebee Taylor and Dean Christopher Fordham of his action.[2]

Following Friday's letter to the LCME, he and Dr. Harold Wiggers asked Dr. Schofield for help in planning and implementing the medical school. On November 25, Chancellor Jenkins and Dr. Monroe called Schofield to discuss what ECU should do to get under way, and asking for help in finding a dean.[3]

Dr. Schofield asked what they had already done. Chancellor Jenkins described the search committee he had appointed, and Dr. Schofield wanted to know what they had done in terms of satisfying affirmative action requirements. He said they should advertise in many different places—in the *Chronicles of Higher Education*, in the *New England Journal of Medicine*, in the *Journal of the AMA*, the New York *Times*, and black newspapers in New York. They should also write to deans and directors of medical schools, consulting the AMA directory for names.

Jenkins said that they would also like his recommendations for possible deans. Schofield said that he would pass the request along to his associates so that he could not be accused of favoritism. He said that they should write to him requesting names of consultants who could visit the ECU campus on a regular basis to advise on what should be done. Dr. Monroe should also get in touch with Dr. Glen Leymaster of the AMA.

Dr. Monroe mentioned that President Friday had proposed thirty students for admission in September, 1975, but he felt there should be some alternative, such as moving admission of the first class to September 1976. To get ready by 1975 would not be impossible, but would rush things. Would it be possible for the LCME at its June meeting to consider the 1975 opening? If it was possible, when should a site visit be scheduled? It would take several months to get ready for it.

Dr. Schofield replied that for consideration at the June meeting, a visit would have to occur in late March or early April. It could be canceled up to the last minute if ECU was not ready. However, they probably could not get a dean that quickly, even though they had already begun the search. The Christmas holidays would interfere, and they would be lucky to identify anyone by late January or early February. He suggested that they not keep the option open too long, but allow only a limited time for candidates to decide. Some prospects would tend to put off decision.

Dr. Monroe asked about the current requirements for provisional accreditation. Dr. Schofield said the dean should be there before a consultant visit. The faculty had to be strengthened, substantive progress made in recruiting basic science faculty, and some clinical people should be there before they could start the first year. Since they were going to go straight through a four-year program, they had to go beyond basic sciences from the beginning. When the provisional accreditation team came, they would want to see what had been done, and what plans had been made. How much curriculum planning had to be done? Dr. Monroe wanted to know.

First, there had to be a facilities plan. Would all the clinical training be done at Pitt Memorial Hospital, or would they build a teaching hospital to accommodate 200 students? Monroe said there were several possibilities: buy the new PCMH; buy and refurbish the old hospital; build a new 200-bed teaching hospital; try to develop an affiliation with the county hospitals, new and old. They did not know which was best. Schofield advised them that they did not need to decide right away, but should take their time about it.

Dr. Monroe said that President Friday's approach was that the LCME should decide, based in a two-year independent school aimed at becoming a four-year school, but he did not think that sounded right. If they intended to go for a four-year school, then toss aside

Friday's idea, Schofield said. Since they had been authorized to move to four years, they should not try to enroll the first class in the fall of 1975. They would have trouble. The LCME would not let the program begin until it was ready. "You might be miracle workers," he said, "but to get a dean, clinical chairmen, building, and legislative funding by April—I don't think you can do it. If you hold the starting time to 1976, it would be better."

Schofield said they should proceed as they wanted to, and when they were ready, let the LCME know. Approval came when the charter class was enrolled. The committee would consult frequently with the new dean, and go over the third and fourth year plans with him at great length, along with everything else. The normal time it had taken the medical schools started since 1960 to get going had been about twenty-seven months. The last nine averaged twenty-five months. Even September, 1976, would be cutting it close—but the LCME would tell them if they were not ready.

Dr. Monroe asked Dr. Schofield about Dr. Harold Wiggers, who was moving to Greenville in the spring. Schofield said that he was a solid man. Even if he had not built any new school, he would be good on relationships. He said he would have confidence in Wiggers, but that they should let the new dean decide about him. If the dean wanted to do it all, then let him, and let others come in periodically as consultants.

Monroe asked about admissions and scheduling again. If they postponed opening, would it be possible to operate for a year without students? Schofield repeated that he did not see how they could start in 1975.

Chancellor Jenkins asked about continuing as they were then going, sending students on to Chapel Hill and keep the one-year program to provide continuity. Schofield thought they should keep everything in Greenville, even though, as Jenkins remarked, the public might not understand. As the school made its new start, the administration should talk about a new hospital. One school, the University of South Florida in Tampa, had built an ambulatory family care center on their campus, and had no inpatient facility of its own. The school used the veterans hospital across the street for beds, breaking with the Johns Hopkins model.[4]

The main question was not how many beds, but how much clinical capacity was available; how many patients flowed through the community hospitals. The LCME would see if it was sufficient, see how many people the hospitals could accommodate per class, and so on. That would be better than deciding that a certain fixed number of beds was needed. In any case, it must be a hospital suitable for teaching. PCMH might have to make some changes, and they should bring in consultants quickly to decide about this.

Monroe asked if there was any point in checking about federal funding, and Schofield said that there was nothing available at the time. The support program was defunct, although Congress might give one more year for capitation grants. The summer before, there had been only $100 million in building funds available, and many schools standing in line. ECU should get its congressmen to work on new legislation. The Comprehensive Health Manpower Training Act of 1971 was up for renewal, and they should enlist their senators and representatives to move it along. It could mean a million dollars a year when the school reached full enrollment.[5]

The conference call closed with Dr. Schofield's urging that they should not rush things, and promised to send a letter stating explicitly that it appeared that 1975 would be an unrealistic date. He said he would like to take a report of their conference, and a copy of the Board of Governors' resolution to the LCME at its next meeting. Chancellor Jenkins asked him to send two letters, one recommending potential candidates for the dean position, and the other about the scheduling of opening the school. Dr. Schofield agreed, and said he would add a list of possible consultants. The question of clinical facilities needed to be resolved as soon as possible. The dean's search committee should ask each candidate's opinion on the subject. He added, "I'm weary of boy deans. Get a mature man. It is tough to start a med school."[6]

The authorization to develop a four-year separately accredited medical school in Greenville had not removed UNC-CH's obligation to provide the LCME by January 1, 1975, with a progress report on the one-year school. UNC Dean Fordham transmitted a summary prepared by Dr. William Cromartie of the progress that had been made under his direction in reorganizing admissions, teaching, examinations, and faculty participation. Dr. Cromartie also gave an account of Dr. Sylvanus Nye's resignation, followed by that of Dr. A. B. Fatteh, which had wiped out the pathology department, so that the UNC medical school Department of Pathology had to provide most of the pathology teaching.

Fordham's cover letter emphasized the Board of Governor's decision to transform the ECU school into a four-year, degree-granting medical school. He asked the LCME to accept the progress report as covering the remainder of the academic year at the end of which the one-year program would terminate along with UNC's responsibility and authority. On December 17, President Friday forwarded Dean Fordham's letter and the enclosed report from Dr. Cromartie to Dr. James Schofield, sending copies to the president of the Board of Governors and the chancellors of ECU and UNC.[7]

Chancellor Jenkins wrote to President Friday on January 8, following up a conversation Friday and Robert Holt, ECU Vice Chancellor and Dean, had the previous day. Jenkins confirmed that Dr. Wiggers and Dr. Schofield were in agreement that it would be unwise to attempt to have an accreditation site visit aimed at provisional accreditation in time to enroll students in September, 1975. ECU's part in land purchase negotiations had been completed, and the renovation of Ragsdale was to begin very soon. However, the survey visit, which would have to be in March or early April, would give only two months to accomplish the planning that had to be done for the four-year school before the site visit, and to recruit a dean and full-time clinical department heads. Further, the visit and the LCME's action might occur before the General Assembly had acted on the Board of Governors' funding requests. Even if the results of the visit were extremely positive, the committee would probably refuse accreditation because of the lack of an assured budget for operation and facilities.

Chancellor Jenkins's considered judgment was that it would not be practical to aim for provisional accreditation in spring, 1975, to admit students that fall. Rather, he wished to admit the first class in September, 1976, a timetable that he felt could be met successfully. The General Assembly would have acted on funding, interim facilities would be ready, the site for building purchased, and architectural planning virtually finished. What would be more important to the LCME was that the dean and his key faculty would be ready to receive the site visitors.[8]

President Friday reported to the Board of Governors on January 10 that Vice Chancellor Robert Holt had notified him that ECU would not seek an accreditation site visit for the school's proposed four-year medical school during 1975, so that entrance of the school's first class would have to be delayed until at least the fall of 1976. The deferral was to enable the medical school staff to continue planning and recruitment of faculty.

Friday said that ECU Chancellor Jenkins had decided that planning and other steps could not be accomplished in time for a 1975 visit. "I think he has made the right decision and a wise decision," he said, "and everyone counsels that you should take as much time and spend as much energy to plan and recruit faculty as possible . . . before seeking accreditation." [9]

On April 15, President Friday told Chancellor Jenkins that Dr. Harold Wiggers had familiarized him with developments at ECU in planning for personnel, program development, and facilities for the new medical school. Friday said that the usual procedure followed in beginning new medical schools was to ask the LCME for a Letter of Reasonable Assurance (LRA) that the program would be accredited. He said that he and Dr. Wiggers had agreed that this procedure should be followed, and that both of them had conferred with Dr. James Schofield about it. The LRA procedure would give the UNC President a way to give the Board of Governors reasonable assurance that the ECU program would be accredited. He was sure that Dr. Schofield would help in developing a procedure and schedule for obtaining the LRA at the appropriate time, making it possible to recommend to the Board of Governors to allocate permanent construction funds or obtain necessary appropriations for capital improvements.[10]

Evidently, there was a misunderstanding. Dr. Wiggers realized that he had not made his view of the situation regarding obtaining a LRA clear to President Friday. He had agreed that it would be a good approach, if feasible, but had thought it was clear that, from his experience and from conversations with Dr. Schofield, it would be useless to attempt such a procedure.

Dr. Wiggers and Dr. Monroe immediately telephoned Dr. Schofield, and he stated very clearly that for ECU to request a LRA from the Liaison Committee would be a precedent-setting request. He also said that the only reason the LCME used the procedure of reasonable assurance was to meet requirements of federal statutes that denied allocation of construction money until accreditation had been reasonably assured. This procedure, he said, was already an "overwhelming and expensive burden for a voluntary agency, such as the LCME, in addition to its heavy schedule of regular accreditation activities."

In any case, the request could not be considered before the June 25, 1975, meeting of the LCME, at which time Schofield said he would advise against acceding to it, since otherwise it would set a precedent impractical for the committee to follow. In particular, to undertake it for every medical education program in the fifty states based on non-federal funds would be impossible. He opposed it on philosophical grounds as well as practical ones.

Chancellor Jenkins said that Dr. Wiggers would secure written confirmation of Dr. Schofield's reaction, and forward a copy of the reply when it was received.[11] Dr. Schofield's answer came on May 8.

He said that he thought the best way to summarize the telephone conversation with Drs. Wiggers and Monroe would be to review what he usually answered to inquiries concerning accreditation of new medical schools.

Schofield noted that the survey of the resources needed to develop a new school, the number and quality of people, academic programs and facilities, had become more and more difficult as start-up grant funding and construction resources had become limited, and as the climate had changed in regard to accreditation itself. Most of the academic medical centers built during the past twenty years had involved funding from different sources, including the federal government. Federal agencies required some guarantees regarding accreditation before they would allocate specific grant funds, and the LRA procedure had been set up in response to federal requirements. A full survey team visit, usually preceded by staff visits, and the favorable judgment of the full committee after studying the survey team report were generally prerequisites for determination that accreditation could be reasonably assured. The LRA pertained to an evaluation of the entire situation: faculty and staff already secured, curriculum planning, availability of students, temporary facilities, funding for new facilities and operating costs, and other factors.

The LCME had been asked for LRA's by proposed medical schools sponsored by the Veterans Administration, but the procedure in such cases was just getting under way. To request a LRA for a state-funded school, to assist in planning and funding, was a new proposition which the LCME would have to consider, the next meeting at which this could be done being, as he had said, on June 25, 1975. If, against Schofield's recommendation, the committee should agree to undertake the LRA procedure for the University of North Carolina, he judged that there would have to be an informal staff visit first to decide when there might be a complete survey team visit.

So, the Letter of Reasonable Assurance route was not a likely one. Still, President Friday requested a visit to get "advice and counsel at the present stage of development of ECU School of Medicine and approaches being taken in planning." [12] On June 20, President Friday notified Chancellor Jenkins that Dr. Schofield and Dr. Leymaster had confirmed their plans for such a visit. They had invited Dr. John Deitrick, former Dean of the Cornell School of Medicine, to assist in the consultations. [13] Dr. Deitrick, something of an elder statesman of the medical education establishment, was Acting Director of the Associated Medical Schools of New York and New Jersey, and had been dean at Cornell University School of Medicine during the 1940's when Dr. Laupus was completing his internship and residency at New York Hospital, Cornell Medical Center.

Dr. William Laupus, who had become dean of the medical school on July 1, was told just before the July 4 holiday that the meeting was to be held, and that he was to attend. This unofficial meeting was to take place on Monday, July 7, with ECU officials in Greenville, and on Tuesday with UNC officials, ECU officials, and legislators in Chapel Hill. Schofield had asked for information on the plans that had been developed, and a collection of planning materials had been sent to him to distribute to the other visitors.[14]

Only a short time before, Dr. Schofield had written for the LCME to refuse issuance to the incipient East Tennessee State University medical school a Letter of Reasonable Assurance preliminary to actual accreditation. The ETSU school was also a second state-funded institution in a state with one already established medical school. It resembled the school at ECU in many ways, both in the nature of political opposition to its founding, and in the deficiencies that had to be overcome for it to be an accredited program. It had no teaching hospital of its own, but depended on community hospitals and a VA hospital located nearby. It had not yet recruited an adequate faculty, and had not planned and built its physical facilities.[15]

The Greenville meeting was held in a conference room at the ECU School of Medicine offices in the east tower of the Biology Building. It began at 9:30 in the morning and resumed after lunch had been served, to end about 3:30 that afternoon. The medical school was represented by Dr. Monroe, Dr. Wiggers, and Dean William Laupus, who had come in from Richmond a day or two earlier so he could be briefed as far a possible on what had gone on before he accepted the deanship. As he looked over the agenda that had been prepared for the meeting, Dr. Laupus did not anticipate how distressing his first involvement in the ECU-Chapel Hill battle would be. He did see that all he could expect to talk about was what was to be done in the future, since he had not been involved in planning up to that point.[16]

When the three visitors came in, they were silent and showed no signs of friendliness. Dr. Schofield announced at the start that the meeting was an unofficial site visit to find out what had been planned and what had been done toward the projected school. He emphasized that it was the LCME's responsibility to keep informed about each stage of development at ECU. He distributed the formal agenda, which was soon forgotten.

Dr. Monroe spoke first, saying that it would not be fair to call on the new dean, since he had just arrived and was not yet fully informed about developments. He gave a progress report on the status of the four-year program. Dr. Laupus remembered that about a half an hour into his report, which was "a detailed but not burdensome presentation of the accomplishments of the schools one-year program in existence from 1972 through 1975, and the planning which had taken place since Dr. Wiggers's arrival in early January 1975, Dr. Deitrick began to show evidence of impatience and began to question Monroe and Wiggers about research, funding, foundations (both local and national) to support research, etc. Deitrick repeatedly interrupted Monroe's presentation with irrelevant questions and remarks. He was on a tirade, repeating himself frequently and appearing to be more angry and less in control as the morning wore on. Schofield and Leymaster participated to a limited degree and controlled themselves much better than Deitrick, who was the angry old man of organized medical education personified, one who had built up a great accumulation of scores to settle with the non-traditional schools of the 60s and 70s, which not so incidentally had paid little heed to his advice and dire warnings. What had been at best expected by us to be an unpleasant but endurable expression of negative impressions of the school's future turned into a bitter, rancorous display of temper by an aging, still arrogant, patrician medical educator."[17]

Deitrick first criticized the floundering that had gone on as ECU attempted to set up a one-year school, then a two-year school, and finally a four-year school. The squabbling between ECU and UNC, he said, had led to confusion and even chaos, so that there could be no rational, step-by-step development.

Then he asked how such an inadequate institution could hope to establish a medical school. There was no foundation for research, which was essential for the success of any medical school—no laboratories and no money to acquire them. He did not believe that a medical school could succeed unless it was research-oriented.

Dr. Monroe interrupted to mention the faculty members, Drs. William Waugh, Sam Pennington, Lynis Dohm, and Hisham Barakat, who had received grants and were carrying on creditable research, along with their teaching. Deitrick ignored this rebuttal as a triviality, and continued to censure ECU for refusal to cooperate with UNC-CH, and to denigrate everything that had been done. Occasionally, Schofield and Leymaster chimed in with their own critical, but less rancorous, comments.

They ate lunch in virtual silence when it was brought in at noon.

The ECU group, with a great deal of self-control, managed to get through a short afternoon session much like that of the morning. At the end of the meeting, Dr. Schofield reminded them that they had been invited to the next day's meeting in Chapel Hill. He made it clear that they were expected to attend.[18]

The next day, Chancellor Jenkins and Drs. Laupus, Monroe, and Wiggers drove up to Chapel Hill for a lunch meeting at the Carolina Inn. They were received with southern cordiality and warmth, which somewhat calmed their uneasiness about being there. Unfortunately, Deitrick, Schofield and Leymaster were disinclined to be civil. It soon became clear that the previous day's disagreeable meeting had been a rehearsal for the full-dress performance.

There were about twenty persons at the gathering, including legislators and members of the UNC Board of Governors and the General Administration, along with the delegation from Greenville.[19] President Friday announced that the meeting had been set up to hear from the LCME representatives about their views on the ECU medical school. He then turned the floor over to Dr. Deitrick, who repeated, with added flourishes, his derogatory report on the ECU program. He reviewed the uncertain objectives, the administrative problems and friction which, he said, were well known to the audience. He cited the absence of planning or financial support for research, and of any architectural plans for basic science and clinical departments, which should be connected physically with the hospital. He emphasized, in particular, the shortcomings of developing an affiliation with the new Pitt County Memorial Hospital.

PCMH was not planned for a teaching hospital, was not fully accredited by the Joint Council on the Accreditation of Hospitals, and the tentative agreement between it and the medical school did not give adequate authority to the university to carry out vital hospital functions. He said that all the PCMH staff should have academic appointments, that the university should have the right to choose all potential staff members for submission to the hospital board, that all the physicians employed by the hospital should be subject to university salary scales, and that an ambulatory care facility with physicians' offices should be developed. As soon as full-time clinical department chairmen could be recruited, the school should set up residency programs. Deitrick's final recommendation regarding the hospital was that the university should consider taking over from the county the debt incurred for building the new hospital, and the responsibility of operating it. There should also be an affiliation with some other hospital in the area so that the medical school would not have to depend on a single clinical facility.

When the meeting was over, there was little socialization. Laupus said, "Some diehards among the anti-ECU-School of Medicine support group had seemed elated, others were stunned by the savagery and ferocious nature of the personal attacks by individuals representing a national accreditation body, however 'unofficial' the nature of their visitation, and most simply withheld judgment until later reflection." [20]

After the meeting, the *Raleigh News & Observer* briefly interviewed Leo Jenkins. He had no doubts about anything involved in the medical school program, including the timetable and the curriculum. He said, "There will be a medical school in the East, and we're not going to be deterred by every rabbit that runs across the highway." [21]

The ECU foursome left Chapel Hill glumly, but they were all furious. For a long time, as they were driving back, no one spoke. Then Laupus and Wiggers agreed that Deitrick's presentation was not worth discussing. Laupus remarked that he had never been through any experience in his life as humiliating as that day, but that he did not want it to color his relations with UNC. What the incident had done was to intensify his wish to succeed in a task he thought could be done, if he was given a free enough hand so he could meet his responsibility.

Senator Ralph Scott, who was also at the meeting with the accreditation officials, told the *Raleigh News & Observer* reporter that according to the LCME, it would not be advisable to try to admit anybody until 1977. He said that Dr. John Deitrick, who was a consultant to the accreditation officials, had recommended that ECU buy the entire Pitt Memorial Hospital. He said that Deitrick thought it very important for medical school personnel to control the personnel in the hospital rather than sharing its administration with the hospital board of trustees. "But," Scott added, "it was just a suggestion."

When asked whether another delay might affect the school's funding, Scott said that there had to be some signs of progress. He was not sure that the Board of Governors was "hot on it" even yet. "I have a feeling that if you're not for something, you just delay and delay and delay," he said. And President Friday was working under the Board's direction. In reply to the suggestion that the medical school might buy the new Pitt County Hospital for a teaching hospital, Jack Richardson, PCMH administrator, said he doubted the county would be willing to sell the hospital if ECU wanted to buy it.

"There seems to be a lot of pride in the hospital right here," he said.

President Friday would not answer specific questions about the meeting with the LCME representatives. He said that whatever was needed to achieve accreditation would be undertaken. Concerning the appropriation, he said, "We've still got to go on and build a faculty and do everything we've been saying. The money has been appropriated, and it will be spent as requirements indicate to build the right kind of program. [This] was not a site visit for any accreditation process. It was a preliminary consultation to assist Dr. Jenkins and me in assessing where we are as we set out to implement the legislative action."

Senator John T. Henley, D-Cumberland, who was also at the Chapel Hill meeting, said that the LCME officials were bothered by ECU's tight time schedule for hiring faculty and building facilities. The *Raleigh News & Observer*'s "reliable source, who asked not to be identified" said that concerns of the accreditation officials created the probability that there would be no entering class in 1976. The newspaper repeated most of this interesting story the next day, with the wire services and many newspapers across the state picking it up. Everyone, it seemed, was worried about the possible delay in the ECU medical school's opening at the time planned.[22]

Dean Laupus, after reflecting on the events of July 7 and 8 and the effect they might have on the future of the medical school, concluded that the LCME visit could be put to good use. He thought that President Friday had seemed embarrassed even as Deitrick was still talking. Laupus was determined that the disagreeable visit would be the last occurrence of outrageous official behavior toward the ECU School of Medicine. The incident could be helpful in marking the separation of the past history of the endeavor to set up the school, when others were responsible, from the present and future of the school, which had become his personal responsibility. He resolved that, as far as possible, emphasis should be given to what had still to be done, and not to explaining the actions that had taken place in the past struggle.

The next week, Dr. Laupus called Dr. Schofield and said he was taking at face value his statement of willingness to support the efforts in Greenville. He asked to meet with him at his Washington office, and talk about where the school should go. When they met, Laupus told Schofield that he wanted quality programs as much as the LCME did. He had entered the situation at ECU without prejudice, and hoped for reciprocation and a chance to make a fair start in a new situation. He asked for Schofield to meet with him at least once a month to discuss what was being done at the medical school, until there was no longer a need for such meetings. During the next three to four months, Laupus went to Washington once each month for a Friday meeting to review progress toward accreditation.[23]

On Wednesday after the LCME visit, ECU Chancellor Jenkins felt impelled to make a public pronouncement about the possible delay in the school opening. He said that he was confident the medical school could open in the fall of 1976, if it got full cooperation from all concerned. "Our new dean, Dr. William Laupus, agrees that the job can be done if he and his staff are given the opportunity to exercise the responsibility any medical school dean should have. This includes the responsibility and the authority to deal directly with the accrediting agency and its staff. "I remain confident that we will be able to develop the medical school on the schedule which was recommended by President Friday and the Board of Governors, on the schedule mandated by the 1975 General Assembly within the funds appropriated by the General Assembly," Jenkins said. [24]

Dean Laupus said on July 29 that the projected date for admitting the first class at ECU medical school, September 1976, was a reasonable target for the admission of the first students. A great many things, however, would have to be brought together in order to meet that deadline.[25]

If it reached the goal, ECU could ask for accreditation from the LCME by late Spring or early Summer 1976 at the latest.[26] The first class would be admitted on a contingency basis, to transfer to Chapel Hill if accreditation did not come through. Laupus was completely confident that the school would be accredited if it asked for accreditation, but ECU would not request it until the school was ready. As they worked toward that goal, there would be regular consultations with members of the LCME to review progress.

The Family Practice residency program should begin in July, 1976, and those in other primary care areas—pediatrics, obstetrics-gynecology, internal medicine, and psychiatry—in 1977 and 1978. The school would have twenty-five or thirty students at the beginning, and ultimately eighty to a hundred.

Laupus said, "We have a mandate from the legislature to focus our attention toward family practice and primary care. Programs such as this are greatly needed throughout the country. We are training our sights on this particular area."

He observed that the school was not starting from scratch. The great amount of planning and work that had been going on for a number of years provided a definite advantage. He added, "It would surprise many critics how thorough and comprehensive this planning has been."

Dean Laupus said that when the General Assembly finally approved funds for the four-year school, the morale of the present faculty members, who were very loyal and hard working, had improved a great deal. Before then, they had been in limbo. He noted that a number of outstanding people were being considered for positions in the medical school The present thirteen faculty members would be increased until about thirty-five were on hand by the time the school was accredited, and these would be the faculty for the first two years.[27]

UNC officials released a letter from Dr. John E. Deitrick, LCME consultant, who had visited ECU the summer before with other committee officials. Deitrick proposed purchasing the entire hospital, and strongly recommended a cooperative arrangement with another hospital, to prevent the medical school from being dependent on only one clinical facility.[28] Laupus later said that the problems Deitrick raised had been resolved in negotiations with LCME officials. "I wish you would burn that letter, because it is completely out of date—water over the dam," he said.[29]

Dr. Harold Wiggers, Senior Consultant to the Dean of the ECU medical school, had replied to Dr. Deitrick on July 14, thanking him for his identification of problems facing ECU in meeting accreditation requirements. He also raised a critical question: Why had the survey reports Deitrick cited failed to mention the many accomplishments that the school had made in working toward its goals? Wiggers reproached Deitrick for making it appear to an audience of Board members and legislators (in which there were opponents to the medical school project) that ECU officials and faculty had failed to recognize the nature of accreditation requirements and had made little progress towards meeting them.

The gist of Deitrick's report, Wiggers said, had been to list things yet to be done, emphasize the difficulties of doing them, and state how improbable it was that provisional accreditation could be met in 1976. The report gave the impression that Deitrick came to bury them rather than stimulate and assist them.[30]

In an address delivered in Raleigh on Tuesday, November 25, to Wake County alumni of ECU, Chancellor Leo Jenkins reviewed the ten-year struggle to gain approval of the new medical school. His speech gave the opposition media an opportunity to renew their assaults on him and the ECU campaign. The Associated Press reported, "ECU Chancellor Leo Jenkins, speaking to alumni here on Tuesday, said that if the "bureaucracy" (UNC General Administration or the LCME) do not raise obstacles, the medical school will admit medical students in the fall of 1976. 'We still predict that ECU will graduate its first class of medical doctors in 1980,' he said."[31]

In an interview with a reporter from the *Raleigh News & Observer*, Jenkins said the attitude of the newspaper toward ECU was unfair. He said that an editorial stating that he was looking for a scapegoat for possible delays in operation of the medical school was sophomoric. "I'd be foolish to refer to my boss as a bureaucrat," Jenkins said. He denied he had made the bureaucracy remark, and that ECU, UNC officials and accreditation officials were getting along beautifully.[32]

The flap originated in a November 25 news release by the ECU News Bureau about the speech Jenkins was scheduled to give that night.[33] The release had been based on a set of notes Jenkins did not use, and when he spoke he did not refer to the General Administration and the LCME. When ECU News Director, William Shires, read the notes to a reporter over the telephone, there was, after the remark about bureaucracy that Jenkins actually made, a separate reference to "the UNC administration and medical school accrediting agencies." The connection between this phrase and the "bureaucracy" remark had been parenthetically inserted by the AP, on the basis of the *Raleigh News & Observer* story. A parallel story distributed by UPI had been based on the ECU news release.

A *News & Observer* reporter attended Jenkins's speech, and reported to the newspaper's metropolitan desk, where the story was altered to attribute the "bureaucracy" remark to the ECU News Bureau. The story, as released, failed to mention that, according to its own reporter, Jenkins had not actually made the remarks contained in the news release.[34]

Chancellor Jenkins, as usual, took advantage of an opportunity to return media fire and mount a counter-attack. On Wednesday, November 26, he said to a reporter that neither the *News & Observer* report nor the ECU news release justified the editorial that the newspaper subsequently published. He said he had intended to say only that "the very machinery of this thing can be slow . . . not in the sense of calling somebody an inefficient bureaucrat." The process of establishing a medical school requires meeting legal rules, negotiating with architects, land purchases, construction, and other things, and "all of that is the machinery of government." He said further that the *News & Observer* had failed to report the summary of ECU's accomplishments included in his speech. He believed that the medical school "could be a 'model for the whole country,' through its focus on primary care and its cooperation with other agencies to deliver health care to 800,000 people in eastern North Carolina."

He also mentioned that the ECU school would cooperate with the UNC-CH medical school, which would be responsible for the "more bizarre programs."

"The *News & Observer* did not report those remarks," Jenkins said. He added, "Omissions can be just as sinful as the other way around." He accused the *News & Observer* of purposefully ignoring that ECU football player Jim Boling had been named to the second string All-America Team that week.[35] The newspaper did report Boling's honor, but did not display it prominently enough to satisfy Chancellor Jenkins.

Also on November 26, Chancellor Jenkins wrote to President William Friday, enclosing a copy of the official news release that ECU had sent out about the November 25 speech. He said that the news release did not reflect his actual comments, and was misreported by the newspapers. He expressed his appreciation for the backing which the University administration had given him, and mentioned his embarrassment at the misunderstanding that the erroneous report had caused.[36]

President Friday called Dean Laupus and advised him to ignore the newspaper controversy, and Laupus wrote him that he had made inquiries locally that indicated Chancellor Jenkins had not made the remarks attributed to him. He mentioned his appreciation of the assistance and support he had received and would continue to need from the General Administration and the Board of Governors. He said that he hoped to provide in a few days a report of the progress that had been made.[37]

President Friday wrote to the members of the Senate Appropriations Committee informing them that Chancellor Jenkins had called to tell him that the *Raleigh News & Observer* story was in error, and to inform them of developments in the implementation of Section 46. He outlined the progress made toward affiliation with PCMH and accreditation of the medical program at ECU.[38]

During the two weeks when Jenkins's speech to ECU alumni in Wake County was a sensation, most of the state's newspapers joined in the clamor with news stories and editorials. The uproar reached from the villages and small towns to the legislature. The reports of Dr. Deitrick's misgivings about ECU's accreditation and the Chancellor's efforts to pooh-pooh them gave both opponents and supporters a grand opportunity to voice their loyalties.

[1] The LCME was established in 1942 as a joint venture of the American Medical Association and the Association of American Medical Colleges. While licensing of physicians and regulating standards of medical practice are in the hands of the various states, the LCME develops criteria, approved by its two parent organizations, for both basic medical science and clinical training of doctors. Its legitimacy as an accrediting agency has been questioned. The anti-competitive practices of the AMA, which substantially influenced the Liaison Committee's policies and operation, led to an attack by the Federal Trade Commission in 1976 on the Committee, following the Committee's application for continued acceptance as a nationally recognized agency to accredit US medical schools. See Schofield, *New and Expanded Medical Schools*, p. 17; copies of correspondence between the FTC and the AMA, November 1976, in ECU School of Medicine Files, Folder "Accreditation - Med School." [Accreditation Folder]. The LCME continues to be recognized as the monitor of quality in medical education in the United States and Canada.

[2] Letter from Presient Friday to Chancellors Jenkins and Taylor, and Dean Fordham, November 19, 1974, in Accreditation Folder.

[3] Transcript of telephone conversation between Chancellor Leo Jenkins, Dr. Edwin W. Monroe, and Dr. James R. Schofield, November 25, 1974, in Accreditation Folder.

[4] Since its founding in the 19th century, the medical school at Johns Hopkins University combined a basic science curriculum of two years with two years spent in the hospital which was operated by the medical school. The combining of science and research with hospital practice became a model for medical schools, notably the University of Rochester and Vanderbilt University Schools of Medicine, as well as Duke University School of Medicine, founded in 1927 with a dean recruited from Hopkins. Cf. Paul Starr, *The Social Transformation of American Medicine* (New York: Basic Books, 1982) pp. 115-116; J. R. Schofield, *New and Expanded Medical Schools, Mid-Century to the 1980s* (San Francisco: AAMC and Jossey-Bass, 1984), p. 111; James F. Gifford, Jr., *The Evolution of a Medical Center: A History of Medicine at Duke University to 1941* (Durham, NC: Duke University Press, 1972).

[5] In 1971, Congress passed P. L. 92-157, authorizing up to

$1,270,000 as a capitation grant for medical schools to construct new buildings, for newly developing schools, and for conversion of two-year programs to full M.D. Curricula. If previous enrollment had been less than 100, and the enrollment increased by 10 students or 10%, $2,500 could be awarded for each first-, second-, and third-year student, and $4,000 per graduate. In 1975, the total possible grant had increased to $1,380,000, although no school ever received the full amount. Further information may be found in Schofield, *New and Expanded Medical Schools*, pp. 23 ff.

[6] Transcript of November 25, 1974 telephone conversation.

[7] Letter from William Friday to Dr. James Schofield, December 17, 1974, with enclosures, in Accreditation Folder.

[8] Letter from Chancellor Leo Jenkins to President William Friday, January 8, 1975, in Accreditation Folder.

[9] *Chapel Hill Newspaper*, January 10, 1975.

[10] Letter from William Friday to Chancellor Leo Jenkins, April 15, 1975, in Accreditation Folder.

[11] Letter from Chancellor Leo Jenkins to President William Friday, April 18, 1975, Accreditation Folder.

[12] Letters from William Friday to Dr. James Schofield and Dr. Glen Leymaster, June 10, 1975, Leo Jenkins Archives.

[13] Letter from William C. Friday to Leo W. Jenkins, June 20, 1975, copy in Accreditation Folder.

[14] *Ibid.*

[15] Note from William Friday to Leo Jenkins, July 10, 1975, with enclosed clipping from *The Knoxville Journal*, Knoxville, Tennessee, July 2, 1975, in Accreditation Folder.

[16] Account of the LCME "unofficial" meeting of July 7-8, 1975, by Dr. William E. Laupus, written on November 13, 1975, in Accreditation Folder.

[17] Laupus, *op. cit.*

[18] Dr. Laupus recalled this as the first time he learned they were expected to attend the Chapel Hill meeting.

[19] Attendees, besides President Friday, the ECU group, and the LCME visitors, were legislators, Senator John Henley, Senator Ralph Scott, and Representative Jimmy Love; board members, William A. Dees, Jr., Adelaide Holderness, Julia Morton, Victor S. Bryant, Dr. Hugh Daniel, Dr. Wallace Hyde, William Johnson, and David J. Whichard II; General Administration members, Vice

President Raymond Dawson, Vice President Felix Joyner, Vice President John Sanders, and Assistant to the President for Governmental Affairs, former Representative R. D. McMillan, Jr. (the president's legislative lobbyist). Names from President Friday's letter of August 8, 1975, forwarding to the attendees a copy of Dr. Deitrick's written report on the July 7 and 8 meetings, approved by Drs. Schofield and Leymaster, ECU School of Medicine Files, Accreditation Folder.

[20] Laupus, *op. cit.*

[21] *Raleigh News & Observer*, July 9, 1975.

[22] *Raleigh News & Observer, idem.*

[23] Laupus, *op. cit.*

[24] *Fayetteville Times*, July 10, 1975.

[25] *Greenville Daily Reflector*, July 30, 1975.

[26] If accreditation was granted by then, the medical school might become eligible for $1 million in federal funding over four years, beginning in 1976.

[27] *Greenville Daily Reflector, idem.*

[28] Letter from John E. Deitrick, M. D., to William C. Friday, LL.D., July 10, 1975, in Accreditation Folder.

[29] *Raleigh News & Observer*, November 15, 1975.

[30] Letter from Harold C. Wiggers to John Deitrick, July 14, 1974, in Accreditation Folder.

[31] Associated Press, November 25, 1975. The article appeared in a number of papers, and in various versions.

[32] "Jenkins claims N&O Errors in Med Goal Story," by Steve Adams, *Raleigh News & Observer, December 4, 1975.*

[33] ECU News Bureau, November 25, 1975, "Jenkins Says ECU 'Confident' of Meeting Med School Deadline," ECU School of Medicine Files, Folder "Jenkins Correspondence."

[34] *Raleigh News & Observer*, December 4, 1975.

[35] *Raleigh News & Observer, idem.*

[36] Letter from Leo W. Jenkins, Chancellor, to President William Friday, November 26, 1975, in ECU School of Medicine Files, Folder "Jenkins Correspondence."

[37] Letter from William E. Laupus, M. D. to Mr. William Friday, President, The University of North Carolina, November 26, 1975, in ECU School of Medicine Files, Folder "Jenkins Correspondence."

[38] Letter from William Friday, President, to Senators J. J. Harrington,

John T. Henley, Kenneth Royall, Jr., Ralph Scott, Livingstone Stallings, and Representatives John Gamble, Jr., Jay Huskins, Horton Rountree, and Thomas Sawyer, November 26, 1975, in ECU School of Medicine Files, Folder "Jenkins Correspondence."

Chapter 20
The Health Sciences Library

A recurrent concern of site visitors of the Liaison Committee on Health Education to the ECU campus was the lack of an adequate medical library. The report of the site survey of the program under development conducted in October, 1970, described a three-phase plan for establishing a Health Affairs Library. The plan projected a collection of 2,000 monographs and texts during Phase I (1969-71), and subscriptions for 250 journals; during Phase II (1971-73), the collection would reach at least 5,000 volumes and 600 journal subscriptions; and during Phase III (1973-75), 15,000 volumes and 900 subscriptions, with at least ten years of back files for all journals.[1] The report concluded that, in spite of some progress in gathering teaching materials, including audiovisuals, a great deal still had to be done. The Phase II goals, it said, would be reasonably adequate for a beginning medical school, but a library limited to the size outlined in Phase I would be a serious handicap.[2]

Phase I began in September, 1969 when Mrs. Jo Ann Bell (Dr. Jo Ann Bell after 1980) was hired to start what was then the School of Allied Health Library. The General Assembly had funded the School of Allied Health and Social Professions, with a building to house it. The plan was to begin developing a complete health sciences library that would serve the School of Allied Health and eventually a School of Medicine.

As late as the LCME's official site visit in January, 1973, the committee still found the library facilities inadequate. The two and a half miles between the medical school and the library and the small space accommodating a large number of students were unacceptable. At that time, the collection contained 19,000 volumes, and the library subscribed to 750 journals. Another 7,500 books were held in the Joyner Library, ECU's main library, and 110 more journal subscriptions maintained there.[3] The committee's judgment appears retrospectively to have been a product either of bias or superficial examination of the library's operation, since it had more than reached the Phase II goals previously judged by the LCME as "reasonably adequate for a beginning medical library." In fact, it had already surpassed Phase III in books, and exceeded Phase II objectives for journal subscriptions.

It was true that about a thousand students in the health sciences were being served in a space of about 2,200 square feet. As Dr.

Jo Ann Bell, the director of the library said, she also got comments from her professional colleagues around the country, from people who had visited ECU as well as other institutions. They asked, "What do you people there do? People just rave about your library."

It was her opinion that the library staff actually profited from the experience of operating in crowded facilities, with most of the library's collection in storage, and the space so crowded that clients could hardly get to the circulation desk. While the library staff were inconvenienced, and were forced to make numerous trips to their storage areas, they learned to work hard to insure that clients were not discommoded. They had materials in storage in the original storage area, and in the old section of Joyner Library—a majority of the collection was in storage when they moved to the new Belk Building—the Allied Health Building—took place in 1971. Items were retrieved from storage three times a day. While some publications were not immediately accessible, the waiting time did not exceed two to three hours.

Never at any time did the library compare to large libraries that had been in existence since the 1800's or early 1900's. This was not among its goals. There was already a very large medical history collection in North Carolina, at Duke University Medical School, and major medical research libraries there and in Chapel Hill. The aim was to build a strong working collection to support the mission of the school. Essential research materials were important, but it was not vital to have a huge research collection in a school devoted to educating primary care physicians. Not until 1975 was there an operating budget specifically for the library.

Dr. Bell and her staff considered the facilities, or the brute size of the library's holdings, to be less important than the ruling philosophy and goal of making the facilities they had fully accessible and adequate to the specific needs of its clientele. The service approach was what convinced its numerous clients that the Health Sciences Library was the best they had ever used.

From the beginning, it was taken for granted that there was absolutely no reason for the library to exist except to serve the clients. A Ph.D. candidate using the library told Dr. Bell, "I don't know where you are able to get these people and how you keep them so oriented to service, because I've used every major research library in this state and I've never seen anything like this library for service." The staff were so active in their pursuit of service that there were occasional complaints that they were too helpful. If anyone appeared not to know quite what he was doing, the staff were conditioned to approach him and ask whether he needed help. Some users were not accustomed to being bothered when they entered a library, and did not wish to be bothered, so they thought it was an interference to be asked if they needed help.

Dr. Bell said in 1991, "It [the library] was one of the few things the *Raleigh News & Observer* never assailed. They never were able to get anything on us, I guess. That is the only thing I can say about the early years. I hated to read the paper at breakfast, because every day there were articles in the paper about ECU and the Medical School and what was wrong with us. I never could understand why people who were perfectly acceptable when they worked at other institutions were just terrible when they got here. They were no longer worth anything, they weren't capable or competent and it was always a trial to read the paper in the morning. I just about gave it up. One thing that they never got, they never had a negative sentence about us. They occasionally had to mention us, but at least they didn't have anything bad to say about us." [4]

There was, from the start, strong support for the library from the medical community, not only moral support, but donations of library materials. As Dr. Bell said, "As soon as they read about it—every physician anywhere east of the mountains had heard about the Medical School being approved—they decided they would give us materials." There were many donations from the local medical community. [5]

Early on, there were two very large donations. One came in 1970 from Mrs. Donnell Cobb of Goldsboro, the octogenarian widow of a distinguished and nationally known surgeon. Dr. Cobb had graduated in 1919 from UNC in Chapel Hill, received his medical degree from the University of Pennsylvania in 1921, was a fellow at the Mayo Clinic, and had practiced at Wayne Community Hospital in Goldsboro up to his death in 1955. Mrs. Bell went with a truck, accompanied by a couple of men to help her, spent the day talking to Mrs. Cobb, and helping to bring the voluminous materials—some 7,000 pounds of it—down from her attic. The collection included texts and monographs dating back to the 1850's (Dr. Cobb's father had been a physician), and large series of surgical journals running continuously back to the 1920's. Many of the books were of interest for the history of medicine, were valuable, and would have been difficult to purchase at the time.

Another donation came from Dr. Robert Phillips of Greensboro. The very large collection of books and journals turned up on a truck one afternoon about five o'clock. It was a major project finding help to get the books unloaded from the truck and into storage.

These two collections were particularly important early contributions because of their size and makeup. They did not contain current literature, but large collections of retrospective materials that gave the library a good foundation. In addition, there were many gifts of individual titles from physicians, extending from textbooks that they had used in medical school to current journals.

The Medical Center Library of the University of Kentucky had many duplicates of both books and journals in a large storage area. Jo Ann Bell arranged in the spring of 1970 to go to Lexington, and selected everything she thought might be useful for the library. The Kentucky library hired a student with funds from ECU to pack the materials and shipped them to Greenville. When the shipment arrived in Greenville there were twelve tons of it, some that Mrs. Bell had not chosen. Nothing was returned.

In May, 1970, Jo Ann Bell met Henry J. Gartland, Director of Library Services for the V. A. At a meeting of the Medical Library Association. He suggested that ECU might obtain access to the lists of surplus materials from V. A. hospitals. Dr. Ed Monroe wrote Dr. M. J. Musser, Chief Medical Director of the Veterans Administration Central Office and former head of the NC Regional Medical Program, and asked for assistance in building the library's collections by receiving duplicate serials or other materials from V. A. Hospitals around the country. Dr. Musser instructed Henry Gartland to look into the possibility, and the Health Affairs Library was able to complete a number of its back-files from the surplus journals that were made available.[6]

The initial location of the library's administration was in a five by ten foot seminar room in the oldest section of the university's main library, the Joyner Library. It was furnished with a desk and bookcase. When it arrived, the collection from Dr. Phillips was stored in seminar rooms on another floor. Shortly after the accessioning and cataloguing of the collection was begun, the embryo health affairs library moved to an area in an unused cafeteria building near Joyner Library. The disconnected steam tables were used to stack the books and journals on which the solitary librarian was working. Not until the summer of 1970 was there any more staff. At that time, a single clerk-typist was added. In 1971 a second librarian was hired, and the next year two more.[7]

From the cafeteria building, the library moved in 1970 to the new biology building, where it remained until 1971. In the biology building—subsequently to become a part of the Science Complex—the library was located in a room designed specifically for use as a library; it had a few shelves around the wall. After the move to the newly-completed allied health building, a reading room with reference books and current medical journals was maintained in the Science Complex. The staff consisted by then of four professional librarians, an audio-visual coordinator, and two library assistants.

During the ten-year stay in the Belk Building, the library's collections grew to 127,000 volumes, and its journal subscriptions rose to over 1,800. It served the Schools of Medicine, Nursing, and Allied Health and Social Professions, with a satellite in the Medical School Teaching Addition at PCMH when that was completed, until it moved in 1982 to the 33,000 square foot facility in the Brody Medical Sciences Building.[8]

---

[1] Liaison Committee on Medical Education, "Report of the survey of Program Under Development at East Carolina University School of Medicine, Greenville, North Carolina," October 11-13, 1970, p. 7. In ECU School of Medicine Files, Folder "Report of the Liaison Committee on Medical Education, October 11-13, 1970."

[2] "Report of the survey," p. 16.

[3] Liaison Committee on Medical Education, "Report of the survey, The University of North Carolina, Chapel Hill, School of Medicine, Chapel Hill, North Carolina, " January 29-31, 1973, pp. 20-21. In ECU School of Medicine Files, Folder "Liaison Committee on Medical Education, 1973-74."

[4] Interview with Dr. Jo Ann Bell, December 11, 1991.

[5] Bell interview

[6] Letters from Edwin W. Monroe to M. J. Musser, June 2, 1970; letter from Henry J. Gartland to Edwin W. Monroe, June 10, 1970.

[8] School of Medicine, East Carolina University, *Catalog,* published by Dean of Admissions, School of Medicine, East Carolina University, Greenville, NC. Library data from issues 1971-73 (preliminary) to 1981-1982 (Vol. 72).

Chapter 21
Accreditation Granted

Since the derivative accreditation of the medical school had been lost in separating from the University of North Carolina School of Medicine, it was necessary for the ECU school to meet on its own the requirements of the Liaison Committee on Medical Education. One essential was the LCME's acceptance of the affiliation agreement with Pitt County Memorial Hospital. There were still a number of department heads to be hired, and much planning to be done for facilities.

After LCME members Drs. James Schofield and Glen Leymaster, and their consultant, Dr. John E. Deitrick, had made their informal visit to the Greenville campus, the latter wrote to President Friday about the problems he had observed at ECU and identified four difficulties: (1) the lack of architectural plans for the basic science and clinical departments of the medical school; (2) PCMH's lack of accreditation; (3) both the absence of approval from the Division of Comprehensive Health Planning of the NC Department of Human Resources for the proposed changes in the hospital under construction, and the deficiencies in the tentative affiliation agreement, which gave "very little authority to the university for some vital functions of the hospital;" (4) the apparent absence of provision for facilities and financial support for research activities in the new school.

As noted earlier in Chapter 19, Dr. Harold Wiggers wrote in mid-July, 1975, to Dr. Deitrick, protesting the one-sidedness of his evaluation of progress at ECU. However, ECU medical school officials and faculty, recognized that, although informal, the report on the deficiencies of their program represented the position the LCME would take. By September, plans had been made and bids let on modifications in a former dormitory building, Ragsdale Hall, to provide for the Dean's office and the offices and student laboratories for the Departments of Pathology, Pharmacology, and Physiology. Additional space had been provided in the Biology Building for Anatomy, Biochemistry, and Microbiology. Student study carrels and an audiovisual center had been planned for Whichard Hall, a building adjacent to Ragsdale.

The accreditation for PCMH was restored on August 15, 1975, and modifications in the hospital's plans to include teaching facilities were approved by the state office of Comprehensive Health Planning on September 22. After the attempt to obtain equal representation between the medical school and the county on the Executive Committee of the hospital's Board of Trustees failed, Chancellor Jenkins had agreed to one-third representation on the hospital Board of Trustees and three-sevenths representation on its Executive Board. He said he believed that this would, along with some other changes in the agreement, protect the University's interest, while not encroaching excessively on the responsibilities of the county to its taxpayers.

Although no funding for research had been obtained, the recruitment of well-qualified faculty, both basic science and clinical, was going on at a brisk pace, and search committees had identified possible chairmen for seven departments. One of the most important needs, planning for buildings to house the medical school, was being met. The plans were to be completed during the next two years. The buildings would house the library, basic science and clinical teaching facilities, an ambulatory care center, and additional beds for PCMH.

On December 16, Dean William Laupus wrote to the faculty of the School of Medicine that a consultation visit of the LCME executives had been suggested for February, 1976. Although this would be a visit preliminary to a full-scale site visit, certain things needed to be done to get ready for it. The renovation of Ragsdale Hall had to be well along toward completion. The site planning should be completed up to the stage of preliminary schematic drawings for the medical school buildings on the land purchased near the new PCMH, including the basic medical education, clinical science, library, and ambulatory care facilities.

There had to be substantial progress toward recruiting three basic science and five clinical department chairmen and other faculty members. The curriculum for the four-year school should be developed as far as the faculty on hand could do it, with a minimum of two years completed and an outline of the last two years ready for consideration by clinical chairmen when they arrived. The plan for the family practice residency must be ready for submission to the review agencies. The General Administration of the University should provide assurance for the development of Ph.D. programs in the basic sciences. Finally, there should be space for the interim ambulatory care facilities.[1]

Dean Laupus was negotiating with the PCMH Board of Trustees and the Pitt County Commissioners to lease a wing of the old Pitt County Memorial Hospital once the move to the new building had taken place. This space would provide interim offices and examining rooms for clinical faculty while construction of the new medical school facilities was going on.

In a Christmas interview by a reporter from the *Greenville Daily Reflector*, Dean Laupus said he still hoped that students could be enrolled in the medical school in the fall of 1976. The accreditation team would point out "deficiencies as they see them," he said, and decide whether an official visit should be made in the spring, after which it would be determined whether accreditation should be granted or not.[2] He did not mention publicly his concern about the loss of a possible federal grant that would give the school $250,000 a year for four years, if the liaison committee failed to accredit the school before the funding law expired that fall.

After the LCME team made an unofficial consultation visit to ECU in February, 1976, decisions about the number of students and other matters critical to the new school would be made. Laupus said that the LCME had the authority to determine how many students could be enrolled. "Although the legislation establishing the school limits the number of first year students to forty, the number is decided by the LCME. They tell you how many you can enroll. I don't see any difference between thirty and forty students," he said. "It's a shame to deprive kids of an opportunity to go to medical school if there is a place for them." He did not anticipate any problem in securing qualified students once the school was accredited.

He was still holding on to the prospect that first-year students could begin between September and mid-December 1976 and still move into their second year by September 1977. Residency programs would begin after the new PCMH was finished and clinical teaching facilities were available.

"We are working together with the architects . . . meeting with them on almost a weekly basis to finalize additions," Laupus said. The school was also very actively engaged in recruiting faculty, with three basic science chairmen, five chairmen of clinical departments and some additional science teachers still needed. Medical school personnel were expected to occupy Ragsdale Hall, as an interim facility, by the end of February.[3]

On January 15, Dr. Dean Hayek, ECU medical school assistant dean for administration, told members of the Washington, NC, Rotary Club that officials of the school were hopeful that the first class in the four-year school would be enrolled by fall.[4] Hayek was the medical school's liaison with the architects, as he was later with the building contractors for the 450,000-square-foot medical sciences building. He was also heavily involved in faculty and staff recruitment, along with his duties as chairman of the admissions committee. Dean Laupus was to say some years later that without Dr. Hayek the medical school would have taken much longer to build, and would have cost much more than it did.

On January 17, 1976, William A. Dees, chairman of the UNC Board of Governors announced that UNC and PCMH in Greenville had signed a final version of an affiliation agreement to use the hospital as a teaching facility, after working out differences on representation on the hospital board and hospital staff regulations. UNC President Friday said the signing "concludes all major pending business as far as the board of governors is concerned in terms of allocating funds and getting the construction projects under way for the medical school." [5]

Like rumbles of thunder in the distance after a storm has passed, there were still reverberations from Raleigh and west of Raleigh. Representative Carolyn Mathis of Charlotte, whose attempt had failed in the 1975 legislative session to postpone the funding of the ECU medical school through the bond issue referendum she proposed and the General Assembly passed, had still not given up. She urged Governor James E. Holshouser, another medical school opponent, to call for a special legislative session in 1976 to consider merging a $32 million ECU medical school appropriation with a statewide bond referendum to fund higher education. She told reporters that she had also discussed the matter with House Speaker James C. Green, who had not rejected her suggestion, but had questioned whether there would be enough time to take it up. [6]

A public hearing was scheduled in Raleigh at two o'clock on January 27 to consider the AHEC-funded Family Practice Center proposed to be built near the new PCMH. The 30,000 square-foot building was estimated to cost $1.8-1.9 million, and it was planned that building would begin within the next three or four months.

Dr. Monroe, ECU Vice-Chancellor for Health Affairs and president of Eastern AHEC, said most of the space in the center would relate to the family practice residency training program. Some space would provide for the EAHEC administrative offices.

Joel Vickers, deputy director of the EAHEC, said that temporary quarters were being built at a cost of about $72,000. The temporary facility, located on the ECU campus next to the Biology Building where most of the medical school faculty worked, would house about $25-30,000 worth of equipment and furnishings, Vickers said. [7]

Pitt County Commissioners sold almost forty-one acres of land to the state for the ECU medical school, at a price of $195,000, the original cost of the land plus a small additional amount per acre for improvements. The parcel of land was located adjacent to that on which the hospital was being built. The county had bought it several years before as part of a ninety-seven acre tract for the site of the new hospital at a price of $390,000. On February 9, C. G. Moore, ECU's Vice Chancellor for Business Affairs, turned over a check for the purchase to Burney Tucker, chairman of the board of commissioners.[8]

Rumbles continued to be heard out of the west. When it met on Friday, February 13, 1976, the Advisory Budget Commission rescinded $13.3 million in capital improvements money, but did not touch the approximately $28 million in construction funds allocated the year before to develop the ECU medical school. This brought about an objection from a member of the commission, Republican Representative Cass Ballenger from Catawba County. He thought it was unacceptable that the East Carolina medical school funds had not been included in the review. "And we don't have anything to say about that, do we?" he asked. State Budget Officer, S. Kenneth Howard answered him that because it was appropriated by a special bill and not as part of the regular appropriation bill, the money could be touched only by an separate act of the General Assembly. It was out of the hands of the commission.[9]

Ballenger said that the ECU medical school expansion funds should be cut, in spite of opposition from the Democratic-controlled Senate. He also said he anticipated the legislature would be called into special session in March by the General Assembly's Appropriations Conference Committee to deal with the $70 million anticipated deficit caused by revenue shortfalls.[10]

In Greenville, a Family Practice Clinic was instituted in a double-wide house trailer on the grounds of the old county hospital, to open March 1, when Dr. James Jones and one medical resident would begin to provide general medical services. The structure had room for four offices, and could accommodate more than four residents on a rotating basis. Hospital and medical school officials hoped that the new service would take some of the non-emergency traffic away from the emergency room, and provide a family doctor for people in Pitt County who had been unable to have one.

On February 17, the Board of Trustees of PCMH approved establishing a joint policy committee called for by the affiliation agreement between the hospital and the ECU medical school, to be composed of five members of the board of trustees and five from ECU, including the vice chancellor for business affairs, vice chancellor for health affairs, dean of the School of Medicine, and two members appointed by the ECU chancellor. They also appointed the Dean of the School of Medicine as an ex-officio member of the Board of Trustees executive committee.

The Trustees asked Charles Gaskins of the County Commissioners to suggest amending the hospital charter to say that a member of the hospital medical staff recommended by that staff be appointed to the hospital's Board of Trustees.

Representatives of the Joint Committee on Hospital Accreditation visited on February 24, to assess the hospital's compliance with recommendations about deficits in the handling of patient records and some other matters made by a site visitor of the Joint Committee on Hospital Accreditation in 1975.[11]

At its meeting on February 27, the UNC Board of Governors recommended fourteen persons for appointment to PCMH's Board of Trustees. The trustees were expected to name the state representatives as well as two additional county appointees to the board at the next meeting of the Pitt County commissioners, for staggered terms. The new appointments increased the board's size from nineteen to thirty-five members, with sixty percent local and forty percent state representation. The Pitt County commissioners confirmed the appointments at its next meeting.[12]

On Monday, March 1, Drs. Edward S. Petersen and James Schofield of the Liaison Committee on Medical Education came for a consultation visit to the ECU campus. The next day, UNC President William Friday came to Greenville to meet with the representatives of the LCME and with ECU officials. Before the meeting, Friday toured the new PCMH building and Ragsdale Hall, the temporary site of the medical school, which was still being renovated. He said that he and the others concerned were doing all they could to keep the medical school expansion program on schedule. He hoped the state's financial crisis would not affect the progress of ECU's medical program. He said he had heard nothing that would indicate any funds would be cut from medical school appropriations.[13]

On Tuesday, Drs. Petersen and Schofield met again with Dean Laupus, and the three held discussions with the chairmen of the basic science departments. Afterwards, the visitors met with Jack Richardson, administrator of PCMH. They returned for more discussions at the medical school. They complimented the faculty and administration of the school on the accomplishments they had made.

However, they stressed that the school was still not prepared for accreditation.

The request for accreditation of the Family Practice Residency by the Liaison Committee on Graduate Medical Education had been turned down because it had been submitted prematurely, before an adequate faculty had been recruited. It was necessary to remedy this. A chairman for the Department of Internal Medicine was urgently needed. Applications for residencies in Internal Medicine and Pediatrics would not be submitted until the fall, when sufficient faculty would be on hand, and the PCMH facilities ready for use.

After completing a new requirement of the LCME, an institutional self-study and analysis, Dean Laupus was to request in October that an accreditation site survey should be scheduled for the last half of November, making it possible for the Liaison Committee to review its findings at its February, 1977, meeting.[14]

Toward the end of August, Dean Laupus made a progress report to Dr. Schofield, asking for the site visit be scheduled in November. Dr. Schofield answered that he was concerned about the completion and occupancy of the new PCMH. Since it was not scheduled to begin admitting patients until after Christmas, 1976, he believed that it would be better to postpone a site visit to January, 1977. Another consideration he mentioned was that the Committee had already set up a heavy load of surveys for November and December.[15]

On October 15, Dean Laupus, after consulting with Chancellor Jenkins and President Friday, wrote to Dr. Schofield asking him to schedule the site survey visit in January, as he had suggested, "in time for the LCME to grant the school provisional accreditation at its April 5-6, 1977 meeting. Laupus said he was pleased with the steady progress that the school had been making, with the Family Practice Residency provisionally confirmed, and residencies in Internal Medicine, Pediatrics, and Psychiatry applied for, new chairmen for the departments of Internal Medicine and Microbiology already at work, and appointment of chairmen for the other clinical departments imminent. All but two of the basic science faculty had been recruited. Laupus concluded his letter, "I trust that you and the LCME will sense both the high quality which is being built into our program and our deep commitment to succeed in this endeavor."[16]

Dr. Harold C. Wiggers announced on January 18 that a four-man accreditation team from the LCME was visiting ECU. He said, "If the survey team's evaluation is favorable, the accreditation of the ECU Med School will be on the agenda of the April meeting of the

LCME. We feel that great progress has been made and we will be equipped to handle first-year students by this fall."

According to Wiggers, the school could enroll a maximum of forty students. The LCME would probably recommend an initial enrollment of twenty-eight to thirty-two students. The facilities at Pitt Hospital would not be ready by the fall of 1977, but this would cause no problem, since they would not be needed by the medical students for two years. The Family Practice Center would be available to incoming students, since it should be ready by June or July.

The LCME's team, which began their visit on Sunday, January 16, 1977, and planned to stay in Greenville to January 19, was made up of Dr. Andrew Hunt, dean of Michigan State Medical School; Dr. John Kemp, dean of the University of Toledo School of Medicine; Dr. Ira Singer, an internist from Nebraska and director of medical research for the AMA (who served as secretary for the team); and Dr. John Stetson, dean of the University of Florida at Gainesville Medical School.[17]

The accreditation group from the LCME left Greenville on Wednesday. Dr. Raymond Dawson, vice president for academic affairs for the UNC system, was questioned about the visit, and said that the decision about provisional accreditation was expected in April. He declined to speculate on the outcome of the LCME's deliberations. He said that ECU had received the funds it requested and had recruited many faculty members, including key department heads. Nearly seventy positions were funded in the budget.[18]

On Thursday, January 20, ECU Chancellor Leo Jenkins issued a statement saying he expected students to be enrolled in the medical school in September. He based his confidence on conversations with the accreditation team from the LCME during its three-day site visit in Greenville. He said he was very pleased by the verbal report given by the accreditation site team before they left. He was sure that the Liaison Committee on Medical Education would approve accreditation at its meeting in April and would be an affirmative report.[19]

On Friday, February 11, the UNC Board of Governors' Planning Committee approved ten changes requested by the hospital staff to the ECU-PCMH affiliation agreement that had been signed on December, 1975. There was considerable discussion of the changes, and two board members had reservations about them. William A. Johnson was concerned about an amendment that gave the medical staff executive committee veto power over any plans that would duplicate hospital services. George Watts Hill objected to all the changes, as he had to the original agreement, because he said the university was compromising too much.

Dean Laupus told the Board of Governors that the question about duplicating services was moot because the medical school would not want to duplicate hospital services. He also told the planning committee that the medical staff of the hospital would take it personally if the amendment about duplication of services was turned down. The planning committee approved the amendment, but stipulated that the veto power should be given to the chairman only and not to the full executive committee.

The planning committee also had reservations about a change saying the university could not impose any requirements that would restrict practices which met accreditation standards, because they were concerned this stipulation would lock the medical school into low standards. The rule, Laupus said, would apply only to medical staff members who were not on the ECU faculty, and he did not anticipate its causing problems for the school.

The amendments were sent back to the PCMH board of trustees for a vote on the changes in wording made by the planning committee. The final step would be for the UNC Board of Governors to vote on the amendments if there were no further changes.[20]

After the board meeting, Dean Laupus commented that the changes made by the UNC Board of Governors Planning Committee were not major, and that he and others were pleased the agreement had held up so well. He said that the dean of another medical school anticipating affiliation with an existing hospital had requested a copy of the ECU-PCMH agreement, after being referred by an accrediting agency which found the local agreement a model one.[21]

Governor James B. Hunt, speaking on March 26, at the dedication of the new Pitt County Memorial Hospital, said the facility represented a true partnership between local and university officials. Hunt pledged that the General Assembly would restore the $3.8 million for the 114-bed tower for medical school clinical instruction.[22]

Chancellor Jenkins announced at a news conference on Thursday, April 7, 1977, that the ECU School of Medicine had received accreditation and would admit its first class of twenty-eight students in August. He said that the Liaison Committee on Medical Education had met Tuesday and Wednesday and approved provisional accreditation for the school, as expected. Jenkins said he expected a full written report within two weeks. The initial class would be enlarged to thirty-two students in the fall of 1978. Later increases would have to be approved by the LCME, and the maximum size of classes would depend on the UNC Board of Governors.[23]

On Monday night, June 20, the Senate approved a $7.9 million budget for 1977-79. Included in it were $3.82 million for the bed tower at PCMH.[24] According to Felix Joyner, vice-president for finance for the UNC system, this money was all that ECU was scheduled to receive during the biennium starting July 1, unless a special tax bill passed. He also said that the medical school would have some real problems if the General Assembly in its spring, 1978, session revised that part of the budget for the second year of the biennium and eliminated the funding. The budget included $3.5 million in new operating money for the medical school in 1977-78. More than $5 million had been requested for the second year, but the university could expect no more than continuation of the $3.5 million. Unless at least $2 million was appropriated for 1978-79, it will be difficult to add new faculty.

Pitt Representative Horton Rountree was questioned about the budget, but had nothing very encouraging to say. "The way things are moving now," he said, "we just can't say the money will be there for the second year of the biennium. A lot of stuff has been cut out (of the first year budget) to be reviewed next time." There had been a resolution to end the session on June 30 and re-convene May 31, 1978, just after the primary, for a four or five week session. Legislative committees would continue to work and be prepared for a short session dealing primarily with budgetary matters.[25]

Not all the rumblings had died down, and only the most naive observer could expect that they would. The tensions that had energized the struggle to establish the four-year medical school were still present, though somewhat muted. Now, with accreditation approved and the initial installments of funds for construction on their way, all the major obstructions had been surmounted. The school's administration and faculty were ready at last to begin final preparations to receive the first class in the fall of 1977.

[1] Memorandum from Dean William C. Laupus to Faculty, School of Medicine, December 16, 1975, in ECU School of Medicine Files, Folder, "Accreditation—Med School."

[2] *Morganton News Herald,* December 26, 1975. Written by Stuart Savage, *Greenville Daily Greenville Daily Reflector,* for the Associated Press.

[3] Associated Press Interview of William E. Laupus by Stuart Savage.

[4] *Washington Daily News,* January 17, 1976.

[5] *Raleigh News & Observer,* January 17, 1976.

[6] *Kannapolis Independent,* January 21, 1976.

[7] *Greenville Daily Reflector,* January 20, 1976

[8] *Greenville Daily Reflector,* February 9, 1976.

[9] *Raleigh News & Observer,* February 14, 1976.

[10] *Hickory Daily Record,* February 17, 1976.

[11] *Greenville Daily Reflector,* February 26, 1976.

[12] *Greenville Daily Reflector,* March 2, 1976. The Board of Governors recommended: Raleigh Carver of Elizabeth City, chairman of the Pasquotank County Board of Commissioners; Greenville attorney James T. Cheatham; Mrs. Donald Diechman, a New Bern auto dealer; Burroughs-Wellcome Greenville plant manager, Henry G. Leslie; Bill Neal, Roanoke Rapids businessman; Nancy Norwood, Goldsboro; Louis Renn, Jacksonville, a real estate agent and Onslow County Board of Commissioners' chairman; Dean Rich, Raleigh, NCNB eastern region trust officer; William R. Roberson, Washington, a former member of NC House of Representatives and Chairman of the Board of WITN-TV; Norfleet Sugg, Pinetops, executive of Planters Bank and Trust Company of Rocky Mount; Hal H. Tanner, Sr., Goldsboro, publisher of the *Goldsboro News-Argus*; Mrs. Martha Walston, Wilson, member of the Wilson City Council; Dr. Charles Watts, Durham, medical director of NC Mutual Insurance Co.; and Dr. Jesse Williams, Fayetteville, director of the Cumberland County Health Department. *Greenville Daily Reflector,* February 27, 1976.

[13] *Greenville Daily Reflector,* March 2, 1976.

[14] Letter of William E. Laupus to William C. Friday, June 30 1976, in ECU School of Medicine Files, Accreditation Folder.

[15] Letters from William E. Laupus to James R. Schofield, August 23, 1976, James R. Schofield to William E. Laupus, August 26,

1976, in ECU School of Medicine Files, Accreditation Folder.

[16] Letter of William E. Laupus to James R. Schofield, October 15, 1976, ECU School of Medicine Files, Accreditation Folder.

[17] *ECU Fountainhead,* January 18, 1977.

[18] *Chapel Hill Newspaper,* January 19, 1977.

[19] *Greenville Daily Reflector,* January 20, 1977.

[20] *Chapel Hill Newspaper,* February 13, 1977; *Greenville Daily Reflector,* February 14, 1977. The five amendments were duly approved without alteration, and became part of the affiliation agreement.

[21] *Greenville Daily Reflector,* February 17, 1977.

[22] *Raleigh News & Observer,* March 27, 1977; *Greensboro Daily News,* March 27, 1977.

[23] *Greenville Daily Reflector,* April 7, 1977.

[24] *Hickory Daily Record,* June 21, 1977.

[25] *Greenville Daily Reflector,* Monday, June 27, 1977.

Chapter 22
The Medical School Opens Its Doors

The end of 1976 had approached with two major obstacles still to be surmounted. With the signing of the affiliation agreement and its approval by the UNC Board of Governors and the PCMH Board of Trustees, the first hurdle was out of the way. That signing practically insured that the school would be accredited, since the other requirements had been or were being met: curriculum development, teaching facilities, the library, and faculty recruitment. When, in April, the full Liaison Committee on Medical Education approved provisional accreditation, and the initial installments of funds for construction on their way, all the major barriers had been negotiated. The school's administration and faculty were free at last to begin final preparations to receive the first class of medical students in the fall of 1977.

PCMH did not move into its new facility just after Christmas, as had been planned, but by the end of March had made its transfer from the old hospital building. The hospital's 377 beds were adequate to begin supporting clinical teaching, as well as to provide for medical research. The administrative offices of the medical school and the offices of the clinical faculty were to be located in the School of Medicine's "teaching addition" to the hospital, flanked by the existing bed tower and the one that was to be added by the medical school to provide additional facilities for clinical teaching. On June 21, 1977, the state Senate approved $3.82 million for the bed tower.[1]

A building to house the Eastern Carolina Family Practice Center and the Eastern Area Health Education Center was being constructed between the hospital and the site where the medical sciences building was to be located. The Family Practice Center was to provide accommodations for medical students and residents who had targeted primary care, the principal objective for which the School of Medicine had been established. The Center was opened with a formal ribbon-cutting in June, and was thrown open for business in December. There were already seven residents in training in family practice in July, when the first twenty-four residents joined the hospital's house staff.

The construction of the medical sciences building did not actually begin until 1979. The lowest cost estimate received in 1978 was $33.91 million, $8.91 million more than the funds that had been budgeted by the General Assembly. After strenuous efforts, led by Dr. Dean H. Hayek, who continued to work closely with the architects and engineers, ways were found (including leaving some laboratories and other areas to be finished later on) to bring the cost down to $26 million. The building was dedicated on October 29, 1982, named the Brody Medical Sciences Building in honor of the Brody family of Greenville and Kinston, who had made a $1.5 million grant to the East Carolina University Medical Foundation.

Renovations to provide space for the medical school in Ragsdale Hall had been completed in 1976, and had been occupied, along with temporary accommodations in two trailers, by members of the administrative staff. Before the medical students arrived, additional space was found in Whichard Building, adjoining Ragsdale.

The search for faculty, especially clinical faculty, expanded. The effect on the social life of the faculty and administrators already present was most salutary. There were a lot of dinners with prospective faculty members.[2] As Dr. Robert E. Thurber, professor and chairman of physiology from the earliest, one-year medical school days in 1970, said, "Attracting good faculty was not difficult. Getting them here for a visit often was. Except for a few who were flown to South Carolina by mistake, most visitors arrived at the old Kinston airport, usually at night. The ride into Greenville provided two unforgettable sights: the lights of the DuPont plant and the wide-screen action at the North 11 porno drive-in theater." [3]

A few representative appointments were made during 1977. On May 5, the appointment of Dr. Walter J. Pories, chief of surgery at Cleveland Metropolitan General Hospital, as professor and chairman of surgery at the ECU School of Medicine was announced. Dr. Pories was professor of surgery at Case-Western Reserve University School of Medicine, and a founder of Cancer Center, Inc., a cooperative venture of Case-Western Reserve and Cleveland Clinic Hospital.[4] On June 19, the chairman of the Department of Family Practice, Dr. James Jones, announced that Drs. C. Christopher Bremer, Joseph E. Agsten, and Rose Pully, all of Kinston, had been added to the department's clinical faculty. These were practicing family physicians, who would teach and observe medical students and residents.[5] Drs. Robert Shackelford and Hervey Kornegay, family physicians of Mount Olive, were also appointed to the clinical faculty of the Department of Family Practice.[6]

Drs. Joseph W. Litten, Donald R. Hoffman, and Leo Robert Hanrahan, Jr., were selected as members of the faculty of the Department of Pathology.[7] Dr. Eugene D. Furth, chairman of the Department of Internal Medicine,[8] announced that Dr. Spencer Raab and

Dr. Mary J. Raab were coming from the University of Arkansas to join the departmental faculty. Dr. Spencer Raab was to head the Oncology Section of the Department, and Dr. Mary Raab to be a member of the Hematology Section.[9]

In mid-August the *Chapel Hill Newspaper* announced that ECU School of Medicine would open its first class, "officially ending a fight for a four-year medical school that began more than a decade ago when the school's two-year med school was started."[10] The battle was "officially" over, indeed, but there remained discontents that seemed to be permanent. As late as 1992, President Friday was still dissatisfied with the decision that had been forced on him. In particular, he believed that it had been a mistake to enter into an agreement to use facilities at Pitt County Memorial Hospital for teaching, rather than having the medical school establish its own teaching hospital. He said, "I didn't have any doubt about the need for the hospital that had to be there. I think we made a bad decision in how we set it up administratively—it ought to be a part of the University and ought to have been from the beginning."

He said of the long struggle between Chapel Hill and Greenville over the ECU School of Medicine, ". . . the thing that I regret most about it was the politicalization of it. It was not settled as an academic question, never was from the beginning. And I tried desperately to keep the University of North Carolina out of politics. It's in the political process because it's a public institution, but it never should take sides, choose up or draw. . . . You pay a terrible price in the public mind, though, when you go at an issue politically, I don't care which side you're on. You also draw strength away from the main campus. For example, here at Chapel Hill, when the decision was made to go to four years, I don't think they built a building on the main campus for seven years, because all the money had to go into the medical school."

Before making his decision to give up the joint planning effort, Friday had talked with Senator Ralph Scott, telling him that the months of fruitless striving showed there could be no satisfactory solution on educational grounds. He told Scott, "It is clearly going to be resolved politically, so tell me what you want to do. Because, I said, there's no point carrying this on any further. We've carried it on for months. There's a weariness out in the state that's bad for East Carolina, it's bad for the University. People are fed up with hearing all of this bickering, and we've got to bring it to an end." There was a clear possibility that all their exertions had been wasted. As he said,

"I just saw it all unraveling." He thought that Chancellor Jenkins also realized this in the end, because things had gone too far, there had been too much tension on both sides, and too much acrimony. [11]

It is doubtful that anyone on the Greenville campus failed to realize that the offensive public conflict had to end. There were efforts to seek understanding, and some forgetfulness. Chancellor Jenkins said, "Bill Friday and I are very good friends and he had a role to play and I had a role to play. It was his role to follow the power structure on his campus. And the power structure on his campus gave him a strong signal that they did not want a medical school at East Carolina. So, he'd have been rather foolish to go behind their back and help me get a medical school. Probably would have cost his job even. So, therefore, he did not join in, in terms of being a friend of our project or helping us with our project." [12]

In an interview that appeared in the *Greenville Daily Reflector* on Sunday, August 21, 1977, Dean Laupus said, "The relationship with Chapel Hill is now cordial. They don't interfere with us, and we don't interfere with them. I've never felt the hostility. Once the decision was made by the legislature, and the school became a fact, the people—the faculty—in Chapel Hill seemed to accept it and say, get on with it." [13]

Regardless of any trace of harsh memories, the opening of the new school was taken as an opportunity to celebrate. The names of the charter class of medical students were published. The newspapers of the state were awash with news articles and editorials about the occasion, as both the Associated Press and United Press International carried the story. Most of the students entering the medical school were written up in their local papers.

Dr. Dean H. Hayek, Dean of Admissions, said the school had received 350 applications, 280 of them North Carolinians. Only twenty-eight students were admitted, all of them residents of North Carolina who had expressed interest in family practice or other primary care fields, and also in practicing in the state after their graduation. Five members of the charter class were minority students. [14]

The Admissions Committee was made up of thirteen persons, including Dr. Hayek. The admission requirements were quite conventional for a medical school, apart from the emphasis on interest in primary care, and the limitation to North Carolina residents. In its decisions, the committee considered grade point average, Medical College Admissions Test scores, and letters of recommendation from college faculty members and friends.

Each applicant was required to write an essay explaining why he or she wished to study medicine. Two members of the committee examined the entire application and two other members examined the essay of an applicant. Dr. Hayek said that this stage of the process was considered to be an objective evaluation. A subjective phase consisted of separate interviews of the applicant by two committee members who had not been involved in the objective phase. The findings of the six examiners were presented to the entire committee for discussion, evaluation, and a final decision.

The interviewers considered the applicants' personalities, and "what we foresee as the student's ultimate impact on medical practice, such as will he remain to practice in North Carolina, and what are his attachments to the state," Dr. Hayek said. 'Attachments' included relatives living in the state, or whether spouses were from North Carolina. Every reasonable attempt was made to find students who appeared likely to remain in the state when they started their practices.

Dr. Zubie W. Metcalf, Jr., a member of the committee, said that he and the other members considered extracurricular collegiate activities, as well as employment experience. Dr. Metcalf was Director of the Center for Student Opportunities in the School of Medicine, which had been set up to assist minority and disadvantaged students who experienced academic or personal problems. The staff of the Center also worked with counselors in high schools, junior colleges, and community colleges to recruit promising students. Dr. Hayek added, "If the applicant is poor as a pauper, his or her work is every bit as important as participating in sports or clubs and fraternities." He also said that a second-year class was to be added in the fall of 1978, and each year subsequently a class would be added until 1980, so that when the first class graduated, there would be a full four-year program.[15]

On Monday, August 22, 1977, the first class of medical students reported to Ragsdale Hall for orientation, and on Tuesday classes began there and in the Science Building a short walk across the campus.[16] No time was lost in starting work in gross and microscopic anatomy and biochemistry, as well in the psychosocial aspects of medical practice, emphasizing normal growth and development in our society. From the beginning there were weekly conferences in primary care, which focused on the most common diseases encountered by primary care physicians. Later in the first year would come neurosciences, microbiology, physiology, and pathology (which would continue into the second year).

The second year would continue with pharmacology, more microbiology and biochemistry, courses in laboratory and physical diagnosis, genetics, reproduction and growth, biostatistics, and an introduction to surgery. Surgery courses were slated to go on through the third year, with the addition of internal medicine, family practice, obstetrics and gynecology, psychiatry, and pediatrics. During the fourth year, there would be clinical rotations in internal medicine, family practice, and sub-specialties of surgery and medicine. Two hours each week through both third and fourth years would be devoted to weekly clinical correlation clinics, at which the clinical faculty would present cases.[17]

A short while after the arrival of the first class of medical students, an interview of Dr. Edwin Monroe was published in a special edition of the *Greenville Daily Reflector* celebrating the dedication of a new addition to the hospital. Dr. Monroe gave a résumé of the history of the struggle to establish the ECU School of Medicine from the time he joined the campaign.

Monroe and Dr. Robert Williams, an ECU political scientist, had spent several months in 1964 investigating the health manpower situation in North Carolina, especially its eastern counties, and relating their finds to the national situation. During 1964 and 1965, Dr. Leo Jenkins traveled to wherever in eastern North Carolina he could find an audience for his message about health care needs that were not being met.

Monroe said that when the controversial plan to build a two-year medical school at East Carolina was overruled by the Board of Higher Education in 1965, it was abandoned temporarily, and ECU settled for a one-year medical program. This was started, with twenty students, in the fall of 1972. Later, after the restructuring of higher education in the state, the college approached the UNC Board of Governors about adding another year to the program.

The Board set up a committee—called the "Jordan Committee" after its chairman—to study the idea. After some months of study, the committee recommended that the school at Chapel Hill should be expanded and that the state should provide support for North Carolina students who would attend Bowman Gray and Duke. Concluding that the concept of a two-year school was no longer a viable concept, the committee recommended that a team of experts should be hired to see if the state needed another four-year school. On a recommendation from the panel of out-of-state experts, the Board of Governors placed the one-year program under the control of the dean at Chapel Hill, who was charged to upgrade its quality. The system of Area Health Education Centers recommended by the panel was also initiated.

During this time, the legislature set up the Medical Manpower Study Commission to carry out its own investigation. Dr. Monroe said, "The thrust of their report to the legislature was that the one-year program ought to be expanded to two years and eventually to four years. So the legislature passed an appropriations act and gave us some money to strengthen the one-year program and enlarge it and add a second year. They said the program down here should emphasize family medicine and attempt to recruit minorities."

He then passed over in silence the months of conflict between the staff of the ECU medical school and administrators from Chapel Hill imposed by the national accreditation group for medical education. He went on to tell about the 1974 recommendation by President William Friday and the Board of Governors that a four-year school be developed. And to say that the legislature agreed to appropriate funds to reach more than $40 million for construction during the 1975-77 biennium. That year the operating budget was nearly $2 million. The way was clear to hire a dean and recruit department chairmen and faculty members.

"We've had to watch it these past few years, but the fight was over in November of 1974 when the Board of Governors recommended approval," Dr. Monroe said. "It's a very significant achievement whereby the hospital and medical school can work together and continue to serve the community. This helped in costs because we didn't have to build an additional hospital for the medical school. I see ahead an orderly development for a complete and comprehensive school of medicine. What this means for Greenville and Pitt County is that it not only provides a school and teaching program but also a comprehensive medical center serving eastern North Carolina.

"I think that whatever service you think of being available at UNC or Duke will be available here," he concluded. "It takes time and a lot of hard work." [18]

[1] *Greenville Daily Reflector,* June 27, 1977. Construction was begun on April 4, 1980, and the tower was completed in October, 1981

[2] Barnes interview, January 15, 1992.

[3] Brody Building dedication issue of *ECU Med Review* (Fall 1982) p. 7.

[4] *Chapel Hill Newspaper,* May 5, 1977; Curriculum Vitae in School of Medicine Files.

[5] *Kinston Free Press,* June 19, 1977.

[6] *Mount Olive Tribune,* June 21, 1977.

[7] *Washington Daily News,* July 25, 1977.

[8] Dr. Furth had been appointed in August, 1976.

[9] *Greenville Daily Reflector,* July 31, 1977.

[10] *Chapel Hill Newspaper,* August 19, 1977.

[11] Friday interview, July 2, 1992.

[12] Jenkins interview, August 31, 1988.

[13] *Greenville Daily Reflector,* August 21, 1977.

[14] The names of the first class are listed in Appendix B.

[15] *Greenville Daily Reflector,* August 17, 1977.

[16] *Greenville Daily Reflector,* August 21, 1977.

[17] *School of Medicine Bulletin,* (Greenville, NC: East Carolina University) Vol. 64, No. 1 (1977-79).

[18] Interview of Dr. Edwin W. Monroe by Keith Mills, Greenville *Daily Reflector* Staff Writer, Reprinted in *Laurinburg Exchange,* September 14, 1977.

Sources

Books

Two books have served as the main secondary sources for this history:

Bratton, Mary Jo Jackson. *East Carolina University—The Formative Years, 1907-1982*. Greenville, North Carolina: East Carolina University Alumni Association, 1986. [Bratton]

Link, William A. *William Friday—Power, Purpose, and American Higher Education*. Chapel Hill and London: The University of North Carolina Press, 1995. [Link]

While these histories are both exemplary for their balance and absence of partiality, the emphasis in each is naturally on the institution which is its main focus. I have leaned heavily on Dr. Link's account in places where I have felt that I was perhaps inclined to favor the ECU point of view too much.

The following volumes were useful for particular time periods or particular subjects:

Clay, James W., Douglas M. Orr, Jr., and Alfred W. Stuart. *North Carolina Atlas*. Chapel Hill: The University of North Carolina Press, 1975.

Crabtree, Beth G. *North Carolina Governors, 1585-1974, Brief Sketches*. Raleigh: North Carolina Division of Archives and History, 1974.

Gifford, James F., Jr. *The Evolution of a Medical Center: A History of Medicine at Duke University to 1941* Durham: Duke University Press, 1972.

Hedrick, Georgette. *Chronology of the ECU School of Medicine, 1964-1976* (with an Addendum for 1977-1985). Xerox. Greenville, 1985. [Hedrick]

King, Arnold K. *The Multicampus University of North Carolina Comes of Age, 1956-1986*. Chapel Hill: The University of North Carolina, 1987. [King]

Lefler, Hugh Talmage & Albert Ray Newsome. *North Carolina - The History of a Southern State.* Third Edition. Chapel Hill: The University of North Carolina Press, 1973. [Lefler]

Powell, William S. *North Carolina Through Four Centuries.* Chapel Hill and London: The University of North Carolina Press, 1989. [Powell]

Roberts, Nancy. *The Governor.* Charlotte: McNally and Loftin, 1972.

Schofield, J. R. *New and Expanded Medical Schools, Mid-Century to the 1980s.* San Francisco, Washington, and London: AAMC and Jossey-Bass Publishers, 1984.

Snider, William D. *Light on the Hill —A History of the University of North Carolina at Chapel Hill.* Chapel Hill and London: The University of North Carolina Press, 1992. [Snider]

Starr, Paul. *The Social Transformation of American Medicine.* New York: Basic Books, Inc., Publishers, 1982.

Newspapers

My most important sources, by far, were daily newspapers, especially the *Greenville Daily Reflector* and the *Raleigh News & Observer.* Besides these, I have referred to the following:

Asheville Citizen

Asheville Times

Burlington Times-News

Chapel Hill Newspaper

Chapel Hill Weekly

Charlotte News

Charlotte Observer

Durham Morning Herald

Durham Sun

ECU Fountainhead

Fayetteville Observer

Goldsboro News -Argus

Greensboro Daily News

Greensboro Record

Henderson Dispatch

Hickory Daily Record

High Point Enterprise

Jacksonville Daily News

Kannapolis Independent

Kinston Free Press

Knoxville (TN) Journal

Laurinburg Exchange

Lexington Dispatch

Monroe Enquirer-Journal

Morganton News-Herald

Mount Olive Tribune

Plymouth Roanoke Beacon

Raleigh Times

Red Springs Citizen

Rocky Mount Evening Telegraph

Rocky Mount Telegram

Statesville Record and Landmark

Tarboro Southerner

Washington (NC) Daily News

Wilson Daily Times

Winston-Salem Journal

Winston-Salem Sentinal

The Leo Jenkins Papers in the East Carolina University Archives and the William C. Friday Papers in the University Archives, University of North Carolina-Chapel Hill have been basic sources, against which the newspaper accounts and interviews have been checked.

Interviews

I have utilized (some as background, without specific citation) the following oral history interviews for which tapes and transcripts are located in the East Carolina University School of Medicine.

> By the author:
> Barnes, Donald W., January 15, 1992.
> Bell, Jo Ann, December 11, 1991.
> Dawson, Raymond, June 10, 1992.
> Fordham, Christopher, May 21, 1992.
> Friday, William C., July 7, 1992.
> Fulghum, Robert 5., November 6, 1991.
> Hardison, Harold, March 26, 1992.
> Huskins, J. P., April 2, 1992.
> Lawrence, Irvin E. Jr., January 22, 1992.
> McNeill, M. Evelyn, March 25, 1992.
> Monroe, Edwin W., January 3, 1992.
> Morgan, Robert B., March 17, 1992.
> Pennington, Sam, January 29, 1992.
> Rountree, H. Horton, October 14,1991.
> Wilson, Glenn, April 22,1992.
> Wooles, Wallace R., November 13,1991.

Dr. Leo Jenkins was interviewed by Paul Crellin (August 31, 1988) and by Dr. William E. Laupus (October 5, 1988). These interviews are on videotape and audiotape.

APPENDIX A
Chronology of Events

MAJOR EVENTS LEADING TO THE ESTABLISHMENT
OF ECU MEDICAL SCHOOL

1962

East Carolina College President Leo Jenkins mentioned to Governor Terry Sanford that a suggestion had been made to establish a medical school in Greenville.

1964

July 20. President Jenkins included a proposal for a two-year medical school in his summary of ECC's long-range plans presented to the General Assembly's Advisory Budget Commission.
October 1. The ECC Board of Trustees passed a resolution setting up a committee to study the medical school proposal.

1965

April 1. State Senator Walter B. Jones, Jr., submitted a bill, co-signed by many eastern senators, proposing establishment of a two-year medical school at ECC. In the house, Representative W. A. Forbes submitted an identical bill.
June. The Senate Appropriations Committee and the House Higher Education Committee approved legislation to create a two-year ECC medical program, with the provision that unless the proposed medical school could be accredited by January 1, 1967, the issue would be referred to the Board of Higher Education.
July. The East Carolina medical school bill passed in both the Senate and the House. Jenkins stated that January 1967 was not a realistic target date. ECC could not meet the accreditation deadline.

1968

January. A School of Allied Health Professions and Medical Education Center were established by the ECU Board of Trustees. Dr. Edwin W. Monroe was appointed Dean.
President Jenkins continued to push for a medical school at ECU.

1969

March. ECU officials the General Assembly asked for $2.46 million to start a School of Medicine.

July. The Senate gave final approval for $375,000 to get a two-year school started.

1970

June. Dr. Wallace R. Wooles was named director of Medical Science and Professor of Pharmacology at ECU, to assist in planning a two-year medical school.

1971

February. The Liaison Committee on Medical Education of the American Medical Association and the Association of American Medical Colleges told Dr. Wooles that the ECU medical school could be accredited by 1972.

May. Bills were introduced in the House and Senate to appropriate $1.8 million to ECU for a one-year medical school.

July. The appropriations bill was enacted by a vote of thirty-seven to four.

ECU started recruiting faculty members, and prepared to receive its first class of student in September, 1972. Three hundred applications had been received to fill twenty seats. The students were to be transferred to UNC-CH at the end of their training at ECU.

1972

June. Governor Robert Scott said he would appoint a five-member subcommittee of the UNC Board of Governors to look into a two-year medical school for ECU.

August. Robert B. Jordan III was appointed head of the committee studying ECU's request to expand its medical school. ECU asked the Board of Governors to expand the one-year medical school to a two-year school by September 1974.

September. The first class of medical students, with twenty members, began their first year of training.

1973

January. The UNC Board of Governors accepted the recommendation of the Jordan Committee that the ECU medical school not be expanded immediately, but that consideration should be directed toward a new degree-granting school of medicine.

February. The Board of Governors decided to submit the ECU medical school question to a five-member panel of out-of-state medical educators.

March. The panel of medical educators were selected, to report to the Board of Governors by September.

April. The AMA and AAMC issued a joint report sharply criticizing ECU and UNC for their bickering and lack of cooperation. As a result of the study, President Friday and Chancellor Jenkins agreed that ECU's one-year medical school was to be placed under the total control of UNC's dean of medicine.

May. The General Assembly's Joint Appropriations Committee tentatively approved setting aside $25 million to use if and when and new medical school was approved.

Dr. William Cromartie, associate dean for clinical sciences at UNC, was named liaison administrator between ECU's medical program and the medical school at Chapel Hill.

September. The consultant's report was turned over to the Board of Governors. The panel suggested that the ECU medical school not be expanded for at least a few more years. They concluded that a medical school at ECU was not the best means of improving health care in North Carolina, and that ECU lacked the leadership, skill, and background to build a viable school.

The UNC Board of Governors voted to accept the consultants' report.

November. The Board of Governors approved an education plan submitted by President Friday. It included funds to upgrade ECU's one-year medical school..

December. The NC Advisory Budget Commission approved $25 million of the $30 million medical education package sponsored by the UNC Board of Governors, and voted to add $7.5 million to the $7.5 million already in reserve for use if the state decided to build another medical school.

The Medical Manpower Study Commission unanimously endorsed a report rejecting many of the consultant team's recommendations, and recommending a new two-year medical school at ECU and expansion of the school's enrollment to thirty or forty as soon as possible.

1974

January. A bill to expand ECU's medical school was introduced into the legislature. The bill called for increasing class size from twenty to forty in the 1975-76 school year and adding a second curriculum in 1976-77.

February. The Joint Appropriations Committee approved the bill to expand the ECU School of Medicine, and voted to include its provisions in the state's regular budget appropriations package.

May. The UNC Board of Governors authorized Chancellor Leo Jenkins to begin planning for a second year for the School of Medicine at ECU.

June. The LCME ruled that ECU expansion plans must be carried out within the framework of the UNC medical school. Dr. Christopher Fordham, Dean of UNC medical school, met with Chancellor Jenkins to discuss expansion plans. A search committee was set up to find a full-time director for the program.

July. Dean Wallace Wooles resigned, clearing the way for Fordham to appoint a new dean for the ECU medical school. Dr. William Cromartie took over as interim director.

August. Twenty students, all N.C. residents, began their first year of medical training—the third class to begin at ECU.

October. A disagreement between medical school planners and PCMH officials temporarily blocked expansion plans for the ECU medical school.

November. Key policy committees of the UNC Board of Governors and President Friday recommended a four-year medical school at ECU.

The Board of Governors approved development of a four-year medical school at ECU and recommended that the 1975 General Assembly appropriate an additional $35.2 million for construction as well as an appropriation for current operations.

The Advisory Budget Commission recommended funding of a four-year medical school at ECU.

Chancellor Leo Jenkins appointed a search committee to select a dean for the school.

December. Dr. Harold C. Wiggers, retired dean of the medical school in Albany, New York, agreed come to ECU as an advisor in planning the medical school expansion.

1975

January. Full funding for the ECU medical school was recommended in the budget presented to the 1975 General Assembly.

PCMH invited ECU medical school faculty to practice medicine and educate medical students as guests of PCMH. Hospital officials said they did not want to see a separate teaching hospital set up by the school.

March. PCMH trustees approved affiliation of the hospital with ECU's medical school. ECU trustees unanimously approved the affiliation proposal. Seven million dollars would be cut from ECU's funding request by the affiliation with PCMH.

June. PCMH temporarily lost accreditation because of more than seventy violations of guidelines of the Joint Committee on Accreditation of Hospital. The violations were the result of deficiencies in the old hospital that would be corrected in the new one.

The General Assembly approved a two-year, $6.5 million operating budget for ECU medical school, and $32 million for medical school construction.

Dr. William E. Laupus was appointed Dean of the ECU School of Medicine.

July. PCMH received provisional one-year accreditation from the JCAH.

September. The Comprehensive Health Planning Section of the Department of Human Resources approved expansion of facilities at PCMH to accommodate the ECU School of Medicine.

December. PCMH and the ECU School of Medicine signed an affiliation agreement on use of the hospital for clinical teaching facilities.

1976

February 9. Land was purchased for the ECU School of Medicine.

October. For the 1977-79 biennium, the UNC Board of Governors included in its budget $9 million for ECU medical school operating expenses and $3.8 million in capital funds for adding patient beds at PCMH.

1977

January. The Liaison Committee on Medical Education made a survey visit to ECU School of Medicine

April. Chancellor Leo Jenkins announced the ECU medical school had received accreditation from the LCME.

August. A charter class of twenty-eight students was admitted to the four-year program at the ECU School of Medicine.

APPENDIX B
The First Class

Class of 1981
of The East Carolina University School of Medicine's
Four-Year Medical Program

Thomas Leary Beatty, M.D.
Karl William Beesch, M.D.
Robert Forrest Brown, M.D.
William Edward Brown, M.D.
Philip Douglas Burton, M.D.
Natalear Rolline Collins, M.D.
Eugene Davis Day Jr., M.D.
Manjul Sharma Dixit, M.D.
Frances Doyle, M.D.
Sigsbee Walter Duck, M.D.
Linda Marie Edwards, M.D.
David Ray Faber II, M.D.
Mary Beth Foil, M.D.
Peter Mercer Johns, M.D.
Robert Spurgeon Jones Jr., M.D.
Brenda Mills Kluttz, M.D.
Kenneth Stuart Lee, M.D.
John Henry Lowder Jr., M.D.
Alan Bland Marr, M.D.
Raymond Bruce Minard, M.D.
George Horace Moore Jr., M.D.
Fernando Rene Puente, M.D.
Daniel Carl Rendleman, M.D.
Bonnie Caulkins Revelle, M.D.
Franklin Robert Sample Jr., M.D.
Tony Preston Smith, M.D.
William Holladay Spivey Jr., M.D.
Michael David Tripp, M.D.

APPENDIX C
Chancellor's Committee

Chancellor's Advisory Committee
(Called "The Committee of 65")

Mr. Hoover Adams, Dunn
Judge S. Gerald Arnold, Fuquay-Varina
Lenox D. Baker, M.D., Durham
Edgar T. Beddingfield, Jr., M.D., Wilson
Andrew Best, M.D., Greenville
Mr. H. Clifton Blue, Aberdeen
Mr. Leo Brody, Kinston
Mr. J. T. Church, Henderson
Donald L. Copeland, M.D., Clinton
George C. Debnam, M.D., Raleigh
The Honorable Claude DeBruhl, Candler
Mr. Henry A. Dennis, Henderson
The Honorable William R. Flowers, Plymouth
Joe Lee Frank, M.D., Ahoskie
Ernest Furgurson, M.D., Plymouth
John R. Gamble, M.D., Lincolnton
Mr. J. Marse Grant, Raleigh
The Honorable James C. Green, Clarkton
Ira M. Hardy, M.D., Greenville
The Honorable Joseph J. Harrington , Lewiston
The Honorable Jesse Helms, Washington, DC
The Honorable John T. Henley, Hope Mills
Dr. Jack Hill, Fayetteville
Mr. Wilbur Hobby. Raleigh
John P. Holt, M.D., Asheville
Mrs. Paxon M. Holz, Swansboro
Lieutenant Governor James B. Hunt, Jr., Raleigh
The Honorable J. P. Huskins, Statesville
Amos Johnson, M.D., Garland
Mrs. Amos Johnson, Tomahawk
Mr. Roddy Jones, Raleigh
The Honorable Walter Jones, Washington, DC
The Honorable J. Russell Kirby, Wilson

Mr. Keith Lamb, New Bern
Mr. Howard Lee, Chapel Hill
Frank H. Longino, M.D., Greenville
William R. McConnell, M.D., Greenville
Mr. Reginald F. McCoy, Laurinburg
The Honorable William D. Mills, Maysville
The Honorable Robert Morgan, Lillington
Philip G. Nelson, M.D., Greenville
Charles P. Nicholson, Jr., M.D., Morehead City
Mr. Joe M. Parker, Ahoskie
Mr. Troy W. Pate, Goldsboro
Mr. Dick Paul, Washington, NC
Mr. Eugene Price, Goldsboro
Coy C. Privette, Kannapolis
Mr. W. R. Roberson, Jr., Washington, NC
The Honorable Horton H. Rountree, Greenville
The Honorable Kenneth C. Royall, Jr., Durham
The Honorable Ralph H. Scott,   Haw River
The Honorable Robert Scott, Raleigh
William J. Senter, M.D., Raleigh
Mr. John Sledge, Raleigh
Mr. D. Livingston Stallings, New Bern
The Honorable Thomas E. Strickland, Goldsboro
Jack Tannenbaum, M.D., Greensboro
Allen Taylor, M.D., Greenville
J. Benjamin Warren, M.D., New Bern
The Honorable William T. Watkins, Oxford
Mr. David. J. Whichard II, Greenville
Jack W. Wilkerson, M.D., Greenville

APPENDIX D
The Founding Faculty

The Founding Faculty of the
School of Medicine at East Carolina University
1970-1975

Dr. Hisham Barakat, Biochemistry
Dr. Donald Barnes, Pharmacology
Dr. Jo Ann Bell, Director of the Health Affairs Library
Dr. Jack Brinn, Anatomy
Dr. Hubert Burden, Anatomy
Dr. G. Lynis Dohm, Biochemistry
Dr. Abdullah Fattah, Pathology
Dr. Robert Fulghum, Microbiology and Immunology
Dr. Dean Hayek, Assistant Dean and Director of Admissions
Dr. Irvin Lawrence, Anatomy
Dr. Evelyn McNeil, Anatomy
Dr. Edwin Monroe, Vice-Chancellor for Health Affairs
Dr. Baxter Noble, Medicine and Physiology
Dr. William Nye, Chairman of Pathology
Dr. Sam Pennington, Acting Chairman of Biochemistry
Dr. Michael Schweisthal, Chairman of Anatomy
Dr. A. Mason Smith, Microbiology and Immunology
Dr. Robert Thurber, Chairman of Physiology
Dr. William Waugh, Chairman of Medicine
Dr. Wallace Wooles, Dean and Chairman of Pharmacology

APPENDIX E
Photographic History

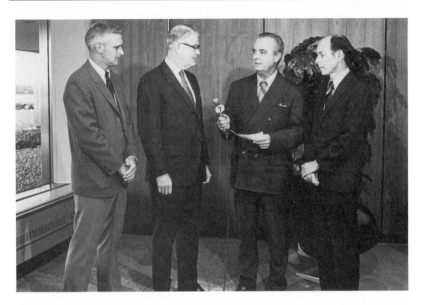

Announcement of the Burroughs-Wellcome Grant, Aug. 2, 1971
Left to Right: Wallace R. Wooles, Harry Leslie, Leo Jenkins, and Ed Monroe

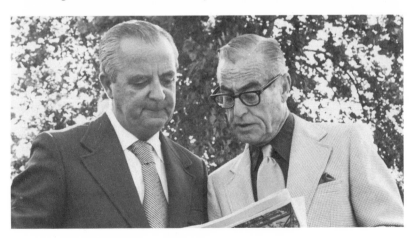

*Dr. Leo Jenkins with Senator Thomas White of the
Advisory Budget Commission, July 19, 1972*

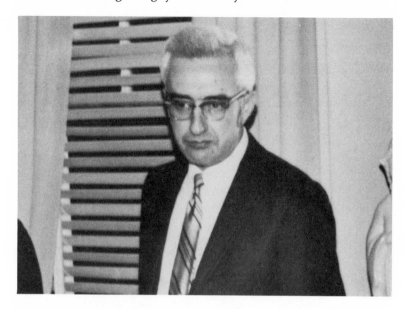

Dr. Dean H. Hayek, Dean of Admissions
ECU School of Medicine

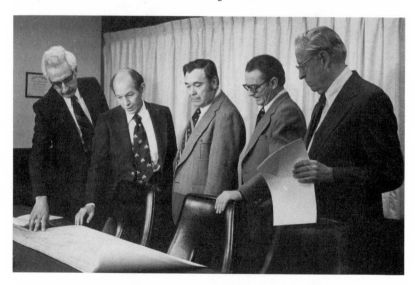

Purchase of land for ECU School of Medicine, Feb. 9, 1976
Left to Right: Dean Hayek, Ed Monroe, Burney Tucker, Gene White, and W.
W. Speight

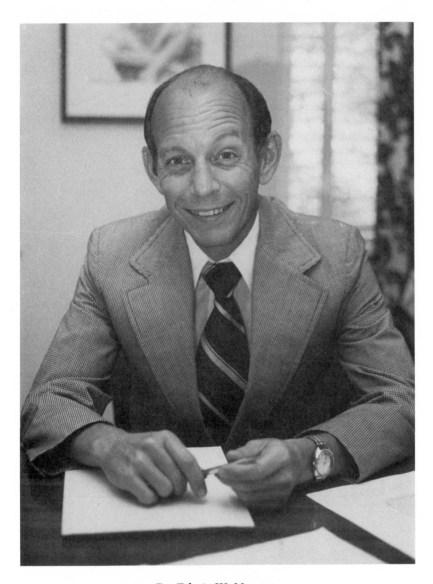

Dr. Edwin W. Monroe
Vice Chancellor for Health Affairs
and President of Eastern AHEC

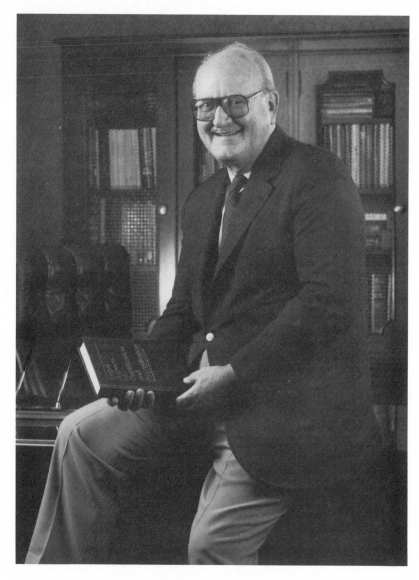

Dr. William E. Laupus
Founding Dean of the Four-Year ECU School of Medicine
and Vice Chancellor for Health Sciences

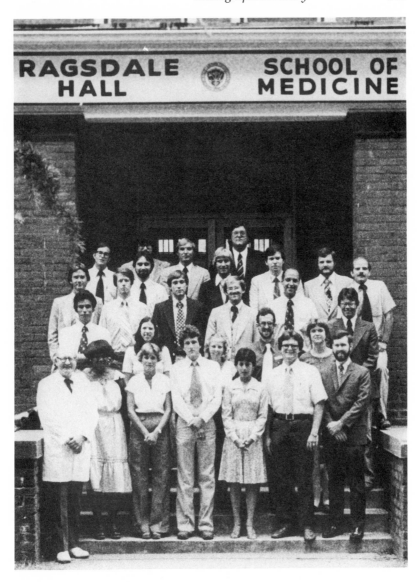

First Class of Four-Year Medical Students
Class of 1981

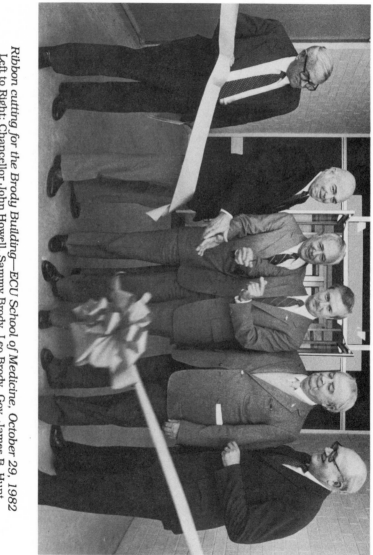

*Ribbon cutting for the Brody Building—ECU School of Medicine, October 29, 1982
Left to Right: Chancellor John Howell, Sammy Brody, Leo Brody, Gov. James B. Hunt,
Chancellor Emeritus Leo W. Jenkins, Dean William E. Laupus*

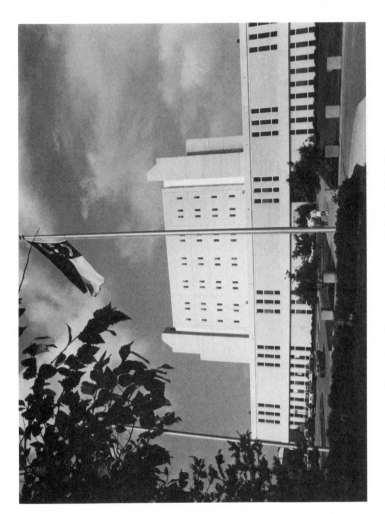

East Carolina University, School of Medicine
The Brody Medical Sciences Building

Index